Smart Healthcare

Digvijay Pandey · Rahul Kar ·
Binay Kumar Pandey · Prabjot Kaur ·
A. Shaji George · Florin Popentiu Vlădicescu
Editors

Smart Healthcare

Fuzzy Logic and AI-Driven Solutions for Patient Care

Springer

Editors
Digvijay Pandey
Department of Technical Education Kanpur
Kanpur, Uttar Pradesh, India

Binay Kumar Pandey
Department of Information Technology
Govind Ballabh Pant University
of Agriculture and Technology
Pantnagar, Uttarakhand, India

A. Shaji George
Almarai Company
Riyadh, Saudi Arabia

Rahul Kar
Department of Mathematics
Kalyani Mahavidyalaya
Kalyani, West Bengal, India

Prabjot Kaur
Department of Mathematics
BIT Mesra
Ranchi, Jharkhand, India

Florin Popentiu Vlădicescu
Department of Control Engineering
and Industrial Informatics
University Politehnica of Bucharest
Bucharest, Romania

ISBN 978-981-95-8827-5 ISBN 978-981-95-8828-2 (eBook)
https://doi.org/10.1007/978-981-95-8828-2

This Springer imprint is published by the registered company Springer Nature Singapore Pte Ltd.
The registered company address is: 152 Beach Road, #21-01/04 Gateway East, Singapore 189721, Singapore

Preface

The rapid evolution of healthcare technologies in recent years has transformed the way medical professionals diagnose, treat, and manage patient conditions. Amid this transformation, fuzzy logic and artificial intelligence (AI) have emerged as vital enablers for developing intelligent, adaptive, and personalized healthcare systems. The edited volume "Smart Healthcare: Fuzzy Logic and AI-driven Solutions for Patient Care" explores the convergence of these computational paradigms, highlighting their capacity to enhance decision-making, automate complex processes, and foster patient-centered innovation across the healthcare continuum.

Traditional healthcare models often struggle to manage uncertainty, imprecision, and the vast heterogeneity of medical data. Fuzzy logic, with its ability to model human-like reasoning and handle vagueness, complements the data-driven precision of AI algorithms, creating a synergistic framework for smart healthcare solutions. This integration enables systems that are not only computationally efficient but also context-aware and interpretable—qualities essential for real-world medical applications where lives and decisions are intricately linked.

This book brings together leading researchers, engineers, data scientists, and healthcare practitioners from around the globe to present cutting-edge research and practical implementations of fuzzy-AI-based systems in patient care. The contributions span a wide spectrum of topics, including intelligent diagnosis and prognosis systems, decision-support tools, medical imaging analysis, personalized treatment design, health monitoring, telemedicine, and predictive analytics for preventive care. Each chapter provides a blend of theoretical insights, methodological advances, and real-world case studies that collectively demonstrate how these intelligent systems can address pressing healthcare challenges.

The goal of this volume is twofold: to serve as a comprehensive academic resource for researchers and students pursuing work in AI and fuzzy systems in healthcare, and to offer a practical guide for clinicians, policymakers, and industry professionals seeking to implement smart technologies in medical environments. By bridging the gap between computational intelligence and healthcare delivery, this book aims to inspire new directions in the design of reliable, ethical, and human-centric intelligent healthcare systems.

We extend our sincere gratitude to all contributing authors for their scholarly efforts and to the reviewers for their valuable feedback. We also thank the editorial and production teams for their continued support in bringing this volume to fruition. We hope this book serves as both a reference and a catalyst for further exploration into how fuzzy logic and AI can collaboratively revolutionize patient care in the era of smart healthcare.

Kanpur, India Digvijay Pandey
Kalyani, India Rahul Kar
Pantnagar, India Binay Kumar Pandey
Ranchi, India Prabjot Kaur
Riyadh, Saudi Arabia A. Shaji George
Bucharest, Romania Florin Popentiu Vlădicescu

Contents

About the Editors

Dr. Digvijay Pandey is currently working as an Acting Head of Department in the Department of Technical Education Kanpur, Government of Uttar Pradesh, India. Before this, he joined TCS in 2012 as an IT analyst and worked on various US/UK/Canada projects until 2016. He is also a faculty member at IERT Allahabad. He has teaching and industry experience of more than 11 years. He works as an editor for a peer-reviewed international journal. He has over ten years of experience in the field industry as well as teaching. He has written 15 books, 92 book chapters and 250 papers that have been published in Science Direct (Elisever)/SCI/UGC/Scopus Indexed Journals and also acts as an editor for a peer-reviewed international journal. He has presented several research papers at national and international conferences. He chaired a session at the IEEE International Conference on Advance Trends in Multidisciplinary Research and Innovation's (ICATMRI-2020). He has four patents that have been published in The Patent Office Journal, and one that is currently being processed in the Australian Patent Office Journal. He serves as a reviewer for a number of prestigious journals, including Scientific Reports (nature Publication), Clinical and Translational Imaging (Springer), ijlter (Scopus Indexed), and a slew of others. His research interests include medical image processing, image processing, text extraction, information security, and other related fields.

Rahul Kar is currently working as a State Aided Teacher of Mathematics faculty of Kalyani Mahavidyalaya, Kalyani, Nadia, West Bengal. He has worked as a guest faculty of Gurunanak Institute of Technology and other 2 colleges. In total he has 5 years of teaching experience. He has published many more than 10 research papers with scopus index. He also working as an editor of 4 national and international journal and reviewer at 5 international journals. He is working as an editor of several mathematics book. He is an annual member of Indian Mathematical Society as well as honorary member of Carmels Research Institute, Dakar, Senegal.

Prof. Binay Kumar Pandey is an Assistant Professor at Govind Ballabh Pant University of Agriculture and Technology in Pantnagar, Uttarakhand, India. He obtained his education qualification in the field of Information Technology, with a focus on Bioinformatics, image processing, and high-performance computing. In 2005, he received his first degree in B.Tech. from IET Lucknow (Uttar Pradesh Technical University, Uttar Pradesh, Lucknow), India. He started working as an assistant professor in the department of information technology at Govind Ballabh Pant University of Agriculture and Technology in Pantnagar in 2010 and has since worked on a wide range of UG and PG projects. He has over a decade of experience in the fields of teaching and research. He has over 70 publications in prestigious journals, including those from renowned publishers Springer, Inderscience, Taylor and Francis (SCIE/Scopus Indexed Journals, and others), as well as three patents published in the Indian official journal of patents and two patents published in the Australian official journal of patents. He is also an editor of scientific books published by international publishers such as NOVA International. He has received numerous awards, including the PM Scholarship, among others. He chaired a session at the IEEE International Conference on Advent Trends in Multidisciplinary Research and Innovation (ICATMRI-2020) on December 30, 2020, hosted by Pankaj Laddhad Institute of Technology and Management Studies in Buldhana, Maharashtra, India, and is a reviewer for SCI/Scopus indexed journals published by Springer, Wiley, Inder Science, Tech Science Publishers, Elsevier, and several others. He is an Associate Editor of SN Social Sciences, a multidisciplinary journal published by Springer Nature and Partners Universal International Research Journal (PUIRJ).

Dr. Prabjot Kaur is working as a faculty in Birla Institute of Technology, Mesra, Ranchi since last 14 years. She is a Ph.D. in Operation Research: Decision sciences. Her interest are applications of Fuzzy logic, Intuitionistic fuzzy sets, MCDM etc. in her area of research amp; other applications. She has several publications in National and International journal of repute. She is guiding and guided several Ph.D. and Master's thesis. She has presented her research papers in several conferences abroad. She has also completed a UGC major research project in Supply Chain Management (Vendor Selection Problem). She has two books to her credit.

Dr. A. Shaji George is a highly respected and accomplished figure in the fields of education and the ICT industry. With over 30 years of experience in designing and deploying large-scale projects, Dr. George has made significant contributions to industry. He has a passion for working with clients to help them overcome complex business challenges, drive innovation, and deliver results. Dr. George is recognized as an expert in the field of ICT and has published over 300 research papers in national and international journals and conferences. He is also the author of 30 books that have been published by reputed international publishers. His extensive contributions to the field have earned him 20 awards, recognizing his outstanding achievements and contributions to the industry. Dr. George is the founder of PU Publications, PUIRJ, PUIIJ and PUIRP International Journal. He has a keen interest in wireless networking, cloud computing, big data analytics, the Internet of Things, and industrial automation systems. He works with clients from a wide range of industries to develop strategies and implement next-generation solutions that transform their businesses.

Dr. George's wealth of knowledge and expertise make him a highly respected and sought-after expert in industry. His dedication to the field of ICT has enabled him to make significant contributions that have helped to shape the industry's future.

Dr. Florin Popentiu Vlădicescu is at present UNESCO Professor to Department of Control Engineering and Industrial Informatics, University "Politehnica" of Bucharest and Co-Chairholder to UNESCO Chair in Information Technologies, University of Oradea. Professor Florin POPENTIU VLĂDICESCU has been a Visiting Professor at:

- Telecom Paris, ENST
- Ecole Nationale Superieure des Mines Paris, ENSMP
- Ecole Nationale Superieure de Techniques Avancees, ENSTA
- ETH—Zurich
- Université Pierre et Marie Curie Paris, UPMC
- Delft University of Technology
- University of Twente Enschede
- Technical University of Denmark Lyngby
- Sultan Qaboos University
- University of Calcutta

He was a member of the Programme Committees for, ESREL′ 95, ′97—′03 and ′10—′12, held in UK, Portugal, Norway, Germany, Scotland, Italy, and Holland, Czech Republic, Greece, France and Finland.Also he was a member of the Programme Committee for ISSAT RQD, 2007, 2014-2022 in Ho Chi Minh City, Vietnam, Washington, Philadelphia, USA and Toronto, Canada, Las Vegas, Nevada, Miami, Florida USA, MA RS-2007–2012, 2014, 2019–2020 in Saint-Petersburg, Russia, WMSCI 2008-2012 in Orlando, Florida, USA, IADIS 2012, in Lisbon, Portugal MCCSIS 2013, held in Prague, Czech Republic, WBC 2014–2018, held Lisbon, Portugal, MCCSIS 2015 and MCCSIS 2020 in Las Palmas de Gran Canaria, Spain and Zagreb, Croatia BDM CC 2013, ICCD 2014, ICCD 2020 and ICCC 2016 held in Bhubaneswar, NABIC 2018, Vellore, December 6–8, India, ICIEECT 2017, Karachi, IMTIC ′15, Mehran University, Jamshoro, iCOMET 2019, Sukkur IBA University, Pakistan, VECoS 2015 and eLSE 2012–2021, held in Bucharest, Romania, ICDSBA 2018, in ChangSha, Hunan, IISA 2017 in Beijing, June 17–18, 2017, ICMIR 2017 in Kunming, China, May 2021, 2017, ICCD 2018 in Guangzhou, China, ICIM 2019–2020, held in Cambridge and London UK, ICIM 2022 EAET 2022, held in Imperial College London, UK, ICIC 2019-20, Mohali, Punjab,India, ICDAM-2020, 18th June 2020, Polkowice Poland and Haryana, India, ICITEE 2019–2021, Changsha, Hunan, China, ICICV 2020-21, Jaipur, India, ICIII 2021–2022, Osaka, Japan, MMBD 2020-21, Beijing, China, IICICT, Wuhan China, CIPR 2021, Kolkata, India, ARCI′21, Chamonix-Mont Blank, France, ISEAE 2021, Changsha, China, ICCIDM 2021, Aitam Andhra Pradesh, India, ISCTIS 2021Guilin, June 4–6, 2021, China, ICIMIR 2021 August 06–08, 2021 in Kunming, Yunnan, China, ICICT 2021 November 26-27, Delhi-NCR, Ghaziabad (UP), India,3DWCT 2022, May 24–26, 2022, DOSCI 2022, March 5, 2022, Lucknow, ICEITSA 2021, December 10–12, 2021, Huaihua,

China, ICCM, December,19–20, 2020, Bhubaneswar, India, ICDAM, June 26, 2021, Polkowise, Poland, SSEM, April 15–18, 2022, Changsha, China.

He has been invited in October 2014 to joint Steering Committee for Erasmus Mundus Action 2 Leading Mobility between Europe and Asia in Developing Engineering Education and Research (LEADERS) project as the representative of the University of Oradea, for the period 2014–2018. Prof. Florin POPENTIU VLÃDICESCU has published over 200 papers in International Journals and Conference Proceedings is author of one book and co-author of 4 books and co-editor of 4 books published by Springer. He has worked for many years on problems associated with software reliability and has been co-director of two NATO research projects involving collaboration with partner institutions throughout Europe. He is on advisory board of several international journals, Reliability: Theory amp; Applications, IJCS, ARIV and Microelectronics and Reliability (1988–1996) published by Pergamon Press/Elsevier and Sukkur IBA Journal of Computing and Mathematical Sciences (SJCMS) published by Sukkur IBA University. He is reviewer for ACM Computing Reviews, Neural Computing and Applications, IJCSIS, and Associated Editor to IJICT Guest Editor for International Journal of Distributed Systems and Technologies (IJDST), Special Issue on Innovations in Distributed Computing and Applications. Also he is a member of ENBIS, IEEE Reliability Society, IEEE Senior Member (SMIEEE). Dr. Florin POPENTIU VLÃDICESCU has been elected Fellow of the Academy of Romanian Scientists in 2008.

He is EU Expert for the H2020, ID EX2002BO39599, ALL EU Programme and Quality Agency for Higher Education (Academic Information Centre). His Research ID is E- 5787-2010. Also in 2009 he has been nominated UNESCO Expert in the field of Higher Education, Research and Knowledge. Prof. Florin POPENTIU VLÃDICESCU is currently Visiting Professor at quot;ParisTechquot; which includes the quot;Grandes Ecolesquot; The ATHENS Programme, where he teaches courses on Software Reliability. He also lectures on Software Reliability at International Master of Science in Computer Systems Engineering—Technical University of Denmark. Prof. Florin POPENTIU has been Keynote Speaker to ICCRT 2017 Karachi, IEMIS 2018 and iCOMET 2019, Sukkur IBA University, Pakistan, ICCD 2018 in Guangzhou, China,, WICT 2018 in Kochi, ICIC 2018 in Mohali, Punjab, India.

More information can be find on the following web pages:http://imm.dtu.dk/~popen/http://imm.dtu.dk/~popen/list.html

Enhancing Patient Care Management with AI and Fuzzy Systems

Kali Charan Modak, Sanju Mahawar, Shishir B. Nuti, Suhasini Vijaykumar, K. I. Pavan Kumar, Aradhana Sahu, and Hussein Basim Furaijl

Abstract This study examines an innovative approach to patient care management through integrating solutions that address imprecision with advanced computing technology. The discussion begins by examining current challenges in patient care, including elevated patient volumes, fragmented data, and the necessity for rapid, tailored decision-making, followed by the introduction of innovative concepts that integrate adaptable cognitive processes with data-informed analytical methods. The systems help to accurately determine the degrees of truth, management of the intrinsic uncertainty in clinical data, highlighting the role of the predictive modeling and deep pattern recognition in a facilitating the early diagnosis, risk stratification, and personalized therapeutic recommendations. Important uses included a real-time monitoring

K. C. Modak (✉) · S. Mahawar
IPS Academy, Institute of Business Management and Research, Indore, India
e-mail: kali.modak@gmail.com

S. Mahawar
e-mail: sanju746@gmail.com

S. B. Nuti
4th year MBBS student at BGS Global Institute of Medical Sciences, Bengaluru, India
e-mail: shishir.nuti@gmail.com

S. Vijaykumar
Department of Computer Applications, Bharati Vidyapeeths Institute of Management and Information Technology, Navi Mumbai, India

Bharati Vidyapeeth Educational Complex, Pune, India

K. I. Pavan Kumar
KLEF College of law, Koneru Lakshmaiah Education Foundation, Vaddeswaram, India
e-mail: principal.law@kluniversity.in

A. Sahu
Department of Computer Science and Engineering, Rungta College of Engineering and Technology, Bhilai, India
e-mail: aradhanasahu236@gmail.com

H. B. Furaijl
Collge of Pharmacy, University of Al-Ameed, Karbala, Iraq
e-mail: h.alfrejee@alameed.edu.iq

D. Pandey et al. (eds.), *Smart Healthcare*, https://doi.org/10.1007/978-981-95-8828-2_1

system that evaluate the vital signs and available lab data during all the time, as well as automated the diagnostic tools that determines the medical images and a patient histories. The integration of these technologies not only allows for more accurate predictions and treatment planning, but it also makes clinical decision-making more open by providing explainable, rule-based outputs. This hybrid approach will assist healthcare professionals to make the important use of their available resources, improve patient outcomes, and to reduce the chance of making numbers of mistakes. The study also able tackles the problems that come with existing traditional systems, such needing a lot of the data and having to retrain them often by showing the way of the combining data-centric models with systems that can able to handle uncertainty leads to solutions that are more adaptable, efficient, and easy to use. The combination of the Internet of Medical Things (IoMT), telemedicine, and explainable decision support tools calls for greater study to improve these models so they can meet the needs of modern healthcare settings as they change.

Keywords Patient care management · Fuzzy logic · AI · Diagnosis · Healthcare efficiency · Real-time monitoring

1 Introduction

The patient care management is considered essential for coordinating services, optimizing treatments. Several issues arise due to increasing patient populations, funding limitations, and the complexity of medical treatments. These issues are required to be addressed to improve healthcare efficiency and patient happiness. An aging population and chronic diseases are straining healthcare systems making patient care management difficult. As hospitals and clinics are often overcrowded, delaying diagnosis, treatment, and follow-up, therefore, healthcare providers struggle to maintain efficiency and quality as demand rises. The shortage of trained medical experts makes it challenging to provide tailored care to each patient. The healthcare data fragmentation is another issue and patient histories are typically inconsistent due to medical record fragmentation. In the dearth of EHR interoperability, healthcare professionals are unable to exchange information. This leads to redundant testing, misdiagnoses, and postponed treatments. The lack of integrated data management makes the clinicians unable to make educated decisions and adversely affects patient outcomes. An effective care management is often hindered by cost and the healthcare organizations sometimes lack budgets to invest in new medical technologies and infrastructure. Growing operational expenses and the costs of medications and treatments impact both providers and patients. The less fortunate individuals have restricted access to quality care due to financial constraints. The issues include patient engagement and adherence to treatment protocols. Many individuals fail to follow recommended regimens due to a lack of understanding and financial limitations, which are considered obstacles or challenges in accessing healthcare. The lack of access to medication and follow-up appointments deteriorates health outcomes elevates hospital readmission rates. The most serious cases necessitate rapid response and effective resource allocation within healthcare systems. The delays in life-saving therapies normally occur, due to shortages in ICU beds, staff, and medical equipment. The response process needed enhancement to reduce preventable fatalities.

1.1 Technology in Improving Healthcare Efficiency

The technological advancements have transformed the healthcare industry, by simplifying the procedures which reducing operational inefficiencies. By incorporating digital technology, it is possible to achieve faster diagnosis, better patient monitoring, and more effective treatment options. Nowadays, the healthcare demands are on the rise rapidly and technology is crucial for optimizing service delivery and resource management. Automation is considered as a one of the most significant methods though which technology has alleviated administrative burdens and minimized human error. An automated processes that cut down the paperwork in hospitals allow medical staff, to spend more time providing patients with the required care. Systems like computerized physician order entry (CPOE) reduce the possibility of dangerous drug interactions and facilitate error-free prescription handling. The automated billing and claims processing also improve the financial operations by reducing payment delays and improving hospital revenue cycles. Normally, the improvements in medical diagnostic have also transformed healthcare efficiency in more effectively. The medical diagnostics methodologies such as computed tomography (CT) scans, high-resolution magnetic resonance imaging (MRI), and three-dimensional (3D) imaging are examples of modern medical imaging techniques that offer more detailed information that can be utilized for the early and precise diagnosis of illness. AI-assisted image recognition helps radiologists find abnormalities more quickly and improving patient outcomes that helps to cutting down on diagnostic time. These developments increase the likelihood of successful treatment for conditions like cancer, neurological disorders, and cardiovascular problems by increasing the rate of early detection. Supply chain optimization is another aspect of healthcare efficiency. An AI-powered intelligent inventory management systems uses to predict the demand for pharmaceuticals supplies that can help hospitals cut waste and also improve supply reliability (Burton et al., 2019). The RFID (Radio-Frequency Identification) and blockchain-based tracking technologies make medical logistics more transparent with help of preventing the supply chain from handling fake medications and guaranteeing the timely delivery of essential supplies. The use of remote patient monitoring (RPM) has significantly increased efficiency as well as decreased readmissions to hospitals that offered ongoing care for the chronic illnesses. Medical devices that continuously monitor the vital signs such as blood sugar, oxygen levels, and heart rate make the medical professionals to take preventative measures as soon as possible. A continuous evaluation can help patients having a conditions like diabetes, heart disease, or hypertension who don't need to be hospitalized, as frequently which eases the strain on healthcare facilities. The new opportunities for enhancing surgical accuracy and medical education have been made possible due to the use of the virtual and augmented reality (VR/AR). Before the start of executing intricate procedures on actual patients. Students and healthcare professionals may further develop their skills in a secure environment by utilizing virtual reality (VR) simulators. The use of virtual reality enhances surgical precision and reduces risks by superimposing digital information onto the patient's anatomy. Information security protocols have safeguarded sensitive patient information despite enhancing efficiency. The aims of authentication with multiple factors, secured databases, and AI-driven threat detection systems involve safeguarding private data and ensure compliance with regulations such as HIPAA. The public's confidence in telehealth services and electronic health records relies on a secure virtual framework.

1.2 *AI and Fuzzy Systems in Healthcare*

A considerable component of the revolution in medical care supply can be linked to the implementation of sophisticated computer techniques. This evolution has help to enabled more accurate diagnostics, and enhanced choice-making that help to aid professionals in formulating more informed judgments. Such advanced tools analyze vast amounts of clinical data and identify complex patterns. Emerging medical technologies exhibit enhanced precision and adaptability with integrating computational intelligence and uncertainty management processes. The ability of sophisticated algorithms for computation to analyze extensive datasets and detect early indications of diseases is a crucial attribute of these systems. Conventional medical treatments predominantly depend on the human competence; nevertheless, this knowledge may be limited by temporal constraints and subjective judgment at times. Contemporary algorithms should swiftly analyze patient histories, diagnostic scans, and laboratory findings to detect potential health risks prior to the onset of severe symptoms. This enables timely intervention, ultimately resulting in less problems and an enhancement overall the patient's general health. The ability to manage ambiguous and flawed medical information represents another crucial element. The overlap of symptoms among many health conditions affects the attainment of definitive outcomes by rule-based methodologies. The integration of varying levels of risk, magnitude, and probability constitutes a method by which computational models designed to understand uncertainty provide a more adaptable approach (Yang et al., 2019). This tool can be particularly beneficial whenever accurate measurements be unavailable or when medical practitioners have to consider several factors in therapeutic decision-making. To enhance accuracy as well as adjust to unexpected variations throughout operations and these systems evaluate sensory feedback in real-time systems. The automated methodologies employed by the pharmaceutical research expedite drug development by identifying potentially beneficial compounds and assessing interaction possibilities. This reduces the time required enabling the implementation of innovative medicines in clinical environments. This is particularly evident in the management of chronic illnesses. The remote monitoring devices have benefited from the implementation of contemporary computing methods. The biosensors and wearable devices constantly compute several critical parameters that included the heart rate, glucose levels, and oxygen saturation. The versatile models evaluate variations contextually, differentiating, by using a typical alterations and preliminary warning signals. This contrasts with models that depend solely on predetermined threshold values. The outcome confirm that the critical warnings receive prompt action that help to reduce the incidence of superfluous alarms. These technologies are establishing a foundation for a new paradigm of precision medicine. This shift toward personalized healthcare not only enhances patient outcomes and also optimizes resource allocation available in the medical facilities. This effort is being facilitated by the integration of sophisticated analytical abilities and flexible decision-making structures (Secinaro et al., 2021). As a result, healthcare providers are better equipped to make informed decisions that directly impact patient outcomes. Furthermore, this shift toward personalized care enhances the efficacy of treatments and fosters a more patient-centric approach.

2 AI and Fuzzy Systems in Healthcare

2.1 Fuzzy Logic and Fuzzy Systems

Fuzzy logic is a computer method that helps people make decisions when things aren't clear or certain. Fuzzy logic lets inputs have different levels of truth, but classical binary logic only lets inputs be true or false. This makes it easier to think about things in different ways. This method works best in systems that are hard to define or that have a lot of related factors that affect the results. Fuzzy logic uses fuzzy sets, which let you be a part of more than one group instead of just one. A fuzzy system can tell you that a temperature is not just hot or cold, but also mildly warm, fairly hot, or very cold. This is because things aren't always clear in the real world. This method is very useful in many areas because it helps people analyses and respond to changes in the environment in a more human-like way. A normal fuzzy system has four main parts: fuzzification, a rule base, an inference engine, and defuzzification. Fuzzification uses pre-set membership functions to turn exact numbers into fuzzy values. There are a lot of "if-then" statements in the rule base that come from experts which tell the system what to do. The inference engine normally uses these rules to figure out the inputs mean and give the right answers. The next step is defuzzification that turns the fuzzy outputs back into real-world numbers. Fuzzy logic is used a lot in AI, automation, and smart control systems right now. It can also improve how businesses work by changing parameters in real time based on how things are changing. It makes robots more adaptable by allowing them to move more precisely when they can't predict what will happen next. The fuzzy logic is also used in everyday things like car control systems and household appliances to make them easier to use and work better together. One of the best things about fuzzy logic is that it can deal with unclear and vague information. It works like human reasoning because it lets people make decisions even when the facts aren't clear or complete. This is very helpful to find out what's wrong with someone, how dangerous something is, or what the weather will be like (Jiang et al., 2017). The Fuzzy logic is becoming more common in machine learning, neural networks, and optimizations algorithms. This makes systems that are smarter and can change to fit different situations. It can be stay important for a lot of new uses, because it can balance strict computational logic with the complexity of the real world (Lee et al., 2021).

2.2 AI and Fuzzy Systems in Healthcare

Artificial intelligence in healthcare system uses a modern computing methods, like machine learning, deep learning, and natural language processing to perform an analysis of the complex clinical data and help people make decisions. This technology utilizes a lot of structured and unstructured data available in electronic health records, medical imaging, genomic data, and patient-reported outcomes, to find patterns and also predict how diseases will progress, and suggest personalized treatment plans. Artificial intelligence can improve the patient care by making diagnoses more accurate, treatments more specific, and administrative tasks more efficient. AI automates a routine task and cuts down on human error that the healthcare workers focus on getting patients involved and making difficult clinical decisions. AI-driven systems can be able to find early-stage tumors and microfractures in imaging images that people might miss and making it easier to get treatment on time and improve the net outcomes. AI-powered predictive analytics can perform analyses at a patient's risk factors and predict what outcome, which helps the doctors take steps to avoid problems. AI algorithms analyze patient data in order to create individualized treatment plans that take into account of genetic predispositions, lifestyle factors, and environmental influences. The personalized methods normally help to make the treatment more effective, reduce side effects, and make the best use of resources. Artificial intelligence speeds up the process of finding new drugs and conducting clinical trials. This expands healthcare research and development beyond just clinical uses. Traditional research methods require substantial time and financial investment, whereas machine learning algorithms can pinpoint promising therapeutic targets and predict pharmaceutical efficacy from large datasets. The natural language processing can also obtain a lot of useful information from the large amounts of medical literature and patient feedback that can help to improve a medical practices and policies. The artificial intelligence is actually used to automate scheduling, billing, and supply chain logistics for the patients in hospital. This makes a healthcare delivery systems much better and also cuts down the incur administrative costs. AI helps data-driven healthcare systems to deal with a too much information by turning the raw data into a useful insight that improves the treatment outcomes. Because AI can learn and change, its healthcare applications are always changing. With each new dataset, machine learning models get better at making predictions and are more reliable. Healthcare is always changing because new diseases are always coming up and the demographics of patients are always changing. Because of this, education is always necessary. There are many benefits to using AI in healthcare, but there are also big problems with data privacy, ethics, and regulation (Graham et al., 2019). These issues need to be fixed to make sure that AI systems protect patient privacy and get the most out of clinical benefits. By improving accuracy, efficiency, and personalization in patient care, it improves clinical outcomes and the delivery of healthcare. Artificial intelligence is set to change healthcare in a big way, from diagnosing and treating patients to managing administration and doing research. This will make the system more efficient, cost-effective, and focused on patients (Ojo et al., 2024).

3 AI in Patient Care Management

3.1 AI-Driven Diagnosis and Decision Support Systems

AI-powered diagnostic along with decision-making tools are now changing the medical field, by making clinical decision-making more accurate and more efficient. By using machine learning, deep learning, and natural language processing together, it is possible look at a lot of medical data, such as genomic information, electronic health records, and medical images. One of the most important uses of AI in a diagnosis is in medical imaging. The deep learning models can considerably identify the illnesses that included cancer, pneumonia, and neurological disorders. Basically, the artificial intelligence algorithms are designed to perform analyses on radiological images, like X-rays, MRIs, and CT scans. In order to find problems that human radiologists not able to detect. This method helps find a problem in very early stage and able to make patients' lives better. AI used in decision support gives a medical staff real-time advice based on symptoms of a patient's, medical history, and treatment standards. Clinical decision support systems (CDSS) use AI and hospital data to make personalized treatment suggestions, predict how an illness will progress, and cut down on medical mistakes. AI helps with triage by putting the most important cases at the top of the list in emergencies. Chatbots and virtual assistants powered by artificial intelligence help with initial diagnosis and keeping patients involved, which makes these procedures easier for medical staff. These technologies combine artificial intelligence with traditional knowledge to help people make better decisions. This improves patient care and makes healthcare facilities, like hospitals and clinics, run more smoothly (Chakraborty et al., 2023).

3.2 *Predictive Analytics for Patient Outcomes*

Artificial intelligence-driven diagnostic and decision-making technologies are together revolutionizing the medical field by performing improvement in the metrices such as accuracy, efficiency, and speed of clinical decision-making. These systems analyze the medical data that includes genomic information, electronic health records, and medical imaging. One of the most significant applications of artificial intelligence in diagnosis is inside medical imaging. Deep learning models may also help to accurately diagnose diseases including cancer, pneumonia, and neurological disorders. The objective of artificial intelligence algorithms is to analyze radiological images to identify the anomalies that may be missed by human radiologists. This approach can be enhanced an early detection and improve patient health. The artificial intelligence in decision support provides a medical personnel member a detailed real-time recommendation that is based on a patient's symptoms, medical history, and also the treatment standards. The clinical decision support systems are used to amalgamate artificial intelligence with hospital information and also provide personalized therapy recommendations, forecast illness progression, and minimize a medical error. The AI assists in this whole triage process and prioritizing the most critical cases in emergency situations. Artificial intelligence-driven chatbots and virtual assistants helps to facilitate the initial diagnosis and the patient engagement, which normally helps to reduce the burden on medical staff during these procedures. These technologies also ensure that the enhanced decision-making by integrating artificial intelligence with the conventional expertise. This enhances patient care and operational efficiency in healthcare facilities, including hospitals and clinics (Chakraborty et al., 2023).

3.3 *Recommendations for Individualized Treatment*

These personalized treatment recommendations make use of sophisticated data analytics to tailor medical care to the specific characteristics of each individual patient. These systems provide precise and effective treatment plans. It also enhances patient outcomes by integrating genetic information, medical history, lifestyle factors, and real-time health data. Such an approach allows for an accurate and efficient treatment plan to be developed. The field of oncology is considered one of the most important applications of customized medicine in the present time, and in this field, AI-driven models examine the genetic profile of a patient to make recommendations for targeted therapies. Oncologists are able to establish the most effective treatment combinations. It is also limiting unwanted effects with the use of this method. In a similar manner, predictive algorithms are used in cardiology. This predictive algorithm is used to evaluate risk variables such as blood pressure, cholesterol levels, and lifestyle habits. These recommendations aim to create tailored strategies for preventing and treating heart disease. The machine learning models are going to be helpful in optimizing medication programs. This is because the models can predict how a patient will react to a specific prescription. This guarantees, that the dosage is as effective as possible and also to lowers the danger of unwanted drug reactions. The decision support systems powered by artificial intelligence enable medical professionals to make dynamic adjustments to therapies based on real-time patient data. This enhances the overall management of the chronic diseases, such as diabetes and hypertension. The personalized treatment enables healthcare practitioners, to provide care which is more precise, efficient, and patient-centered. Moving away from a one-size-fits-all strategy ultimately leads to improved medical results (Joshi et al., 2022).

3.4 Virtual Health Assistants and Chatbots

The chatbots and virtual health assistants are used to revolutionize the patient interaction. By offering immediate access to an appointment booking, symptom assessment, and medical advice. These artificial intelligence (AI) tools use a machine learning and the natural language processing (NLP) together to communicate with patients, respond to health-related enquiries, and assist medical professionals with daily duties. The preliminary diagnosis and triage are to be considered two important areas where the virtual assistants are usually used. A chatbot is used to receive a patient's description of their symptoms, thereafter evaluates it, and then suggests potential explanations, self-care advice, or medical help. By identifying a non-urgent case and referring an emergency patient to the right care unit. This will be lessened the overall workload for a medical staff working in a healthcare center. Through the process of symptom monitoring, medication reminders, and lifestyle advice, chatbots can also be used to enhance the management of chronic illnesses. Real-time coaching is provided to the patients suffering with diseases like diabetes or hypertension to ensure that the treatment plans are followed. The chatbots for mental health have also help users by providing a crisis intervention service, emotional support, and a cognitive behavioral therapy (CBT) procedure. In addition to assisting patients, the virtual health assistants expedite the administrative duties like appointment scheduling, medical record retrieval, and insurance-related enquiries. These AI-powered solutions are be used to improve a healthcare delivery, cut down on a wait times, and give patients greater control over their health by increasing their accessibility and efficiency.

4 Fuzzy Systems in Patient Care

4.1 Handling Uncertainty in Medical Diagnosis

Managing uncertainty in a medical diagnosis has presented a significant difficulty in contemporary healthcare due to the intrinsic variability and the ambiguity of clinical data. Often, a patient's symptoms only partially match a binary classification of conditions that are usually present or absent. This uncertainty basically originates from the multiple factors, including a discrepancy in patient reporting, inaccurate measurement instruments, and an insufficient medical history. The conventional diagnostic methods frequently depend on inflexible thresholds and dichotomous decision-making that can be oversimplify intricate medical situations and risk a misdiagnosis. The excellent method for the addressing of this ambiguity is the utilization of the fuzzy logic. In contrast to traditional methodologies, fuzzy logic does not impose a rigid binary decision but rather allocates varying degrees of membership to different diagnostic criteria. For example, instead of categorizing a symptom as merely mild or severe. Fuzzy logic enables clinicians to assess the intensity on the continuous spectrum and also refined depiction that encapsulates the intricacies of a patient's situation. Fuzzy logic is used to enable more precise diagnostic assessment methods. The Fuzzy logic is considered as an essential element in medical imaging for managing the noisy and a frequently ambiguous data that are produced by a modalities like MRI, CT scans, and ultrasounds. Fuzzy segmentation algorithms are used to allocate incremental membership values to pixels, thereby precisely outlining a boundary between various tissue types, even when those boundaries are not explicitly specified. This feature is crucial for differentiating between normal tissue and abnormal regions, such as tumors or lesions, where conventional approaches may fail due to overlapping intensity data. The use of fuzzy logic in hybrid models, combined with machine learning approaches, markedly improves the diagnostic process. Although the machine learning algorithms are proficient in analyzing extensive datasets and also uncovering the concealed patterns. But it frequently functions as black boxes with complete restricted interpretability (Pandey & Pandey, 2025). By incorporating a proper fuzzy logic that provides these systems with a visible, rule-based framework. This combination facilitates ongoing learning from fresh data, while preserving the adaptability to manage confusing or incomplete information (El-Douh et al., 2023).

4.2 Fuzzy Logic in Medical Imaging and Pattern Recognition

The use of fuzzy logic in medical imaging and pattern recognition has brought about a revolution in diagnostic analysis by solving the problem of dealing with the inherent uncertainty and variability of image data. It does this by assigning degrees of membership to pixels, which makes intricate segmentation and accurate tissue categorization much easier to do. By using this method, the detection of small anomalies is improved, and the differentiation of overlapping tissue features is accomplished more efficiently. The use of fuzzy algorithms into medical imaging systems allows for the processing of noisy data and ambiguous boundaries, which ultimately results in images that are clearer for diagnosis. Fuzzy logic helps with pattern recognition by examining gradual changes, which ensures improved early disease diagnosis and provides more precise and interpretable outcomes for clinical decision-making, ultimately leading to an improvement in overall patient care. Finally, fuzzy logic helps improve overall patient care. Application of Fuzzy Imaging & Patterns are as shown in Fig. 2.

1. *Continuous Fuzzification*: Fuzzy logic assigns a spectrum of membership values to each pixel rather of a simple binary classification. This is in contrast to the traditional method of binary classification. This method is able to capture tiny gradients and variations in tissue characteristics, which enables a more detailed picture of anatomical structures to be created. It assists in identifying between gradual changes in tissue types, which is particularly significant when distinguishing between healthy and pathological parts of the body.
2. *Dynamic Threshold Adaptation*: Two examples of dynamic threshold adaptation are as follows: Adjustments to segmentation thresholds are made automatically by the system in response to fluctuations in local intensity. With the help of this dynamic adaptation, sections that have fluctuating levels of brightness or contrast are accurately identified. This method improves the precision of boundary recognition in complicated images by reducing the number of misclassification mistakes that frequently occur with fixed threshold approaches. This is accomplished by adapting thresholds to different sections of the image at different times.
3. *Effective Noise Reduction*: The elimination of random noise and the reduction of image artifacts are both significantly facilitated by the utilization of fuzzy approaches. A reduction in the impact of spurious fluctuations is achieved by the system by the assignment of varied degrees of significance to the values of those pixels. Consequently, this leads to images that are cleaner and more reliable, which in turn improves subsequent analysis such as the characterization of tissues and the detection of anomalies.
4. *Enhanced Detail Extraction*: A better detection of small textures and subtle edge characteristics inside medical images can be achieved through the use of the fuzzy logic technique. When it comes to precisely diagnosing minor anomalies or early indicators of clinical illnesses, this enhanced detail extraction is absolutely necessary. The distinction of intricate structures is made possible in locations where conventional approaches could miss differences that are clinically significant despite being seemingly insignificant (Ahmad et al., 2023).
5. *Anomaly Detection*: Fuzzy systems are able to recognize unusual patterns and deviations by analyzing degrees of membership across several features. This is referred to as "anomaly detection." Because of this skill, it is possible to detect potential pathological changes at an earlier stage, such as the growth of tumors or the degradation of tissues. Fuzzy logic makes it easier to implement timely

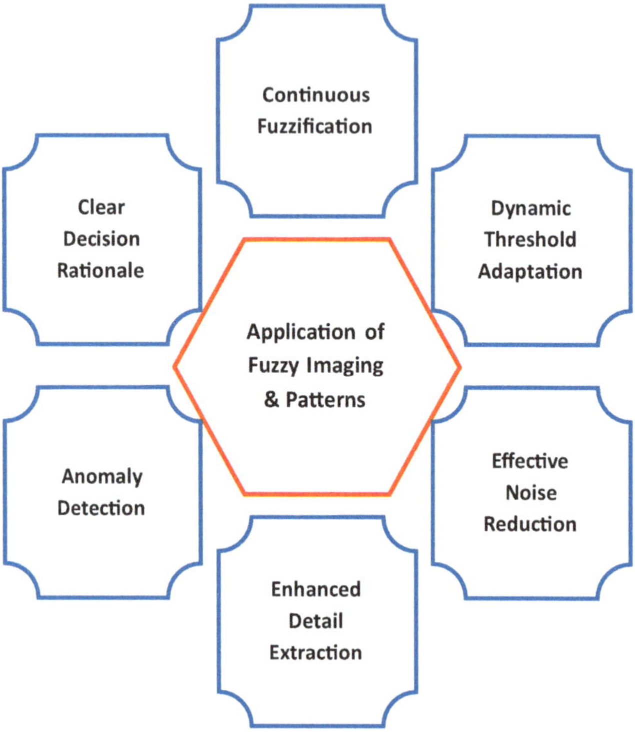

Fig. 2 Application of Fuzzy Imaging & Patterns

treatments and conduct additional diagnostic evaluations by highlighting regions that constitute a considerable departure from the typical patterns.

6. *Clear Decision Rationale*: The decision-making process under fuzzy logic is transparent and based on rules, which is one of the advantages of fuzzy logic. Each output is derived from specific rules that offer a clear justification for the classification or segmentation result. These rules are utilized to produce each output. As a result of this transparency, doctors are able to more easily comprehend the data, validate the process, and accept the suggestions made by the system, which ultimately contributes to improved clinical decision-making.

5 Integration of AI and Fuzzy Systems in Healthcare

The hybrid AI-fuzzy models show a substantial progression in a contemporary healthcare decision-making system. These models combine an analytical capability of the sophisticated machine learning algorithms along with the adaptable human-like reasoning of a fuzzy logic. The conventional data-driven systems basically depend on extensive, a well-organized datasets and intricate neural networks to identify the patterns and provide predictions. It frequently encounters difficulties, when confronted with inadequate or unclear clinical data. Conversely, a fuzzy logic proficiently manages ambiguity by interpreting the inputs as degrees of truth instead of a binary value. A Hybrid models, by integrating these two methodologies may provide the advantages of a both elevated accuracy and the interpretability, hence it improving a diagnostic precision and the treatment planning. In these hybrid systems, a machine learning element is to be evaluate large quantities of both organized and unstructured medical data, including imaging, laboratory results, and patient histories. This investigation establishes the basis for early disease identification, risk assessment, and predictive analytics. Simultaneously, the fuzzy logic components engage to analyze ambiguous or imprecise information such as subjective symptom descriptions and qualitative clinical observations employing expert-defined rules and membership functions. The Patient-reported a descriptor such as a mild or severe are assessed by using a fuzzy set that enabling the system to produce subtle insights that enhance a patient triage and a personalized care plan. This dual-layered strategy is guarantees that the given recommendations are statistically sound while simultaneously addressing the intrinsic variability in a clinical situation. The advantages of AI-fuzzy integration surpass those of conventional healthcare systems. A significant benefit of a AI-fuzzy integration is the improvement in a diagnostic precision that utilized the integration of a meticulous data analysis and adaptable reasoning. A hybrid models can normally use to identify a nuanced illness indicators that, the traditional methods may miss. This results in more dependable forecasts, particularly in situations when swift decision-making is essential, such as in emergency or intensive care environments. These models are also providing a tailored treatment suggestions by consistently adjusting to a fresh patient data and clinical results. The capacity to adapt treatment programs in a real-time diminishes the probability of an adverse medication reactions, and also enhances the efficacy of therapeutic measures. A significant advantage is the enhanced transparency in the decision-making process. The conventional AI systems are frequently regarded, as a black boxes due to their provision of outputs without any transparent justifications. Conversely, the fuzzy logic element of hybrid models provides clear and the rule-based reasoning that practitioners can readily comprehend and verify (Sreedhar et al., 2025). This transparency fosters the trust among healthcare providers and also facilitates the ongoing enhancement of the systems (Kumarganesh et al., 2025). Additionally, a hybrid models exhibit greater adaptability and sustain a strong performance, while encountering limited or low-quality data and necessitate less frequent retraining than exclusively AI-driven systems. This versatility is especially beneficial in dynamic clinical settings, where the patient situations may swiftly alter. The amalgamation of a AI and the fuzzy logic within a hybrid models made up a robust decision support framework that will be enhances clinical processes [17], optimizes resource distribution, and markedly elevates patient outcomes. These systems exemplify a patient-centered methodology, that guaranteed the healthcare provision in an accurate and flexible, particularly in response to the intricate nature of medical practice.

6 Conclusion

New computational approaches and fuzzy logic can alter patient care management. We showed how data-driven algorithms efficiently process large clinical data to provide accurate diagnoses and personalized treatment plans, while fuzzy logic handles uncertainty and subjectivity in real-world medical situations. These methodologies combined into hybrid models improve diagnostic accuracy and interpretability, overcoming constraints in rule-based decision-making systems. These hybrid models use large datasets and powerful pattern recognition to diagnose and stratify diseases early and allocate healthcare resources more efficiently. Fuzzy logic also interprets ambiguous symptoms and imprecise data to provide more sophisticated patient assessments and dynamic treatment modifications. This integration improves diagnostic precision, treatment planning, and real-time patient monitoring, which helps manage chronic illnesses and reduce hospital readmissions. Fuzzy systems rule-based explanations help doctors validate and comprehend procedures, which increases decision-making transparency and trust. Potential impact on patient care management is significant. These hybrid solutions accelerate clinical workflows, eliminate medical errors, and improve patient outcomes by enabling a patient-centric approach. These systems' continuous monitoring and adaptive capabilities provide more tailored care, which is especially useful in emergencies and severe chronic conditions. Rigid data analysis and flexible reasoning let doctors make better, faster judgments, improving healthcare. To address data quality, system scalability, and smooth connection with healthcare infrastructures, future studies must refine these hybrid models. These systems need multidisciplinary collaboration between physicians, researchers, and technologists to improve adaptability and precision. More clinical studies and real-world validations will improve model performance and increase healthcare professional acceptance.

References

Ahmad, S., Masood, S., Khan, N. Z., Badruddin, I. A., Ahmadian, A., Khan, Z. A., & Khan, A. H. (2023). Analysing the impact of COVID-19 pandemic on the psychological health of people using fuzzy MCDM methods. *Operations Research Perspectives, 10*, 100263.

Burton, R. J., Albur, M., Eberl, M., & Cuff, S. M. (2019). Using artificial intelligence to reduce diagnostic workload without compromising detection of urinary tract infections. *BMC Medical Informatics and Decision Making, 19*, 171.

Chakraborty, S., Raut, R. D., Rofin, T. M., & Chakraborty, S. (2023). A comprehensive and systematic review of multi-criteria decision-making methods and applications in healthcare. *Healthcare Analytics, 4*, 100232.

El-Douh, A. A., Lu, S., Abdelhafeez, A., & Aziz, A. S. (2023). Assessment the health sustainability using Neutrosophic MCDM methodology: Case study COVID-19. *Sustainable Machine Intelligence Journal, 3*, 1–10.

Graham, S., Depp, C., Lee, E. E., Nebeker, C., Tu, X., Kim, H. C., & Jeste, D. V. (2019). Artificial intelligence for mental health and mental illnesses: An overview. *Current Psychiatry Reports, 21*, 116.

Jiang, F., Jiang, Y., Zhi, H., Dong, Y., Li, H., Ma, S., Wang, Y., Dong, Q., Shen, H., & Wang, Y. (2017). Artificial intelligence in healthcare: Past, present and future. *Stroke and Vascular Neurology, 2*, 230–243.

Joshi, S., Sharma, M., Das, R. P., Rosak-Szyrocka, J., Żywiołek, J., Muduli, K., & Prasad, M. (2022). Modeling conceptual framework for implementing barriers of AI in public healthcare for improving operational excellence: Experiences from developing countries. *Sustainability, 14*, 11698.

Kumarganesh, S., Malathi Murugesan, C., Ganesh, N., Santhiyakumari, M., Thangavel, K., Jayaram, K. M., Sagayam, B. K., & Pandey, B.K., & Pandey, D.. (2025). Hybrid plasmonic biosensors with deep learning for colorectal cancer detection. *Plasmonics, 20*(7), 4895–4909.

Lee, E. E., Torous, J., De Choudhury, M., Depp, C. A., Graham, S. A., Kim, H.-C., Paulus, M. P., Krystal, J. H., & Jeste, D. V. (2021). Artificial intelligence for mental health care: Clinical applications, barriers, facilitators, and artificial wisdom. *Biological Psychiatry: Cognitive Neuroscience and Neuroimaging, 6*, 856–864.

Ojo, Y., Davids, V., Oni, O., Odoemene, M., Idowu-Collin, P., & Eyeregba, U. (2024). A multi-criteria approach for evaluating the use of AI for matching patients to optimal mental health treatment plans. *Read. Time, 2024*, 5–9.

Pandey, B. K., & Pandey, D. (2025). Securing healthcare medical image information using advance morphological component analysis, information hiding systems, and hybrid convolutional neural networks on IoMT. *Computers in Biology and Medicine, 185*, 109499.

Secinaro, S., Calandra, D., Secinaro, A., Muthurangu, V., & Biancone, P. (2021). The role of artificial intelligence in healthcare: A structured literature review. *BMC Medical Informatics and Decision Making, 21*, 125.

Sreedhar, C., Suresh Kallam, G. S., Pradeep Ghantasala, S., Anthoniraj, S., Kumarganesh, K. M., Sagayam, B. K., Pandey, B.K., & Pandey, D. (2025). Enhancing healthcare data security using RFE and CRHSM for big data. *Computers in Biology and Medicine, 190*, 110063.

Yang, X., Wang, Y., Byrne, R., Schneider, G., & Yang, S. (2019). Concepts of artificial intelligence for computer-assisted drug discovery. *Chemical Reviews, 119*, 10520–10594.

AI-Powered Scheduling and Workforce Management in Healthcare

Chetan V. Hiremath, A. Vinay Bhushan, and Mahantesh Halagatti

Abstract The healthcare operations are being revolutionized by AI-powered labor management and scheduling. It is used to turn manual and traditional scheduling into a proactive data-driven process. In order to ensure that a labor allocation has been perfectly in line with a changing of the patient demands, this work looks at the application of cutting-edge technologies such as machine learning, predictive analytics, natural language processing, and IoT integration in the optimization of the staffing operations. These systems may be used to reduce administrative overhead and also minimize the danger of understaffing or overstaffing. By using historical data and the real-time inputs to predict peak periods and dynamically build an optimum shift of the rosters. In addition to increasing operational effectiveness and also lowering the overtime expenses. The shift scheduling automation is normally used to encourage a balance in the workload among medical professionals. This approach has been used to prevent burnout and also raise job satisfaction levels overall. By combining the data from several sources, such as wearable technology and electronic health records. A real-time resource allocation capability has allowed for quick reactions to unforeseen events that include emergencies or the abrupt spikes in-patient admissions. The decision-making is being improved by the smooth interoperability of various systems that enable managers to quickly reallocate the resources and that have upheld high patient care standards. The importance of ongoing monitoring and strategic staffing use in creating a robust and adaptable healthcare environment. The future developments in AI technology are expected to improve the scheduling of the precision and broaden the range of linked data sources, which is utilized for opening the door for workforce management systems that are even more flexible and safe.

C. V. Hiremath (✉)
Operations Management, Kirloskar Institute of Management, Harihar, India
e-mail: hirechetan@gmail.com

A. Vinay Bhushan
Department of Analytics, Kirlsokar Institute of Management, Harihar, India
e-mail: avbvinay@gmail.com

M. Halagatti
Operations Management, School of Management Studies and Research, KLE Technological University, Hubballi, India
e-mail: mahantesh.halagatti@kletech.ac.in

D. Pandey et al. (eds.), *Smart Healthcare*, https://doi.org/10.1007/978-981-95-8828-2_2

These innovations' main objective has been to improve the patient outcomes and also foster a more encouraging work environment for the healthcare providers by tackling the issues with data privacy and the ethical considerations.

Keywords AI-powered scheduling · Healthcare scheduling · Workforce management · Predictive analytics · Machine learning · IOT integration

1 Introduction

The Artificial Intelligence (AI) methodology is used to swiftly revolutionized the healthcare workforce management by applying a data-driven methodology for the scheduling and the resource allocation. In a healthcare setting, it is characterized by unpredictable variations in the patient requirements and personnel availability. AI systems have been offering a strategic approach to optimize a set of the staffing levels and also ensure the efficient and effective deployment of the medical experts. These advanced technologies have been amalgamating the historical data, real-time inputs, and intricate predictive analytics to optimize the various multifaceted processes of managing a heterogeneous workforce. A primary function of AI in this field is its capacity to process and evaluate vast volumes of information. An AI algorithm can be used to predict the periods of the high demand by analyzing data from sources such as electronic health records (EHRs), patient intake systems, and external factors like seasonal trends. This predictive capability is used to enable healthcare administrators to modify staffing plans more proactively and also assure the preparedness of the organization for peak periods and also the maintenance of high standards in-patient care (Dave & Patel, 2023). The ongoing learning component of AI is utilized to enhance these predictions. This system adjusts to an emerging pattern and also increases its precision over time. The automated scheduling is considered a vital component of the AI-driven workforce management. The conventional scheduling techniques have been typically dependent on a human input and the rigid procedures that may result in inefficiencies and discrepancies between the staff availability and a patient's requirements. Conversely, AI-driven scheduling systems are to assess numerous aspects concurrently that include the employee qualifications, labor regulations, and historical performance metrics to provide the efficient schedules. This automation has been diminishing administrative burdens. During it is fostering a more equitable distribution of shifts and guaranteeing that each team member has been deployed in appropriate places. The numerous AI systems are used to integrate a natural language processing (NLP) functionality with a more intuitive understanding of scheduling requests and staff input. This functionality has been used to enhance contact between healthcare providers and the available scheduling system. This technique enables rapid adjustments and tailored scheduling solutions. By utilizing real-time monitoring and the adaptive algorithms, AI functions acted as a central command that is used to persistently readjust workforce distribution in response to the changing conditions, including unforeseen sets of staff absences or abrupt increases in the number of patient admissions (Brambilla et al., 2021).

1.1 Efficient Scheduling in Healthcare

The effective scheduling in healthcare is fundamental for delivering superior patient care. It is essential in reconciling patient needs with the availability of an healthcare personnel that is crucial in a field where the delays or deficiencies in a service can led to the significant repercussions. Effective scheduling basically impacts the patient outcomes by guaranteeing consistent staff coverage. An effective schedule management must be ensured that the patients receive prompt assessments, treatments, and interventions, hence minimizing the chance of problems. In emergency rooms or intensive care units, it is found that the appropriate distribution of qualified staff can determine a swift response to the urgent crisis or a life-threatening wait. This not only augments patient safety but also elevates overall recovery rates (Prakash et al., 1914). A notable factor has been affected on the healthcare practitioners. The characteristic of the medical work has been frequently entailing extended hours and high-pressure environments that render the staff's well-being essential. It is also found that the ineffective scheduling may result in overburdened personnel, therefore heightening the likelihood of fatigue and burnout. Through the implementation of effective scheduling systems. The healthcare institutions can allocate workloads more equitably and facilitate enough rest and recovery. This enhances the morale and also decreases the turnover rates; hence, retaining experienced and knowledgeable personnel becomes easier. A healthier workforce has been found, to be more equipped to deliver a compassionate and patient-centered care required in the healthcare environments. Effective scheduling also provides significant advantages in cost control. Normally insufficient scheduling may result in overstaffing during slow periods and understaffing during busy times, both of which can generate superfluous expenses. By synchronizing the staffing levels with patient demand. The healthcare institutions can mitigate the financial strain of overtime compensation and temporary employment. This financial efficiency enhances the overall sustainability of healthcare operations. The contemporary healthcare setting has been dependent on sophisticated technology and an apparatus that includes diagnostic imaging and electronic health records (EHRs). As the staff schedules are found to be effectively synchronized with these resources that help to optimize the use of both human and technological assets, facilitating smoother operations and a more efficient workflow (Joshi et al., 2024).

1.2 AI in Addressing Workforce Management

The AI-driven scheduling is used to transform healthcare workforce management through the integration of predictive analytics and machine learning to enhance shift planning and resource allocation. This sophisticated system has automated the scheduling and also guarantees the real-time staff allocation. According to patient demand and clinical requirements, the combination of IoT and an automated scheduling optimizes the operations to facilitate the dynamic personnel allocation and the effective healthcare scheduling.

These technologies which are shown in Fig. 1, alleviate administrative hassles, diminish errors, and foster equitable workloads, so improving patient care. As healthcare environments get more intricate, such intelligent systems provide scalable, data-driven solutions that enhance operational efficiency, lower costs, and guarantee high-quality care delivery across various medical contexts, leading to improved outcomes.

- *Smart Predictions*: The Artificial Intelligence (AI) systems have been using historical data and real-time patterns to predict the patient influx and demand. These algorithms can be utilized to anticipate increased demand by evaluating seasonal trends, local events, and patient data. This feature has normally allowed for the proactive staffing adjustments to prepare the hospital for rising patient loads. The system may be used to detect a winter respiratory sickness spike, prompting administrators to change plans. The prediction power also accounts for the weather fluctuations and the local health outbreaks, which can greatly affect the patient numbers. More accurate and reliable predictions are made for the system to receive updated data. The smart predictions improve the resource planning, patient wait times, and care quality to optimize the staff numbers to match demand. The AI-driven forecasting has been making the workforce management proactive and laying the groundwork for an effective healthcare delivery.
- *Auto Scheduling*: The AI-powered technologies has been built to efficient shift rosters, eliminating manual scheduling errors and the inefficiencies. These systems build the balanced schedules that suit the facility operational goals and the personnel limits by assessing an employee availability, skill sets, regulatory requirements, and an individual preference. The automation also ensures that every shift is covered by avoiding the danger of the understaffing during the peak times and overstaffing during quieter periods. The system may also be instantly redistributing the shifts for last-minute absences or crises, to ensure the ongoing service. The technique reduces an administrative cost and also promotes the justice and transparency by evenly allocating an employee duty. The managers can focus on the strategic changes, while auto scheduling streamlines the scheduling process that improving patient care and staff happiness. This method improves operational efficiency and personnel well-being in demanding healthcare (Pisapia et al., 2022).
- *Live updates*: AI-driven scheduling solutions is used to allow the real-time shift roster alterations and assuring an uninterrupted coverage during any unexpected events. When staff absences, emergencies arises, or the number of the patient

admissions increase, then the system instantly reassigns the shifts to maintain an optimal staffing levels. The healthcare system requires a dynamic reactivity since every minute matters and delays can harm patient care. The live updates are commonly integrated with a mobile device and the hospital communication platforms to notify each team members of changes quickly. This streamlines the operations and minimizes the administrative strain of the manually tracking and also changing the timetables. The system's quick adaptation is used to provide the continued patient care and the fair workload distribution among staff. The live updates help to improve the facility agility, an operational efficiency, and health outcomes by aligning the staff with the real-time demands.

- *Staff tracking*: The present modern AI personnel tracking systems helps to deliver constant attendance, performance, and the availability information. These systems can track the staff movements and also ensure where they are required via use of digital check-ins, mobile app integration, and the wearable gadgets. The real-time tracking helps to ensure shifts are covered and spot patterns that may suggest chronic lateness or exhaustion. Data is essential for resource allocation and identifying areas that need support or training. Specific tracking enhances payroll processing, lowers administrative errors, and reduces time theft. These methods foster worker trust, responsibility, and efficiency through transparency. AI personnel tracking helps healthcare managers optimize scheduling and retain a reliable, high-performing team, ensuring patient care (Wang et al., 1878).
- *Balanced Work*: The AI-powered scheduling solutions is used to help the healthcare practitioners to balance the workloads. Individual talents, experience, and past performance data are used to schedule shifts to avoid overburdening any employee. This fair allocation reduces burnout, a significant problem in high-stress healthcare settings. Staff are more productive and satisfied when workloads are balanced, improving patient care. The workload is used to monitor and also adjust in real time to correct the imbalances. The fair scheduling produces a friendly workplace, where the individuals feel valued and recognized for their contributions. Overwork stress is normally reduced by the method of the lowering absenteeism and the improving retention. This balanced approach improves the operational efficiency and fosters a sustainable work culture that used to prioritizes patient outcomes and staff well-being.
- *Decision Support*: AI-driven decision support technologies offer healthcare administrators meaningful insights and recommendations for simplified personnel management. These technologies provide evidence-based staff allocation advice by evaluating huge amounts of data from patient records, staffing logs, and regulatory standards. In time-sensitive circumstances, the insights assist managers make swift, educated decisions. Decision support systems may recommend reassigning workers from low-demand regions to high-patient-volume departments. These solutions also have intuitive dashboards that depict critical performance data, helping managers track staffing levels, trends, and problem areas. This real-time analytical tool simplifies complex data into actionable strategies, ensuring staffing decisions meet operational and budgetary needs. AI decision assistance

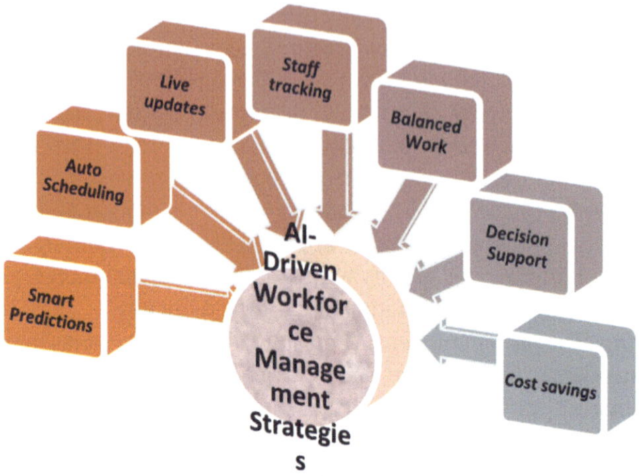

Fig. 1 AI-Driven workforce management strategies

improves patient care, staff satisfaction, and organizational efficiency by giving administrators data-driven insights.

- *Cost savings*: AI-powered scheduling tools match staffing to patient demand, saving healthcare businesses money. These technologies cut overtime pay and agency personnel costs by properly anticipating patient inflows and creating ideal shift rosters. Automating scheduling reduces HR departments administrative workload, freeing up resources for other important tasks. The precision of AI-driven scheduling eliminates overstaffing during slack periods and understaffing during busy times, which can waste money. As machine learning improves demand prediction and resource allocation, scheduling models become more cost-effective. As workers are better deployed to fulfill needs, payroll costs drop and patient care improves. The financial benefits of AI in workforce management help healthcare facilities stay competitive and provide high-quality treatment.

2 Components of AI-Powered Scheduling

2.1 Predictive Analytics for Demand Forecasting

The utilization of historical data and sophisticated algorithms have made the predictive analytics an important component of the contemporary healthcare workforce management. Its main objective is to accurately forecast the demand of the patients. Artificial intelligence systems are used to predict periods of the high and the low patient inflows, with remarkable precision by evaluating huge data sets. These data sets have been included the patient admission rates, seasonal sickness trends, and external influences such as weather patterns and local events. During flu season or unanticipated health emergencies, these models are able to spot early signals of higher admissions that enable the management to modify personnel levels in a proactive manner. By considering this strategy, the risk of an understaffing, during key periods has to be mitigated, and the inefficiencies that result from overstaffing during times of diminished activity are avoided. The predictions are regularly enhanced by the system, through the process of learning from fresh data, which guarantees that the forecasts will be continue to be accurate over time. A dynamic and data-driven approach, this method not only helps improve the distribution of healthcare resources, but it also assists in balancing the workloads of staff members, which in turn helps reduce burnout. In the end, predictive analytics transforms, the workforce planning into a proactive and responsive process that help to improves patient care while also boosting operational efficiency (Townsend et al., 2023).

2.2 *Automated Shift Scheduling and Optimization*

It is found that one of the most important aspects of contemporary healthcare workforce management is the automated shift of the scheduling and optimization. The dealing with complicated variables that include differing staff experience, regulatory work-hour constraints, and rapidly changing patient demand, manually establishing timetables in hectic healthcare environments has been considered time-consuming, prone to errors, and frequently rigid (Marengo & Pagano, 2023). To overcome these obstacles, An AI-driven system uses a complex algorithm that evaluates the various data sources and provides an ideal schedule. The automated scheduling systems can assess the multiple factors by combining data from patient intake systems, attendance logs, and the Electronic Health Records (EHRs). These variables have been included: projected patient volumes, staff availability, individual credentials, and the preferred shifts. As a result, the roster is to be extremely customized to meet the operating requirements of the facility and also guarantees that the appropriate mix of professionals is available whenever the need arises. Additionally, in order to account for unforeseen circumstances like last minute absences or unanticipated spikes in-patient admissions. The system has been dynamically modifying schedules in real time. By dividing duties among various employees fairly, an automated schedule also improves the fairness. This minimizes the burnout and encourages a better work-life balance for healthcare workers by identifying and resolving the possible imbalances using the historical data. When these systems are implemented, then the managers may concentrate on strategic decision-making. The computerized shift scheduling and optimization are used to improve patient care quality and operational efficiency. The essential tool is adjusting to the ever-changing healthcare landscape, and the system's scheduling accuracy increases as it learns from fresh data over time. These automated solutions help create a more robust, responsive, and sustainable healthcare system that benefits both employees and patients by guaranteeing that staffing levels are always in accordance with patient care requirements (Moldt et al., 2023).

2.3 Real-Time Resource Allocation

Real-time resource allocation is considered essential in contemporary healthcare operations that ensure the appropriate deployment of the personnel, equipment, and also the facilities according to current demands. In a dynamic healthcare environment, the influx and urgent circumstances of the patients might change swiftly, which necessitating a prompt reaction. An AI-driven system is essential in this process, as it continuously integrates and analyzes the data from many of the available sources, including electronic health records (EHRs), IoT devices, and real-time operational metrics. These systems have been offering real-time analytics to enable the administrators to rapidly reallocate resources. During a sudden surge of patients in the emergency department, the AI systems can promptly detect underutilized personnel in other departments and recommend the reassignments. Likewise, the systems can oversee the equipment utilization and availability to guarantee that the diagnostic instruments and life-saving items are accessible in critical locations. This responsiveness actually alleviates the delays in-patient care and also prevents the resource waste and bottlenecks. The real-time resource allocation enables anticipatory decision-making. By consistently monitoring important performance indicators such as patient wait times, staff workload, and bed occupancy rates, these systems can be used to anticipate the possible deficiencies before it escalates into significant problems. By doing so, it allows managers to modify a resource allocation even amidst the unforeseen surges or the crises, thus ensuring the continuity of service. Automating this procedure alleviates the administrative load on healthcare administrators and diminishes the likelihood of human error in high-pressure scenarios (Vijayalakshmi et al., 2025). The AI-driven real-time resource allocation can improve the operational efficiency and foster a dynamic, responsive healthcare setting. This enhances the patient outcomes that fosters a balanced workload for personnel, and also ensuring healthcare facilities stay adaptable and efficient in addressing the changing demands of patient care.

3 AI-Driven Workforce Management

Workforce management powered by artificial intelligence has revolutionized the conventional method of staffing. The machine learning optimizes and modifies staffing solutions in real time. For the purpose of ensuring that the healthcare facilities are able to satisfy the ever-changing requirements of patient care, this integrated approach is used to provide support for numerous facets of workforce management. The available digital check-in biometric data and the real-time attendance records are the first steps that the artificial intelligence systems have taken to precisely track the availability of staff members. This all-encompassing data collection serves as the basic foundation for the efficient scheduling, ensuring that the system always has an up-to-date perspective of who is accessible at any given moment in time. Artificial intelligence is able to match the appropriate individuals to the appropriate jobs depending on their experience and the amount of work they are already doing. One of the most important functions of these systems is the assignment of tasks based on skills. Artificial intelligence-driven solutions assign work and shifts to staff members in accordance with their capabilities by examining historical performance, certifications, and unique departmental demands. Not only does this increase efficiency, but it also guarantees that doctors and other medical personnel who are the best qualified are providing treatment to patients. Additionally, continual performance tracking assists managers in identifying areas of weakness in terms of skills and specific areas in which additional training could be advantageous. One further important feature is that it allows for the proactive monitoring of burnout and weariness, respectively. In order to determine that the employees may be at risk of overwork. The artificial intelligence systems track work hours and the shift patterns. The managers receive early signals and are able to transfer the work or change schedules to offer the required relaxation for their personnel. This procedure has ultimately helped to preserve the well-being of the staff and maintain the high standards of patient care. Powerful decision support tools provide actionable insights by means of user-friendly dashboards. It incorporates data on staff performance, patient volume, and operational efficiency. An artificial intelligence has the ability to quickly recommend reassignments and the contingency plans in the event of unanticipated increases in the patient admissions or sudden staff shortages. This helps to ensure that the facility continues to be responsive and has sufficient staffing levels (Shams et al., 2023).

4 AI-Integrated Workforce Management Technologies

4.1 Machine Learning Algorithms

The machine learning algorithms are considered the foundation of AI-driven workforce management solutions. These systems are allowing to learn from the data and to perpetually enhance the scheduling decisions. These algorithms can be utilized to analyze the extensive historical and real-time data to identify the patterns and trends that underpin the predictions of future staffing requirements and resource optimization. The supervised learning methodology has been widely utilized, to predict the patient influx and the requirement of the staffing. The regression models and decision trees are used to evaluate the historical patient numbers. In order to facilitate a precise forecast of the peak and the low-demand intervals. This predictive ability enables healthcare administrators to proactively modify, the workforce numbers to ensure optimal service delivery. The classification algorithm augments this process by categorizing shifts according to workload intensity or risk levels, thereby ensuring that each shift possesses the requisite blend of skills and expertise. The clustering techniques have been used to facilitate, the discovery of concealed patterns in employee performance, absenteeism, and work behaviors. These algorithms help the managers in identifying the abnormalities and potential problems that may not be readily observable. This knowledge can facilitate focused initiatives, such as rectifying chronic understaffing in particular departments or identifying training requirements. The reinforcement learning is a compelling domain in which the algorithm progressively to enhances its performance by analyzing previous scheduling results. These models have been employed in the trial-and-error way to modify the scheduling techniques in real time and adapt dynamically to unforeseen changes such as abrupt staff shortages or increases in-patient admissions. The machine learning algorithms convert workforce management from a static, human procedure into a dynamic and data-driven strategy, and their integration has promoted operational efficiency and cost-effectiveness while promoting a more equitable workload for healthcare personnel, hence enabling improved patient care results (Thomassin-Naggara et al., 2019).

4.2 NLP for Scheduling Requests

The language processing technology has been used to schedule the requests in healthcare revolutions. A staff interaction with a scheduling system translates a colloquial language into automated scheduling commands. This novel technology has enabled healthcare professionals to articulate their scheduling preferences and requirements effortlessly, bypassing complex software interfaces. As the nurse needs to change the Tuesday shift to the Friday morning, and the system autonomously recognizes the critical details such as the particular days, times, and urgency, then it cross-references them with current schedules to ascertain the optimal modification. The technology employs a sophisticated text analysis and the machine learning methods to extract the critical information from each request and also guarantees the accurate interpretation of colloquial or informal language. The technology has been effectively connecting human conversation with digital scheduling. The analyzing context and detecting pertinent an entity such as dates, shift kinds, and employee names. This technique has markedly decreased the administrative burden by typically linked to the manual handling of the scheduling requests. The solution automates the work of a updating rosters in real time and promptly notifies personnel of any changes that eliminates the need for managers to spend hours analyzing emails and texts. This swift adaptability is especially considered vital in healthcare settings. The unforeseen absences or abrupt increases in-patient admissions necessitate prompt modifications that guarantee the appropriate coverage. The system has to process the individual requests while aggregating data from many inputs, allowing it to identify patterns and also forecast future scheduling requirements. Consequently, it is proactive to recommend the modifications that distribute the effort more equitably throughout the team, thereby enhancing work-life balance and mitigating employee burnout. The incorporation of language comprehension for the scheduling demands with an operational efficiency improves overall employee happiness. The employees gain from a more intuitive, user-centric experience that aligns with their inherent communication preferences to facilitate the process of requesting modifications and the offering. The system progressively learns from the interactions. In order to consistently enhance the comprehension of industry-specific terms and the human communication subtleties. This ongoing enhancement, results in the heightened precision and dependability in handling of the intricacies of scheduling requirements. By utilizing the advanced language processing techniques in healthcare scheduling, administrative efficiency is enhanced and staff allocation is optimized, thereby ensuring uninterrupted patient care and effective workforce deployment (Boonstra & Laven, 2022).

4.3 IoT Integration for Real-Time Staff Monitoring

The integration of IoT for real-time staff monitoring is considered as a revolutionizing hospital operation by delivering a continuous, accurate, and actionable insights into the worker actions. The healthcare institutions have been monitoring staff location, movement, and involvement during their duties. By utilizing networked sensors, wearable devices, and smart tracking systems. This integrated network is used to gathers data from many of the sources in real time, such as RFID badges, mobile devices, and environmental sensors to guarantee that, each member of the healthcare team is ideally situated to provide the patient care. The system has been using to tracks the physical location and monitors important performance factors, such as response times, workflow efficiency, and compliance with safety rules. For instance, whenever a staff member enters in a high-risk zone or an emergency is to be identified in a certain region, then the system can promptly notify supervisors and activate the pre-established response protocols, guaranteeing that assistance arrives without delay. This integration improves, the overall operational efficiency by offering a comprehensive perspective on the personnel utilization. The data analytics can use to reveal patterns, such as a peak activity times, prevalent movement bottlenecks, and locations with an inadequate manpower. Armed with these insights, a managers can dynamically modify the workforce levels to optimize the resource allocation, and to rethink workflows to reduce the inefficiencies. Integrating IoT data with current labor management systems enables healthcare firms to automate scheduling, diminish manual supervision, and enhance overall staff coordination. This degree of automation reduces administrative responsibilities and enables managers to concentrate on strategic objectives instead of routine oversight. The real-time surveillance using IoT devices to enhances safety and the regulatory adherence. The solution mitigates the fatigue-related to errors that reduces the hazards linked to the overwork by assuring staff compliance with a best practice and the regulatory norms. It enhances infection control by monitoring movement patterns, which is particularly crucial in settings where reducing cross-contamination is essential. The data collected via IoT devices can enhance the training programs, inform performance evaluations, and influence the future enhancements in operating procedures. The IoT integration for real-time staff monitoring is not merely a technology enhancement but it is a holistic solution that optimizes resource allocation to improve the staff safety, and ultimately increases a patient care outcome. The constant influx of actionable data fosters an agile atmosphere, enabling real-time modifications and ensuring healthcare facilities are consistently equipped to address the demands of their dynamic settings (Hogg et al., 2023).

5 Implementing AI Scheduling

A complete infrastructure has been needed to implement an AI-powered scheduling in the healthcare sector. This design includes a data integration, system customization, model training, deployment, and ongoing development. The process starts with setting up a system, for gathering and integrating data. This system in charge making sure that all relevant information, such as electronic health records, attendance logs, historical schedule data, and real-time patient input, is properly incorporated into one application. This unified data environment is very necessary for the artificial intelligence to make accurate predictions and good scheduling choices. The system's outputs have been depending on the inputs being correct. Thus, it's important to make sure that the data is of the good quality and consistent over this phase. The next stage is to change the scheduling solution, so that it works for the specific demands of the healthcare facility. Each hospital and clinic has its own set of rules for how to run things. These rules normally included the labor laws, supporting certain staffing patterns in a certain department, and also taking into account the requirement and the preferences of each employee. The customization necessitates the proper coordination across the integration of the information technology, human resources, and clinical leadership in order to delineate the specific criteria and the constraints that the AI system must consider. This personalized method makes sure that the schedules that are made follow both internal rules and external regulatory criteria for the organization while also making the best use of the staff. Training the AI models is considered as a big part of the forthcoming third phase. By feeding the machine learning algorithms both historical and the real-time data (Miller, 2022). The system can discover patterns related to the patient inflows, peak demand periods, and staff availability. There are many methods to train models, such as the supervised learning to predict demand and the reinforcement learning to improve the scheduling techniques. The ongoing education is considered as an important part, since it helps the model to adapt to the seasonal changes, changes in the operational rules, and the always changing dynamics of the workforce. This step is done, when thorough testing and validation are performed to make sure that the model will give scheduling suggestions that are accurate and reliable in a wide range of situations (Kumarganesh et al., 2025). The next step after fine-tuning the AI models is to put them into use. At this point, the AI-powered scheduling system will be connected to the current IT systems, which will include the platforms for managing the human resources and the electronic health data. The administrators can be used to assess the system's effectiveness and get user feedback to address the operational challenges through a phased rollout. Typically commencing with a pilot program in a selected department (Praveenkumar et al., 2025). This is done before the system has been used on a bigger scale. During the deployment phase, it is important to make sure that the AI system and other integrated platforms are connected in a way that allows for a smooth flow of data and harmony in operations. An administrators can use real-time analytics and the performance dashboards to keep an eye on crucial metrics like the staffing efficiency, an employee happiness, and the quality of patient care (Pandey & Pandey, 2025). The system is made better by taking into account feedback from both the staff and management. This makes sure that it stays responsive to the constantly evolving field of healthcare.

6 Conclusion

AI-driven scheduling and workforce management is transforming healthcare by automating and enhancing intricate staffing procedures. By utilizing the predictive analytics, automatic shift creation, and real-time resource distribution, the AI-driven scheduling and workforce management are minimizing manual errors and administrative overhead and also ensuring that the personnel levels are optimally aligned with varying patient demands. This leads to optimized resource allocation, economic efficiency, and a more equitable distribution of workload among healthcare workers, ultimately resulting in superior patient outcomes and less staff fatigue. The primary advantages of such systems are diverse. The capacity to forecast patient inflows by using historical and real-time data has been facilitates the proactive planning, and also guaranteeing the adequate staffing during peak periods while preventing overstaffing during quieter times. The automated scheduling reduces the necessity for the laborious human modifications, fostering equity and uniformity throughout shifts. A real-time update and IoT integrations offer an instantaneous visibility into a personnel movements and availability, to facilitating prompt reactions to emergencies or unforeseen staffing alterations. Moreover, a strategic staff allocation, which is driven by sophisticated algorithms, also guarantees optimal personnel-task alignment. Hence improving operational efficiency and elevating employee morale. The future of AI in healthcare has been poised for a significant expansion. The ongoing breakthroughs in the machine learning, data analytics, and integration technologies guarantee, the increasingly sophisticated and adaptive scheduling systems. The future advancements are expected to utilize extensive data sources from wearable technology. In order, to advanced prediction models that will provide enhanced insights into patient care requirements and workforce dynamics. As interoperability among hospital systems advances, The fluid exchange of data will be further augment to the precision and responsiveness of an AI-driven scheduling. The evolving trends in ethical AI and data privacy will be considered as an essential for preserving the trust and security for assuring compliance with the legal norms while providing substantial operational advantages. The use of an AI-driven scheduling transcends a typical technological enhancement and it constitutes a strategic investment in the future of patient care. By converting the conventional scheduling techniques into a proactive data-informed approach. The healthcare organizations can decrease expenses and also enhance the efficiency, while fostering a more resilient and supportive workplace. The use of intelligent scheduling methods helps to facilitates ongoing enhancement and the innovation in healthcare provision that guaranteeing the advantages for both patients and personnel, through a more adaptable and responsive system. By adopting these technologies, it is crucial for the healthcare providers seeking to maintain competitiveness and also provide the outstanding treatment in a progressively intricate and rapid medical environment.

References

Boonstra, A., & Laven, M. (2022). Influence of artificial intelligence on the work design of emergency department clinicians a systematic literature review. *BMC Health Services Research, 22*, 669.

Brambilla, A., Sun, T. Z., Elshazly, W., Ghazy, A., Barach, P., Lindahl, G., & Capolongo, S. (2021). Flexibility during the COVID-19 pandemic response: Healthcare facility assessment tools for resilient evaluation. *International Journal of Environmental Research and Public Health, 18*, 11478.

Dave, M., & Patel, N. (2023). Artificial intelligence in healthcare and education. *British Dental Journal, 234*, 761–764.

Hogg, H. D. J., Al-Zubaidy, M., Talks, J., Denniston, A. K., Kelly, C. J., Malawana, J., Papoutsi, C., Teare, M. D., Keane, P. A., Beyer, F. R., et al. (2023). Stakeholder perspectives of clinical artificial intelligence implementation: Systematic review of qualitative evidence. *Journal of Medical Internet Research, 25*, 39742.

Joshi, G., Jain, A., Araveeti, S. R., Adhikari, S., Garg, H., & Bhandari, M. (2024). FDA-approved artificial intelligence and machine learning (AI/ML)-enabled medical devices: An updated landscape. *Electronics, 13*, 498.

Kumarganesh, S., Malathi Murugesan, C., Ganesh, N., Santhiyakumari, M., Thangavel, K., Jayaram, K. M., Sagayam, B. K., & Pandey, and Digvijay Pandey. (2025). Hybrid plasmonic biosensors with deep learning for colorectal cancer detection. *Plasmonics, 20*(7), 4895–4909.

Marengo, A., & Pagano, A. (2023). Investigating the factors influencing the adoption of blockchain technology across different countries and industries: A systematic literature review. *Electronics, 12*, 3006.

Miller, G. J. (2022). Stakeholder roles in artificial intelligence projects. *Project Leadership and Society, 3*, 100068.

Moldt, J. A., Festl-Wietek, T., Madany Mamlouk, A., Nieselt, K., Fuhl, W., & Herrmann-Werner, A. (2023). Chatbots for future docs: Exploring medical students' attitudes and knowledge towards artificial intelligence and medical chatbots. *Medical Education Online, 28*, 2182659.

Pandey, B. K., & Pandey, D. (2025). Securing healthcare medical image information using advance morphological component analysis, information hiding systems, and hybrid convolutional neural networks on IoMT. *Computers in Biology and Medicine, 185*, 109499.

Pisapia, A., Banfi, G., & Tomaiuolo, R. (2022). The novelties of the regulation on health technology assessment, a key achievement for the European union health policies. *Clinical Chemistry and Laboratory Medicine (CCLM), 60*, 1160–1163.

Prakash, S., Balaji, J. N., Joshi, A., & Surapaneni, K. M. (1914). Ethical conundrums in the application of artificial intelligence (AI) in healthcare-a scoping review of reviews. *Journal of Personalized Medicine, 2022*, 12.

Praveenkumar, T., Anthoniraj, S., Kumarganesh, S., Somaskandan, M., Martin Sagayam, K., Pandey, B. K., Pandey, D., & Sahani, S. K. (2025). Enhanced circuit board analysis: Infrared image segmentation utilizing Markov random field (MRF) and level set techniques. *Engineering Reports, 7*(3), e70029.

Shams, R. A., Zowghi, D., & Bano, M. (2023). AI and the quest for diversity and inclusion: A systematic literature review. *AI and Ethics*.

Thomassin-Naggara, I., Balleyguier, C., Ceugnart, L., Heid, P., Lenczner, G., Maire, A., Séradour, B., Verzaux, L., & Taourel, P. (2019). Conseil, national professionnel de la radiologie et imagerie medicale (G4). Artificial intelligence and breast screening: French radiology community position paper. *Diagnostic and Interventional Imaging, 100*, 553–566.

Townsend, B. A., Sihlahla, I., Naidoo, M., Naidoo, S., Donnelly, D. L., & Thaldar, D. W. (2023). Mapping the regulatory landscape of AI in healthcare in Africa. *Frontiers in Pharmacology, 14*, 1214422.

Vijayalakshmi, S., Pandey, B. K., Pandey, D., & Lelisho, M. E. (2025). Innovative deep learning classifiers for breast cancer detection through hybrid feature extraction techniques. *Scientific Reports, 15*(1), 22212.

Wang, C., Zhang, J., Lassi, N., & Zhang, X. (1878). Privacy protection in using artificial intelligence for healthcare: Chinese regulation in comparative perspective. *Healthcare, 2022*, 10.

Financial Fraud Detection in Healthcare Using AI-Driven Analytics

Toopalli Sirisha, C. H. Sekhar, Nitin Kulshrestha, Divya Sharma, Sharad Gautam, B. Vidhya, and Amal Hasan Jumaa

Abstract The healthcare fraud is now a days emerge as a huge problem that leads to the substantial financial losses that adversity impacts the patient care. The traditional fraud detection methods often fail to keep pace with evolving fraudulent tactics, necessitating the adoption of AI-driven analytics for more effective fraud prevention. The utilization of the artificial intelligence in identifying a number of forms for fraud, such as billing fraud, prescription fraud, telemedicine frauds, and the provider of patient cooperation. The machine learning models, natural language processing (NLP), and anomaly detection algorithms are considered an essential requirement for accurately and efficiently identifying fraudulent activities. As fraudulent schemes are growing more intricate manner. The AI-powered systems facilitate proactive fraud

T. Sirisha (✉)
Department of Management Studies, Sri Venkateswara College of Engineering (Autonomous), Tirupati, India
e-mail: drtoopalli2022@gmail.com

C. H. Sekhar
Department of CSE (AI&ML), GMR Institute of Technology, Rajam, India
e-mail: sekharch.gmrit@gmail.com

N. Kulshrestha
Christ Deemed to be University, Bangalore, India
e-mail: Mymagictimes@gmail.com

D. Sharma
Department of Management, Institute of Technology & Management, Gwalior, India
e-mail: Divya.sharma.mba@itmgoi.in

S. Gautam
School of Management, Graphic Era Hill University, Dehradun, India
e-mail: sharad.gautam20@gmail.com

B. Vidhya
Department of Computational Intelligence, SRM Institute of Science and Technology, Kattankulathur, India
e-mail: vidhyamkumar3@gmail.com

A. H. Jumaa
Al-Nisour University College, Nisour Seq. Karkh, Baghdad, Iraq
e-mail: amal.h.english@nuc.edu.iq

D. Pandey et al. (eds.), *Smart Healthcare*, https://doi.org/10.1007/978-981-95-8828-2_3

detection via continuous learning and real-time analysis. The necessity of a incorporating the AI into legal frameworks is seems to require to guarantee compliance and also preserving the data privacy and the ethical standards. The subsequent study ought to concentrate on enhancing AI models to minimizing false positives and formulating an hybrid detection methodologies. The healthcare sector may substantially reduce fraudulent actions, protect financial assets, and improve the integrity of medical services by utilizing the AI-driven analytics.

Keywords Healthcare fraud · AI-driven analytics · Machine learning · Anomaly detection · Natural language processing · Blockchain

1 Introduction

The financial fraud within the healthcare sector has been find to escalating issue that resulting in substantial monetary losses, which jeopardized the patient care, and the regulatory complications. Fraudulent actions transpire at multiple tiers, including healthcare providers, insurance firms, and patients, leading to escalated medical expenses and misallocation of resources. The intricacy of a healthcare billing, insurance claims, and reimbursement procedures is used to generate the vulnerabilities that fraudsters normally exploited. The billing fraud is considered as a prevalent form of a financial deception in the healthcare, wherein physicians alter the medical codes to obtain an inflated compensation. This encompasses the upcoding wherein a provider invoices for a more costly procedure, than was actually executed, and duplicate billing, where the identical service is billed repeatedly. Phantom billing is one of the deceptive activities in which a supplier's invoice generated for the services that were never performed. These deceptive claims exacerbate healthcare expenses and impose financial burdens on insurance providers and government-sponsored programs such as Medicare and Medicaid. Prescription fraud constitutes a significant problem, frequently implicating healthcare providers, pharmacies, or patients. Physicians may prescribe superfluous pharmaceuticals in return for payments from pharmaceutical firms, while individuals may partake in "doctor shopping" to get many prescriptions for banned narcotics. Deceptive pharmacies may file fraudulent claims for prescriptions that were not really supplied, facilitating drug diversion and illicit resale. Insurance fraud significantly contributes to financial malfeasance in the healthcare sector. Patients may perpetrate identity theft by utilizing another individual's insurance information to obtain medical care, while providers may file fraudulent claims for services that were never rendered. A collaboration that exists between clinicians and patients may result in the orchestrated medical procedures that may produce the fraudulent insurance claims. The proliferation of a telemedicine and the digital healthcare has given rise to a novel form of the fraud. Telehealth fraud encompasses billing for non-existent virtual consultations, exaggerating service durations, or mischaracterizing non-covered services as covered. The digital health platforms and electronic health records (EHRs) pose dangers of the data manipulation, identity theft, and a cyber-related financial offense. The ramifications of a financial fraud in healthcare are extensive, resulting in elevated insurance premiums, which diminished faith in healthcare organizations, and the misappropriation of resources that could have been allocated for authentic patient treatment. The regulatory agencies, such as the Centers for Medicare & Medicaid Services (CMS) and private insurance companies, are nowadays improving the fraud detection systems. As fraudsters employ increasingly a sophisticated method, that healthcare institutions must be incorporate to advanced fraud detection solutions that include AI-driven analytics, to reduce risks and improve financial security.

1.1 Fraud Detection Using AI-Driven Analytics

AI-driven analytics uses machine learning, data mining, and predictive modeling to detect and prevent healthcare financial fraud. Due to the complexity and volume of healthcare transactions, typical fraud detection technologies often miss sophisticated fraud. The AI-based solutions improve the accuracy, efficiency, and adaptability in the detection of the fraudulent patterns. It is found that anomaly detection is a main key of the AI fraud detection tool. To find abnormal trends in the healthcare claims, billing data, and patient records. The machine learning algorithms are used, to examine massive volumes of data. Such findings may include unexpected claim spikes, excessive medical procedures, or suspicious provider-patient interactions. The AI systems help healthcare institutions and insurers investigate these abnormalities and the NLP is another important part of AI-driven fraud detection. Misrepresented or changed medical documents are common in fraudulent claims. Unstructured text data like physician notes, insurance claims, and medical records is analyzed by NLP to find inconsistencies. A more complete fraud detection strategy beyond numerical analysis is possible. The predictive modeling is normally used to identify the fraud before it causes any considerable financial harm. The AI-driven predictive models have learnt from the fresh data, and the model evaluated the past fraud incidents to further improve the detection. These models evaluate claims providers, and patient risk variables, enabling insurers and regulators to detect the fraud. The network analysis which analyzes healthcare system linkages has been used to find the AI-driven fraud detection. The collusion that exists between doctors, patients, and third parties is very common in fraud. The AI can help map these linkages to find the hidden fraud networks, like bogus clinics, identity theft rings, and coordinated billing fraud. Automation and real-time monitoring are used to further improve the fraud detection. AI systems can process massive datasets in real time and alert of questionable activity. This lowers manual audit time and enhances fraud prevention reaction times. AI-driven automation improves claim verification, lowering investigator burden and enhancing efficiency. AI-driven analytics improves through adaptive learning as fraud strategies change. As fraud trends and behaviors change, machine learning algorithms improve their fraud detection. The healthcare sector may improve fraud prevention and financial integrity by integrating AI with blockchain and secure data-sharing systems (Ashtiani & Raahemi, 2021).

2 Financial Fraud in Healthcare

2.1 *Billing Fraud*

Billing fraud is a major healthcare financial fraud. It involves manipulating medical billing and insurance claims to get more reimbursements than due. Healthcare practitioners, facilities, and administrative staff can commit this fraud, causing huge financial losses for insurance companies, government healthcare programs, and patients. Fraudulent billing raises healthcare expenses and burdens insurers and patients. Upcoding, where doctors bill for more expensive procedures than they did, is typical billing fraud. This raises insurance costs and reimbursements. A clinician may bill for a complicated surgery when only modest therapy was done. Duplicate billing the same medical treatment to various insurers or entities is another fraudulent practice. Clerical errors can cause repeated billing, but purposeful duplicate billing is done to get several payments for a single service. Phantom billing submitting claims for medical services, tests, or treatments that were never performed is another deception. False hospitals may manufacture patient visits or laboratory tests to take advantage of patients who don't check their invoices. Unbundling separates medical services that should be reimbursed under one reimbursement code. Despite insurance coverage has been covering them as a single bundled of the treatment, an unscrupulous providers might maximize profits by invoicing each procedure component separately. In another common fraud, some doctors order needless tests, surgeries, and the treatments to boost the revenue. This raises healthcare expenditures and exposes patients to needless treatments. The healthcare service providers can also modify the medical records or diagnostic codes to mask a non-covered procedures for the insurance reimbursement. Such bogus changes distort medical records and raise healthcare costs (Albashrawi, 2016). The billing fraud affects more than the finances. It also raises the insurance prices, and also drains the healthcare resources. The bogus billing can potentially harm patient care by wasting the funds on the bogus claims. The healthcare companies and insurers use AI-driven data, machine learning models, and real-time monitoring to uncover questionable billing patterns. Enhanced auditing, greater compliance, and whistleblower protections help uncover and prevent fraudulent billing, protecting the healthcare system (Ryman-Tubb et al., 2018).

2.2 Prescription Fraud and Drug Diversion

Prescription fraud constitutes a substantial problem within the healthcare sector, encompassing the illicit procurement, dissemination, or abuse of prescription pharmaceuticals. This form of fraud may be perpetrated by healthcare practitioners, pharmacists, or patients, resulting in significant financial losses, jeopardized patient safety, and heightened risk of substance misuse. The deceptive prescribing the practices not only escalate the healthcare expenses, but also exacerbate the increasing issues of a substance addiction that illicit drug trade. A prevalent kind of the prescription fraud is the doctor shopping, wherein an individual's consult that include the many physicians to acquire prescriptions for restricted medications. The patients participating in this activity are frequently fail to declare their current prescriptions. Resulting in the accumulation of substantial quantities of medication that may be utilized for a personal misuse or the illicit resale. Likewise, a counterfeit prescription that represent an additional tactic employed by the scammers. In such instances, an individual's modify the authentic prescriptions or fabricate counterfeit to ones to obtain the controlled substances, frequently via stolen prescription pads or digital forging methods. The healthcare providers have been engaged in prescription fraud by unethical tactics that include the overprescription of drugs. Certain physicians may provide an excessive prescription for the analgesics, sedatives, or stimulants, either due to financial inducements from pharmaceutical corporations or in return of the direct remuneration from the patients (Al-Hashedi & Magalingam, 2021). Fraudulent pharmacies may engage in the prescription fraud by fulfilling a prescription for the fictitious patients or by charging an insurance companies for the medications that were never provided. These actions is exacerbating the financial strain on the healthcare institutions that promote the unlawful distribution of a medications. The drug diversion is intricately associated with the prescription of the fraud that entails the unlawful distribution or abuse of the legally prescribed pharmaceuticals. This transpires when prescribed medications are diverted from their designated medical use to unauthorized persons. This may occur at the multiple stages across the supply chain, including hospitals, pharmacies, and healthcare establishments. An employee in these companies may use the appropriate drugs for the personal consumption or illicit sale. Several patients can illicitly sell their legally acquired prescriptions to the drug dealers or others grappling with this addiction. The ramifications of prescription fraud and drug diversion are found to be extensive and they exacerbate the opioid problem, to elevate healthcare expenditures, and burden law enforcement initiatives aimed at the countering illicit drug distribution. Individuals acquiring pharmaceuticals through deceitful methods face an elevated risk of overdosing and additional health issues. Healthcare institutions and regulatory agencies are deploying sophisticated monitoring systems, including prescription drug monitoring programs (PDMPs) and AI-driven analytics, to identify anomalous prescribing and dispensing behaviors. Enhancing rules, augmenting control of prescribing procedures, and elevating public knowledge are crucial measures in mitigating prescription fraud and medication diversion, thereby safeguarding both patients and the healthcare system (Chaquet-ulldemolins et al., 2022).

2.3 Telemedicine/Digital Healthcare Fraud

The rapid growth of telemedicine and digital healthcare has increased medical access but also fraud opportunities. The telemedicine and digital healthcare fraud involves a fraudulent virtual consultation, remote medications, and the digital billing. The Telehealth abusers may be healthcare providers, patients, or third-party companies that seeking the financial advantage. The fraudulent actions cost insurers and the healthcare systems money and damage the patient trust in digital healthcare solutions. Telemedicine fraud often involves invoicing for unneeded virtual encounters. Some doctors bill telemedicine platforms for unreceived consultations. They may deceive patients about virtual visits or bill for unnecessary services. Providers may schedule automated or recurring virtual appointments with little interaction to boost billing without providing care. Patient deception and identity fraud are also common. Fraudsters may exploit stolen personal information to access telemedicine services and obtain prescriptions or medical benefits. People may share their insurance information with friends and family to receive fake remote consultations and medications. Telehealth platforms with insufficient identity verification are especially vulnerable to fraud. Prescription fraud in digital healthcare is also rising. For financial gain, some physicians write internet prescriptions without medical evaluations. This is especially dangerous with opioids, stimulants, and sedatives. Multiple telehealth providers can be used to buy excessive medication, known as "doctor shopping." Some telemedicine clinics are "pill mills," dispensing drugs without medical proof. Telehealth provider kickbacks are another deception. Some fraudulent companies pay doctors to recommend patients to telemedicine, diagnostic labs, or pharmacies without medical necessity (Da'U & Salim, 2019). Unethical practices raise healthcare expenditures and increase unneeded treatments and prescriptions. Sometimes telehealth providers are part of broader fraud networks that misuse insurance schemes. Remote medical device billing and testing fraud is rising. Telehealth providers may charge for needless medical tests, diagnostics, or remote monitoring. Insurance companies may be billed for unnecessary medical gadgets and services. Fraudsters can also fabricate the test results or medical problems to justify the costly surgeries or treatments on the digital health platforms. Telemedicine fraud threatens the regulators, insurers, and the healthcare providers. Telehealth platforms are using advanced AI-driven fraud detection systems to detect suspect billing trends, unauthorized access attempts, and prescription abnormalities. Preventing digital healthcare fraud requires a stronger identity verification, more compliance requirements, and better cybersecurity. The healthcare business can keep the telemedicine safe, effective, and reliable by the introducing strong oversight measures (Zeng & Tang, 2021).

3 AI-Driven Techniques for Fraud Detection

3.1 Machine Learning Models

The machine learning models as shown in Fig. 1 that is essential for identifying and mitigating the financial fraud in the healthcare. Through the analysis of an extensive data sets, these models can discern trends, anomalies, and the suspicious actions that may be signify the fraudulent behavior. At contrast to the conventional rule-based detection systems, a machine learning models can perpetually learn and adapt, and also rendering them the exceptionally proficient at recognizing changing fraud schemes. These algorithms utilize historical data, claims records, and patient-provider contacts to enhance fraud detection precision and minimize false positives. The supervised learning models are prevalent methodologies in the identification of the healthcare fraud. These algorithms are trained on labeled datasets that comprising both fraudulent and the genuine transactions. The algorithms such decision trees, random forests, support vector machines, and neural networks. This examines the historical fraud incidents to create the predictive models upon completion of training. These models can categorize as a fresh claim and the transactions as either legitimate or possibly fraudulent. The supervised learning excels at identifying the established fraud trends with novel fraud strategies that are absent from the training of the data. Unsupervised learning methods are effective at detecting unidentified fraud patterns without the necessity of labeled data. Clustering methods, like k-means and hierarchical clustering, aggregate comparable transactions, facilitating the identification of abnormalities through deviations from typical behavior. Anomaly detection methodologies, such as isolation forests and autoencoders, discern outliers that may signify fraudulent behavior. These models are advantageous for identifying novel or previously unrecognized fraud schemes, rendering them a significant enhancement to fraud detection systems. Semi-supervised learning integrates components of both supervised and unsupervised methodologies. Due to the scarcity of the labeled fraud data, semi-supervised models utilize a limited number of labeled transactions in conjunction with a substantial volume of the unlabeled data to enhance the accuracy of a fraud detection. This approach improves the efficiency of fraud detection while diminishing reliance on manually annotated datasets (Delamaire et al., 2009). Deep learning models, especially convolutional neural networks (CNNs) and recurrent neural networks (RNNs), are progressively used in the fraud detection, owing to their capacity to analyze an intricate and the high-dimensional data (Delamaire et al., 2009). Convolutional neural networks (CNNs) are proficient in identifying fraudulent patterns within medical imaging and electronic health records, whereas recurrent neural networks (RNNs) are adept at analyzing sequential data, including billing records and prescription histories. The Long short-term memory (LSTM) networks, which is a subtype of recurrent neural networks (RNNs) is use to identify fraud by analyzing temporal patterns in the healthcare transactions and rendering them effective for the detection of the persistent fraudulent activity over time. The reinforcement learning is an innovative method in the detection of healthcare fraud. In contrast to

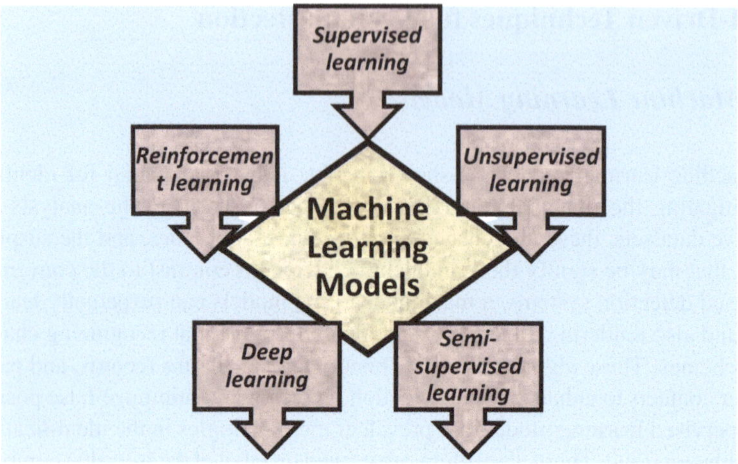

Fig. 1 Machine learning models

conventional models that depend on static datasets, reinforcement learning agents perpetually engage with data environments and acquire effective fraud detection tactics via trial and error. The machine learning models are revolutionizing the fraud detection in a healthcare by increasing the accuracy that diminishing manual labor, and accelerating a response times. Their efficacy relies on high-quality data, an appropriate feature selection, and ongoing upgrades to adapt to changing the fraud strategies (Zhang & Zhou, 2004). By amalgamating several machine learning methodologies, an healthcare institutions can establish resilient fraud detection systems that can protect financial assets, for uphold regulatory adherence, and to guarantee the ethical medical procedures.

3.2 Natural Language Processing (NLP)

The text-based fraud involves a minor inconsistency that are deceptive documentation, or faked records which are need a significant linguistic examination, unlike a structured numerical data. The NLP detects textual anomalies, deceptive patterns, and the inconsistencies to automate fraud detection. By analyzing an unstructured text data from the medical records, insurance claims, prescriptions, and provider notes, Natural Language Processing (NLP) can use to uncover healthcare financial fraud. Entity recognition is considered as a crucial NLP fraud detection application. From unstructured text, Named Entity Recognition (NER) algorithms can extract patient names, provider details, diagnosis codes, treatment descriptions, and billing information. NLP models can identify duplicate claims, mismatched patient-provider relationships, and excessive billing for unneeded treatments by cross-referencing these entities with structured databases. This helps identify fraud like phantom billing, when suppliers bill for services never provided. Medical document and provider communication fraud detection relies on sentiment and semantic analysis. NLP models detect suspect language, tone, and word usage that may falsify or exaggerate medical symptoms. Medical language and cryptic descriptions of pricey procedures are common in bogus claims. NLP can distinguish valid from fraudulent medical narratives using sentiment analysis. Topic modeling and text clustering reveal patterns in vast medical and insurance texts. Based on the thematic similarities, NLP algorithms like LDA and TF-IDF can use to classify medical records and claims. The NLP can highlight the claims from a provider, who routinely use unusual or an expensive process that stray from the industry standards for a further inquiry. This helps to find a provider collaboration and the unnecessary medical billing fraud. Comparing new claims of the previous records allows document similarity to perform analysis to detect the fraud. The NLP models can identify the duplicate or nearly identical claims that are submitted under various patient names or provider data by using cosine similarity, word embeddings, and deep learning-based transformers like BERT. This method helps identify duplicate billing fraud, as healthcare practitioners submit multiple claims for the same operation under different IDs. OCR combined with NLP extracts and analyzes text from scanned medical papers, prescriptions, and invoices to improve fraud detection. Fraudsters falsify dates, treatment information, and billing amounts in written records. NLP-powered OCR may spot discrepancies between digital and physical documents, revealing altered or false claims that manual audits may miss. NLP detects fraud and automates compliance monitoring by checking medical paperwork for regulatory and insurance compliance. NLP algorithms can determine if medical records justify treatments, identify medical code overuse, and indicate non-compliant paperwork. This prevents fraudulent billing and speeds up claim audits for insurers and healthcare regulators. NLP for text-based fraud detection can increase healthcare fraud prevention, reduce financial losses, and strengthen the healthcare system. Transformer-based deep learning models and real-time language processing will improve NLP fraud detection and prevention in digital and traditional healthcare (Phua et al., 2010).

3.3 Anomaly Detection Algorithms

The anomaly detection algorithms are considered as one of the essential things for spotting the fraudulent actions in a healthcare by recognizing atypical patterns or deviations from the standard behavior. These algorithms used to examine an extensive dataset, like as billing records, insurance claims, and electronic health records, to identify the dubious transactions that may suggest as the fraud. In contrast to the rule-based systems that depend on an established criterion. The anomaly detection models may be adjusted to the changing of fraud strategies that rendering them as a proficient in identifying both the recognized and unrecognized fraud schemes. The statistical anomaly detection methods utilize the mathematical models to find a data points that are drastically diverge from the standard one. Techniques such as

Z-score analysis, Gaussian distribution, and percentile-based detection create baseline patterns for genuine transactions. Any of the claim or medical expense that are exceeding a specified threshold is identified as a potential anomaly. Although these methods are straightforward and comprehensible, they may encounter difficulties with the intricate fraud schemes that entail nuanced and non-linear interactions. Machine learning methodologies improve anomaly detection by analyzing patterns derived from past data. Unsupervised methods, like k-means clustering, isolation forests, and autoencoders, are notably efficacious in fraud detection. Clustering techniques, such k-means and DBSCAN, aggregate analogous data points, whereas outliers that do not conform to any cluster or are distanced from cluster centroids are recognized as potential instances of fraud. Isolation forests, a tree-based technique, identify anomalies by isolating infrequent or unexpected transactions with fewer splits than typical data points. Autoencoders, a category of neural networks, are designed to reconstruct standard data patterns and identify transactions exhibiting significant reconstruction errors as probable abnormalities. Deep learning methodologies, specifically Long Short-Term Memory (LSTM) networks and Convolutional Neural Networks (CNNs), augment fraud detection through the analysis of sequential and high-dimensional data. The LSTM networks are considered as a proficient at detecting fraud in the time-series data by identifying an anomalous trend in a patient visits, billing cycles, and prescription records over the time (West & Bhattacharya, 2016). These models can detect anomalies that are based on abrupt alterations in healthcare usage of the trends. Conversely, CNNs examine visual data, such scanned medical records and handwritten prescriptions to identify the discrepancies that may suggest a fraudulent modification to the papers. The integration of various anomaly detection methodologies enhances the precision of fraud detection. Hybrid models combine statistical techniques with machine learning and deep learning to improve the detection of complex fraud schemes. Integrating autoencoders with a clustering technique usually helps to diminish the false positives and identify the nuanced fraudulent tendencies. Anomaly detection algorithms equip with the healthcare businesses with an effective fraud detection capability for mitigating the financial losses and promoting ethical medical procedures. The ongoing improvement of models and real-time monitoring significantly improves their capacity to identify new fraud trends in healthcare transactions (Abdallah et al., 2016).

4 Data Sources and Processing

A combination of a structured and unstructured data obtained from a variety of sources is to be utilized by AI-driven fraud detection in the healthcare industry to successfully identify the fraudulent actions. The structured information that includes the prescription histories, insurance claims, medical billing transactions, and electronic health records (EHRs). The errors like as duplicate claims, excessive billing, and the strange prescription trends can be identified with the assistance of these kinds of the datasets. The additional insights into the potential of a fraud schemes can be gained from the unstructured data, which includes things like clinician notes, diagnostic reports, and patient communications. The new sources of the information that can be evaluated to identify the discrepancies between the reported medical problems and the actual patient health indicators include data from wearable devices and health metrics provided by the internet of things (IoT). The transformation of raw data available into the insights that may be put into action is largely contributed by the data processing. The creation of a more complete fraud detection framework can be accomplished through the utilization of advanced approaches such as data fusion. In order to reduce the number of fraudulent activities that involve identity theft or duplicate billing, automated entity resolution technologies are utilized to link patient records across various healthcare providers. The techniques of anomaly detection make use of statistical modeling and artificial intelligence algorithms in order to identify anomalies from the typical patterns of billing or treatment. Through the ability to continuously monitor transactions, real-time processing capabilities significantly improve the effectiveness of AI-driven fraud detection and it enables the fraud detection models to run efficiently by reducing detection latency and enhancing the responsiveness. The edge computing and the cloud-based artificial intelligence systems are responsible for its implementation. Real-time data streams and predictive artificial intelligence models will need to be integrated in order to maintain robust fraud prevention mechanisms.

5 Emerging AI Technologies

By integrating the cutting-edge techniques that help to improve accuracy, adaptability, and transparency, emerging AI technologies that are dramatically enhancing fraud detection in the healthcare industry. While also preserving the data privacy and the compliance, these technologies are assisting enterprises in the real-time fraud detection.

- *Federated Learning*: This artificial intelligence method allows the several medical facilities and the insurance providers to work together to jointly to train machine learning models without exchanging of the private patient information. Federated AI models used to identify patterns of cross-provider fraud that could otherwise go undetected by enabling the decentralized learning. This approach ensures the adherence to laws such as HIPAA and is especially helpful in detecting a fraudulent claim that span several insurance companies and the healthcare providers.
- *Explainable AI (XAI)*: The conventional AI models based on the deep learning algorithms, sometimes act as "black boxes," making it challenging for the auditors and medical professionals to comprehend the particular claims that are reported as fraudulent. Explainable AI methods that are used to shed light on AI decision-making processes that include SHAP (Shapley Additive Explanations) and LIME (Local Interpretable Model-agnostic Explanations). By assisting a fraud investigator in more confidently and validating a flagged transaction, these techniques

guarantee the transparency and accountability of an AI-driven fraud detection systems.

- *Generative AI for Fraud Simulation*: The researchers are investigating the use of an AI models that include a diffusion network and GPT to produce an artificial healthcare data that can be utilized to train the fraud detection systems. These models aid in making fraud detection algorithms more resilient to the new fraud strategies by producing a variety of the fraudulent scenarios. Furthermore, a generative AI can examine the vast amounts of textual data related to healthcare such as billing records and medications to find discrepancies that can point to fraud.
- *AI-Powered Blockchain Analytics*: The integration of the immutability and transparency of the healthcare transactions, along with the combination of blockchain technology and the artificial intelligence is continuously improving the fraud detection. AI-driven analytics can help to identify irregularities in medication records, insurance claims, and billing trends by using the tamper-proof ledger that blockchain technology normally offers. The Artificial Intelligence (AI)-powered by the smart contracts can be automatically identify and stop fraudulent transactions before as they are performed, by minimizing losses and improving the regulatory compliance.
- *Real-Time AI Monitoring Systems*: The real-time AI monitoring systems uses the continuously examine the healthcare transactions to identify questionable activity as it happens in contrast to the conventional fraud detection techniques that depend on the retroactive analysis. These systems highlight potentially fraudulent claims in the real-time using statistical modeling, deep learning, and the anomaly detection techniques. By preventing fraud before payments are made this proactive strategy can reduces the losses and guarantees that fraud investigators can act more quickly.
- *Reinforcement Learning*: The reinforcement learning used in the AI technique use a model to learn continually via trial and error by being rewarded and the penalized, as in accordance to how well they identify the fraud. The reinforcement learning enables the AI systems to dynamically adjust to the novel fraud schemes, in contrast to the typical machine learning models that depend on the past data. Over time, these models further improve their capacity to identify the new fraud trends and lower the number of the false positives in a fraud detection system.
- *Advanced Biometric Authentication*: To stop identity theft and false medical claims, healthcare systems are incorporating AI-powered biometric authentication techniques like voice recognition, fingerprint scanning, and facial recognition. Biometric AI improves security and lowers the possibility of fraudulent actions, such as phony health records and unapproved invoicing, by guaranteeing that only authorized patients and providers can access medical services (Gyamfi & Abdulai, 2018).
- *Fraud Detection with NLP*: NLP methods are being utilized more and more to examine unstructured textual data (Carneiro et al., 2011), including prescription information, insurance claims, and medical notes. NLP models driven by AI are able to identify questionable trends in textual data, including duplicate claims, fake prescriptions, and needless medical treatments (Pandey & Pandey, 2025). NLP

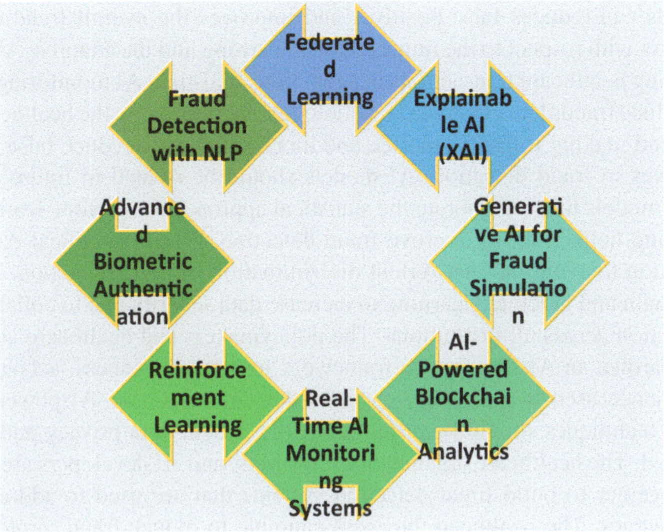

Fig. 2 Artificial intelligence technologies

makes it easier for fraud detection teams to spot fraudulent activity by automating the analysis of massive amounts of medical records (Pandey et al., 2024).

Healthcare organizations and insurers can greatly improve their fraud detection capabilities, lower financial losses, and maintain ethical medical practices by implementing this cutting-edge AI technology which are shown in Fig. 2. AI-driven fraud detection solutions will be crucial to protecting healthcare finances and maintaining patient trust as fraud methods continue to change.

6 Conclusion

Healthcare fraud continues to cause financial losses, legal troubles, and patient harm. Billing, prescription, telemedicine, and provider-patient collusion require enhanced detection methods beyond rule-based systems. Machine learning, NLP, and anomaly detection algorithms are powerful fraud detection and mitigation tools. These proactive tools used to detect fraud in the real time and also ensure healthcare transaction integrity while complying with a data privacy law. The federated learning, explainable AI (XAI), blockchain analytics, and reinforcement learning can further improve the fraud detection accuracy and adaptability. AI-powered biometric identification and blockchain improve fraud prevention by verifying the identities and preventing an unauthorized billing. AI significance in the healthcare fraud prevention evolves as a fraud strategy to get it more sophisticated. Anticipatory AI algorithms are detecting fraud before it causes financial harm. The continuous learning from the developing fraud trends can reduces false positives and improves the overall fraud detection effectiveness with respect to the reinforcement learning and the adaptive AI models. By evaluating healthcare transactions in a real time, real-time AI monitoring systems is use to reduce fraudulent claims. AI technologies are improving the healthcare fraud detection and making it faster, smarter, and more reliable. To reduce false positives and negatives in fraud detection, AI models should be refined in future research. Hybrid AI models that incorporate the statistical approaches, machine learning, and deep learning helps a lot to improve fraud detection. Prioritize ethical AI and the bias reduction to avoid the inadvertent discrimination in fraud detection. By using the blockchain and federated learning to increase data security and to collaborate on fraud detection across all institutions. The policymakers and healthcare authorities must standardize an AI governance framework to assure openness, accountability, and compliance used in the AI-driven fraud detection systems. AI-powered fraud prevention techniques should be promoted while patient data privacy and security are protected. The healthcare organizations, insurers, and AI developers are required to work together to build fraud detection systems that are used to address rising fraud tendencies. The healthcare business can able to reduce fraud, protect financial resources, and provide ethical, high-quality care by investing in AI-driven fraud prevention and tightening regulatory laws.

References

Abdallah, A., Maarof, M. A., & Zainal, A. (2016). Fraud detection system: A survey. *Journal of Network and Computer Applications, 68*, 90–113.

Albashrawi, M. (2016). Detecting financial fraud using data mining techniques: A decade review from 2004 to 2015. *Journal of Data Science, 14*, 553–570.

Al-Hashedi, K. G., & Magalingam, P. (2021). Financial fraud detection applying data mining techniques: A comprehensive review from 2009 to 2019. *Computer Science Review, 40*, 100402.

Ashtiani, M. N., & Raahemi, B. (2021). Intelligent fraud detection in financial statements using machine learning and data mining: A systematic literature review. *IEEE Access, 10*, 72504–72525.

Carneiro, E. M., Dias, L. A. V., Da Cunha, A. M., & Mialaret, L. F. S. (2011, December 11–14). Cluster analysis and artificial neural networks: A case study in credit card fraud detection. In *Proceedings of the 2015 12th international conference on information technology-new generations* (pp. 122–126).

Chaquet-ulldemolins, J., Moral-rubio, S., & Muñoz-romero, S. (2022). On the black-box challenge for fraud detection using machine learning (II): Nonlinear analysis through interpretable autoencoders. *Applied Sciences, 12*, 3856.

Da'U, A., & Salim, N. (2019). Recommendation system based on deep learning methods: A systematic review and new directions. *Artificial Intelligence Review, 53*, 2709–2748.

Delamaire, L., Hussein, A., & John, P. (2009). Credit card fraud and detection techniques: A review. *Banks Bank System, 4*, 57–68.

Gyamfi, N. K., & Abdulai, J. (2018, November 1–3). Bank fraud detection using support vector machine. In *Proceedings of the 2018 IEEE 9th annual information technology, electronics and Mobile communication conference (IEMCON)* (pp. 37–41).

Pandey, B. K., & Pandey, D. (2025). Securing healthcare medical image information using advance morphological component analysis, information hiding systems, and hybrid convolutional neural networks on IoMT. *Computers in Biology and Medicine, 185*, 109499.

Pandey, B. K., Pandey, D., & Lelisho, M. E. (2024). Face mask identification with enhanced cuckoo optimization and deep learning-based faster regional neural network. *Scientific Reports, 14*(1), 29719.

Phua, C., Lee, V., Smith, K., & Gayler, R. (2010). A comprehensive survey of data mining-based fraud detection research. *arXiv*. https://arxiv.org/abs/1009.6119

Ryman-Tubb, N. F., Krause, P., & Garn, W. (2018). How artificial intelligence and machine learning research impacts payment card fraud detection: A survey and industry benchmark. *Engineering Applications of Artificial Intelligence, 76*, 130–157.

West, J., & Bhattacharya, M. (2016). Intelligent financial fraud detection: A comprehensive review. *Computer Security, 57*, 47–66.

Zeng, Y., & Tang, J. (2021). RLC-GNN: An improved deep architecture for spatial-based graph neural network with application to fraud detection. *Applied Sciences, 11*, 5656.

Zhang, D., & Zhou, L. (2004). Discovering Golden nuggets: Data Mining in Financial Application. *IEEE Transactions on Systems, Man, and Cybernetics, Part C (Applications and Reviews), 34*, 513–522.

Edge Computing and IoT for Efficient Healthcare Data Processing

Mallareddy Adudhodla, Niladri Maiti, Naziya Hussain, Akash Jain, Patel Yogeshkumar Jethabhai, Sakthitharan Subramanian, and Hassan Khalid Abozibid

Abstract The hybridization of edge computing along with IoT in healthcare has been used to transform the data processing. These solutions have been used to decentralize the data management that helps to diminish latency, bolster security, and optimize the network capacity. The reduction of the reliance on cloud services has enabled the healthcare organizations to enhance the patient privacy and also

M. Adudhodla (✉)
Department of IT, CVR College of Engineering, Hyderabad, Telangana, India
e-mail: mallareddyadudhodla@gmail.com

N. Maiti
School of Dentistry, Central Asian University, Tashkent, Uzbekistan
e-mail: m.niladri@centralasian.uz

N. Hussain
MPSTME, Mumbai, Maharashtra, India

SVKM's NMIMS Deemed to be University, Chennai, Tamil Nadu, India

N. Hussain
e-mail: naziyahussain@gmail.com

A. Jain
Electronics & Telecommunication, Shri Shankaracharya Institute of Professional Management and Technology, Raipur, Chhattisgarh, India
e-mail: akash.jain@ssipmt.com

P. Y. Jethabhai
Faculty of Computer Science, Shri C.J. Patel College of Computer Studies, Sankalchand Patel University, Visnagar, Gujarat, India
e-mail: yjpatel.fcs@spu.ac.in

S. Subramanian
Department of Computational Intelligence, School of Computing, Faculty of Engineering and Technology, SRM Institute of Science and Technology, Chennai, Tamil Nadu, India
e-mail: tharansakthi@gmail.com

H. K. Abozibid
Al-Zahrawi University College, Karbala, Iraq
e-mail: Ahkaob4@gmail.com

D. Pandey et al. (eds.), *Smart Healthcare*, https://doi.org/10.1007/978-981-95-8828-2_4

ensure the regulatory compliance and optimize system efficiency. The implementation of distributed computing frameworks, energy-efficient AI models, and intelligent task balancing significantly improves scalability and performance. Effective execution necessitates interdisciplinary cooperation among healthcare practitioners, engineers, data analysts, and policymakers. The standardized frameworks and comprehensive cybersecurity protocols are considered crucial for guaranteeing the interoperability and safeguarding data. Progress in federated learning, decentralized artificial intelligence networks, and 5G connectivity will enhance data privacy and real-time analytics. The incorporation of blockchain for secure medical data and energy-efficient AI systems will facilitate long-term sustainability. As digital healthcare advances, investments in scalable and secure infrastructure are essential for sustaining efficiency and accessibility. By utilizing edge computing and IoT, healthcare systems may improve patient care, optimize resource allocation, and foster innovation. Future developments in precision medicine, bioinformatics, and wearable technologies will enhance personalized healthcare solutions, creating a more robust and sophisticated medical environment.

Keywords Edge computing · IOT · Healthcare data · Cybersecurity · Predictive analytics · Interoperability

1 Introduction

Modern healthcare systems collect a lot of information from things like electronic health records (EHRs), medical imaging, wearable devices, and systems that keep an eye on patients in real time. More and more healthcare providers are using digital technology, which has made it easier to get medical information. However, it has also made it harder to process, store, and protect that information. A lot of people use traditional cloud-based solutions, but they usually can't keep up with the speed, volume, and security needs of modern healthcare apps. This is why we need edge computing and the Internet of Things. The amount and speed of the health data are considered as a big problem. Real-time monitoring devices make a lot of data that can be analysed and acted on right away. Intensive care units (ICUs) use real-time data from many sensors to keep an eye on patients' vital signs. If data processing takes too long, it could lead to big mistakes in medicine. Cloud computing is great, but latency can be a problem in situations where time is of the essence, like emergency surgeries, telemedicine consultations, and remote patient monitoring. Privacy and security are also very important issues. In the USA, HIPAA protects sensitive patient information, and in Europe, GDPR does the same. The storing and sending medical data in the cloud have made it more likely that hackers will break into the system, get access to the data, or steal it. Therefore, the healthcare providers must have to follow the rules and keep data safe while data collect, move, process, and store it. There are many places to get the required medical data, and it comes in the different formats and the standards. The medical devices that have use the Internet of Things

(IoT) often use their own protocols, which makes it hard to share data. Hospitals and clinics have a hard time connecting IoT devices, edge computing solutions, and traditional IT infrastructure so that communication is reliable. Computing and infrastructure limitations make it harder to process healthcare data. Many healthcare facilities in rural areas and with low incomes don't have the IT infrastructure they need to process data quickly in the cloud. You need a lot of network bandwidth, storage, and cybersecurity costs to keep cloud-based healthcare analytics solutions going. Edge computing and the Internet of Things (IoT) can help with these problems in a way that is safe, decentralized, and happens in real time. Edge computing makes it easier to handle healthcare data, speeds up response times, and makes things safer by cutting down on the need for centralized cloud systems.

1.1 Real-Time Data Processing

As healthcare has become more reliant on digital technology. There is a greater need for the medical applications that can be used to process data in real time. Modern healthcare systems create a lot of data that needs to be analysed quickly so that doctors can make decisions, keep an eye on patients, and respond to emergencies. Conventional cloud-based processing is good for storing and analysing large amounts of data, but it often has latency issues that can be very important in medical settings. Edge computing and the Internet of Things (IoT) have been used to solve this problem by making it possible to process the data in real time at the site of the treatment, which leads to faster interventions and better patient outcomes. ICUs and emergency rooms need to be able to process data in real time. Medical sensors that track vital signs like heart rate, oxygen saturation, and blood pressure keep an eye on patients who are in critical condition all the time. Delaying the discovery of anomalies could have dangerous effects. Edge data processing enables medical devices to swiftly alert healthcare providers to necessary actions, thereby reducing the risk of adverse outcomes and improving response times. Real-time data processing is essential for the application of remote patient monitoring. Wearable health gadgets and home-based medical monitoring systems are becoming more common. This means that patients with chronic diseases like diabetes, high blood pressure, and heart problems can be watched all the time without having to go to the hospital often. These sensors have been used to send out constant streams of physiological data that needed to be looked at in real time to find any of the related problems (Ai et al., 2018; Alahi et al., 2023). The edge data processing is used to make alarms about any of the unusual situations, like sudden drops in blood sugar levels or arrhythmias, which are sent to concerned healthcare providers or carers right away. This can stop medical emergencies from happening. Telemedicine and robotic-assisted surgeries need data processing with low latency. For the accurate assessments, a remote healthcare consultation has been required for the quick processing of real-time video streaming, AI-driven diagnostics, and sensor-based medical evaluations. In robotic-assisted surgeries, any delay in sending data between the surgeon and the robotic system could cause mistakes in accuracy, putting the patient's safety at risk. Edge computing has made these apps work better by reducing latency and making it easier for the complicated medical procedures to go more smoothly. The real-time data processing is useful for two main things that are predictive analytics and finding diseases early. An edge device can be used the machine learning algorithms to look into a patient's data right on the device and also quickly tell if the illness is getting more worse. The AI-powered diagnostic tools are used to look at medical images like X-rays and MRIs right there in the hospital or clinic. This power makes it easier for doctors to act quickly and speeds up diagnosis. This is especially important for conditions like cancer or stroke, where early detection is key. The real-time data processing has been very useful for the taking care of patients and running of the hospital. The smart hospital management system uses the IoT-enabled devices to keep an eye on the medical equipment, keep track of bed occupancy, and manage supply chains better. The edge computing uses the real-time insights that have been used for the better allocation of the resources, which lets the medical staff focus on taking care of patients instead of dealing with administrative issues. In healthcare, there are many areas where the real-time data processing is needed, such as keeping an eye on patients, using predictive analytics, and the running of the hospitals. Edge computing and the Internet of Things (IoT) provide the infrastructure needed to meet this need by lowering latency, making it easier to make decisions right away, and making healthcare more efficient overall (Arcas et al., 2024a).

1.2 Edge Computing and IoT in Transforming Healthcare

The edge and IoT technologies jointly have revolutionized healthcare through real-time data processing, less latency, and improved patient monitoring, as shown in Fig. 1. Wearable gadgets, biosensors, and intelligent medical apparatus have been continuously gathering essential health care data, which is further processed locally to facilitate expedited decision-making. This integration is used to optimize an emergency response to improve medical imaging diagnoses and facilitates telemedicine through low-latency consultations. Furthermore, it is found that the localized data analysis enhances the hospital resource management by assuring effective equipment tracking and inventory control. By reducing reliance on cloud networks and bolstering security, these technologies foster a more efficient and scalable healthcare system, thereby strengthening patient care and medical decision-making in both urban and remote environments.

- *Real-Time Monitoring*: The wearable and implanted medical devices that has use the Internet of Things (IoT) keep an eye on important signs such as heart rate, blood pressure, oxygen saturation, and glucose levels all the time. These devices collect a lot of health data which needs to be looked at the right away to find any problems. The edge computing processes data on-site that reducing reliance on a cloud system and also ensuring that alerts for critical situations, such as

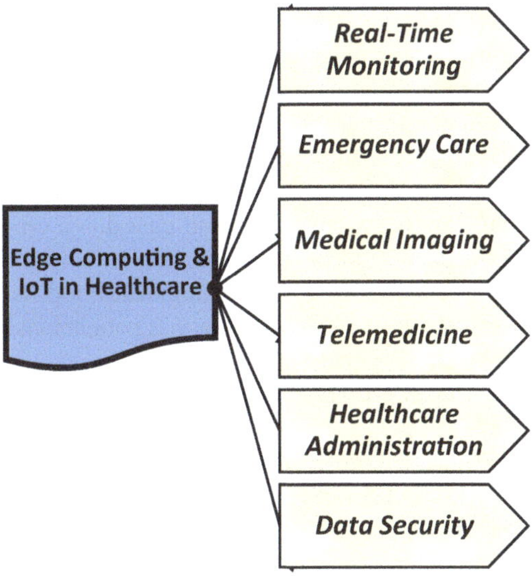

Fig. 1 Role of edge computing & IoT in healthcare

arrhythmias or sudden drops in glucose levels, are quickly sent to healthcare providers. This ability is very important for managing long-term illnesses like diabetes and high blood pressure, as well as for older people who need to be watched over without being able to go to a doctor's office (Arcas et al., 2024b).

- *Emergency Care*: It is very important to get the medical help to right away in emergency rooms and intensive care units. The patients are admitted in critical condition must be checked on all the time to look for the signs of distress. The edge-enabled medical devices must be look at patient data right from it is, which cuts down on the time. It takes to the process and send information to compare the cloud-based solutions. This quick analysis can find heart rhythms that are out of the ordinary, sudden changes in blood pressure, or breathing problems before they become deadly. Edge computing reduces latency, which means that doctors and emergency responders get immediate actionable insights. This improves patient survival rates and makes the work of healthcare workers easier.
- *Medical Imaging*: The conventional medical imaging modalities has been involved the acquisition of a high-resolution images, such as MRIs, CT scans, and X-rays, which are usually processed in centralized cloud systems. The sending of a large image files to the cloud servers may take longer than expected that could affect the decisions about diagnosis and treatment. The edge computing makes the AI-powered diagnostic tools look at images on the spot, and also giving the quick evaluations and cutting down on the time it takes to get results. This is especially helpful in rural areas where network connectivity is not always reliable, making sure that patients get medical care on time. Faster analysis of medical images makes it easier to find important diseases like cancer, stroke, and neurological disorders early on. This is because quick treatment greatly improves patients' chances of recovery.

- *Telemedicine*: Telemedicine has become an important part of the modern healthcare by enabling the patients to talk a doctors from a far flung area through the video conferencing and the AI-enhanced diagnostics. The latency issues are common in the traditional cloud-based telemedicine systems, which lowers the quality of consultations. Edge computing makes telemedicine better by processing video streams, patient data, and AI-driven diagnostics on the spot, which makes the experience smoother and cuts down on latency. This device is very useful in remote or disaster-stricken areas where it is hard to get to expert medical professionals. Edge computing makes it possible to do real-time diagnostics and consultations, which means that patients can get care quickly no matter where they are (Boopathi et al., 2023).
- *Healthcare Administration*: To make sure that patients get the best care and that money is spent wisely. The hospitals need to run well by making the hospitals IoT-enabled infrastructure, that keeps an eye on medical equipment, checks drug stocks, and controls how many beds are available in real time. Edge computing processes data on-site, giving hospital managers real-time information about the availability of resources. This cuts down on the time, it takes to find an important equipment such as ventilators and defibrillators, especially in emergencies. The AI-driven analytics at the edge can also help to predict when supplies will run low, automatically restock inventory, and improve hospital operations. This lets medical staff focus on taking care of patients instead of dealing with logistical problems.
- *Data Security*: In healthcare, protecting patient information is consider as a very important task. There are possible cybersecurity risks with the cloud-based data transmission that include an unauthorized access and data breaches. Edge computing makes things safer by processing important medical information on site, which means that large amounts of data don't have to be sent over networks that might not be safe. Edge computing makes systems less vulnerable to cyber threats and makes sure that healthcare standards like HIPAA and GDPR are followed by only storing and analysing the most important data in centralized cloud systems. Encrypted communication protocols and authentication methods make data protection even better.

2 Architectural Framework

2.1 IoT-Edge Integration in Healthcare

The real-time data processing has been improved by the integration of the Internet of Things-based devices and the edge nodes in the healthcare industry. This leads to the improvements in patient monitoring, diagnostics, and overall healthcare efficiency. The wearable sensors, smart monitors, and implantable biosensors are considered as an example of the Internet of Things (IoT)-enabled medical devices that have been continuously collecting the data on the current health status of a patient (Chen & Ran, 2019). It is necessary to do an immediate analysis of the large amounts of information that are generated by these devices in order to identify irregularities and prevent medical problems. The edge nodes process the data on-site, that helps to cuts down on the latency that comes with cloud-based systems and also make the decisions more quickly. This plan is especially useful in the critical care situations, where the real-time monitoring can help to avoid problems and save lives. Interoperability is considered as an important part of bringing edge technologies and the Internet of Things into healthcare systems. Standardized communication protocols like MQTT and HL7 let medical devices made by different companies send data to edge computing units without any problems. This allows hospitals, rural clinics, and emergency responders to work together well. Also, analytics that use artificial intelligence and are installed on edge nodes can give you predictive insights. These insights can include finding heart disease or breathing problems early, which lets healthcare providers take action before the problem gets worse. Adding the Internet of Things to the edge of the network makes better use of bandwidth and can also make data security better by reducing the need for centralized cloud networks. There is less risk of data breaches and cyberattacks because sensitive patient data is processed closer to where it came from. This technology has made sure that healthcare services are always available in areas with poor internet access. This is especially helpful for healthcare facilities in rural and remote areas (Cicirelli et al., 2021).

2.2 *Real-Time Healthcare Network Topology*

An organized network topology is considered crucial for the real-time administration of the healthcare data, facilitating uninterrupted connectivity among IoT devices, edge nodes, cloud systems, and healthcare service providers. In a standard configuration, medical IoT devices that include the wearables, sensors, and intelligent hospital apparatus incessantly gather patient data. This information has been processed locally at an edge node, therefore diminishing the latency and also enhancing real-time decision-making. The hierarchical network concept that comprises a numerous level has been frequently employed in the healthcare sector. At the device layer, an IoT sensors and medical apparatus are used to collect the patient's important signs and transmit the data to adjacent edge nodes. The edge layer processes, filters, and the analyses of the data prior to the transmitting pertinent insights to the cloud. The cloud layer has been functioning as the primary repository for long-term storage, sophisticated analytics, and the remote access for healthcare practitioners (Deng et al., 2020). A hybrid network structure that has been used to integrate the centralized and decentralized computing ensures a better efficiency. The edge computing alleviates network congestion by processing a time-sensitive data locally, whereas the cloud servers oversee extensive analytics and the historical data storage. This method reconciles the immediate processing requirements along with the comprehensive data management functionalities. Security and reliability are considered as a paramount in the real-time healthcare networks. A mesh architecture has been frequently used for redundancy, which helps in facilitating various routes for data transfer and diminishing the likelihood of a system failure. To protect the patient's important information from the cyberattacks to secure communication protocols, encryption, and authentication techniques have been utilized. The healthcare networks have been used to accommodate an expanding volume of the IoT devices and the data traffic without compromising their performance. 5G and software-defined networking (SDN) augment flexibility, facilitating uninterrupted data transmission between devices and healthcare platforms. By implementing an effective network architecture, healthcare companies can help to enhance real-time monitoring, optimism resource allocation, and guarantee secure, continuous medical services, ultimately resulting in improved patient outcomes and more efficient healthcare operations (Khan et al., 2019).

3 Scalability and Interoperability

3.1 Standardization Issues across Medical IoT Devices

The standardization challenges among the available medical IoT devices have provided considerable difficulties in interoperability, data security, and regulatory compliance. The proliferation of manufacturers has been creating IoT-enabled medical devices that resulted in the discrepancies in the communication protocols, data formats, and integration techniques, obstructing seamless connectivity between devices and healthcare platforms. A significant problem that is found is the absence of compatibility. The various medical IoT devices have the proprietary communication protocols that complicate the integration of numerous systems within a hospital. For instance, certain devices utilize MQTT, and others employ HL7 or FHIR. Resulting in compatibility challenges in the data interchange across edge computing units, cloud storage, and the electronic health records (EHRs). Data security and privacy are considered significant issues owing to the lack of standardized encryption and the authentication protocols. A diverse security implementation across the devices renders the healthcare networks that are vulnerable to cyber threats, heightening the risks of data breaches and illegal access to sensitive patient information. The absence of established cybersecurity protocols has complicated the assurance of comprehensive data protection (Pandey et al., 2021). The regulatory compliance that differs by a country is complicating the global deployment of the IoT-based healthcare solutions. Medical IoT devices must comply with several standards, including HIPAA (USA), GDPR (Europe), and the MDR (EU). The absence of universally recognized certification processes hinders the deployment of the IoT in the healthcare sector. The scalability challenges emerge, because of the discrepancies in network infrastructure, and the IoT device interoperability in a healthcare organization. Certain hospitals that employ an old system have a lack of compatibility with modern IoT devices. This necessitating an expensive update or a middleware solution. The absence of a universal standard makes the expansion of IoT implementations intricate. Nowadays, an industry-wide collaboration has become essential for building standardized protocols, cybersecurity frameworks, and regulatory norms to tackle these set of the difficulties. An international initiative for interoperability and standardization has been augmenting the efficiency, security, and scalability of medical IoT, and hence it is enhancing patient care and healthcare operations.

3.2 Scalability Concerns in Healthcare Networks

The expansion of healthcare networks has been used to meet the growing demands of patients and the improvements in existing technology offers a considerable hurdle in terms of scalability. At the same time that medical institutions are integrating Internet of Things devices, edge computing, cloud systems, and AI-driven analytics, it is becoming increasingly difficult to guarantee continuous data flow, security, and efficiency. The resolution of these issues is found to necessary in order to preserve the high quality of a healthcare services and also simultaneously adapting to the requirements of the future. A growth in the amount of data traffic and congestion on the network is a significant obstacle. The implementation of an Internet of Things-enabled devices, that include the imaging systems, smart medical equipment, and wearable sensors, results in a significant increase in the amount of the data that is collected in real time. The transmission of an excessive amount of data might slow down processing and have an impact on essential healthcare activities if the network infrastructure is not suitable for scaling. The efficient management of this increasing amount of the data load can be facilitated through the use of a high-bandwidth solutions such as software-defined networking (SDN) and 5G networks (2G networks). An additional obstacle that must be overcome in order to scale healthcare networks is interoperability and device compatibility. There are still a lot of hospitals that rely on outdated systems, which might not be able to accommodate modern Internet of Things technologies, which might lead to integration problems. Standardized communication protocols, like HL7 and FHIR, are absolutely necessary in order to guarantee that new and existing devices may communicate to one another without any interruptions. In addition, ensuring that the resources have been distributed evenly between the cloud and the edge is essential for the scalability. In contrast to cloud servers, which are used for managing the long-term storage and large-scale analytics. Edge computing has been provided an efficient method for processing the time-sensitive data locally (Ometov et al., 2022). Keeping the performance of the network at a satisfactory level requires both the effective allocation of workload and the optimization of resources. It is becoming an increasingly important to prioritize the cybersecurity and a data protection because number of connected devices continues to rise. Expanding networks are susceptible to cyber vulnerabilities and data breaches if they do not have a security framework that can be scaled up. In the process of the encryption from beginning to finish. Architectures based on zero trust and threat detection driven by artificial intelligence are help a lot to improve the security. There are still considerable number of the issues regarding the cost and the investment in an infrastructure, particularly for smaller healthcare facilities and rural hospitals that are constrained by budgetary constraints. There are a number of ways that financial barriers can be overcome that includes government funding, public-private partnerships, and cloud-based solutions that are considered as cost-effective. Another significant obstacle is the reliance on a dependable communication in the existing remote regions. It is necessary to implement new solutions such as satellite-based networks, mobile health units, and edge computing hubs in order to guarantee that all individuals have equal access to medical services while expanding healthcare networks to areas that are currently underserved. In order for healthcare facilities to attain scalability, they need to adopt a strategic strategy that incorporates cutting-edge technologies, established protocols, stringent security measures, and financially sustainable models. As a result, expanding networks are guaranteed to continue to be effective, secure, and capable of satisfying the ever-increasing requirements of contemporary healthcare (Pandey & Pandey, 2025).

4 Data Governance and Compliance

The healthcare sector is now prioritizing a robust data that used in governance. Due to the proliferation of an IoT and the edge computing. In order to ensure patient safety, foster trust, and maintain efficiency, it is essential to securely manage extensive volumes of patient data while adhering to legal, ethical, and operational regulations. Healthcare companies must establish robust frameworks addressing privacy, ethics, data security, and legal obligations for AI-driven healthcare solutions. The regulatory compliance has been constituting a crucial aspect of the governance. The healthcare organizations must adhere to the regulations such as HIPAA (USA), GDPR (Europe), and MDR (EU) in order to safeguard patient's rights, data privacy, and security. These regulations are delineated by the appropriate methods for the collection, storage, sharing, and safeguarding of a medical data. As compliance necessitates the implementation of a suitable data management policy. Therefore, a stringent access controls, and auditing mechanisms has been used to prevent unauthorized access and the data exploitation. As medical IoT devices continue to gather confidential health information, obtaining patient consent and safeguarding their data remain paramount. Patients must retain authority over the utilization and dissemination of their personal health information to ensure its protection. This necessitates the establishment of explicit consent protocols and methods for data anonymization. The healthcare governance must incorporate access control and the required data security. To safeguard data and also minimize its exposure to the outsiders. An enterprise must use Role Based Access Control (RBAC) along with multi-factor authentication (MFA), and robust encryption techniques. The blockchain-based storage models and the other innovative technologies that are used to safeguard data integrity and also to reduce the dependence on centralized systems to enhance security significantly. The quality and integrity of data are equally crucial as security for informed healthcare decision-making (Premsankar et al., 2018). The real-time synchronization of IoT devices, edge nodes, and electronic health records (EHRs) along with automatic validation checks and AI-driven verification, ensures that the accuracy of the patient data. This reduces the likelihood of an errors in diagnosis and the therapy. The expansion of a multinational healthcare cooperation increases the security and a regulatory concern around cross-border data transmission. The legal disputes that happen among nations regarding protection of the data legislation, complicate the exchange of healthcare data between countries. Establishing interoperability frameworks and standardized international data-sharing agreements can address these issues. The growing utilization of AI-driven analytics also presents, an ethical concern such as bias, accountability, and transparency. AI models must be trained on diverse datasets. In order to mitigate biases that may occur, due to inequitable treatment or the erroneous diagnoses. The regular audits, ethical AI standards, and transparent decision-making processes are considered as an essential to ensure that AI-driven healthcare is to be equitable and dependable. Implementing robust data governance principles enables healthcare organizations to improve compliance, security, and confidence in digital healthcare systems. Despite advancements in healthcare technology, patient rights remain safeguarded by a meticulously controlled system that ensures the ethical, secure, and efficient management of patient data (Shi et al., 2016).

5 AI and Machine Learning at the Edge

5.1 AI-Driven Diagnostics and Decision-Making

The implementation of an intelligent automation system with a sophisticated data interpretation and an adaptive learning model has been transforming the healthcare industry. AI utilizes deep learning, reinforcement learning, and natural language processing (NLP) to extract meaningful insights from unstructured medical data, such as notes from doctors, pathology reports, and real-time sensor data. This is in contrast of the traditional diagnostic approaches that are rely on the other methodologies. The creating of the comprehensive patient profiles is made possible by using the multi-modal artificial intelligence, which helps to integrates many data sources such as genomic sequencing, radiological images, and electronic health records (EHRs). This is a huge achievement in research and development. For the purpose of improving the diagnostic accuracy. The artificial intelligence now uses to synthesize the various inputs rather than depending on the data from a single source. This is required for the more accurate illness diagnosis as well as determining the progression tracking. Another trend that is emerging in the field of a medical artificial intelligence is the federated learning that enables the healthcare organizations to train AI models in a collaborative manner without sharing any kind raw patient data. This decentralized strategy improves generalizability across a variety of populations while simultaneously enhancing privacy. It ensures that artificial intelligence systems learn from a wide variety of datasets, which helps to reduce bias. By imitating human reasoning, cognitive computing systems that are powered by artificial intelligence are now providing assistance in making complex decisions. These systems have shown the capability to perform the real-time analysis for a treatment plans, taking into account the drug interactions, history of the patient, and also the comorbidities in order to make the prescription for the individualized therapy. Additionally, they adjust themselves on a regular basis in response to new medical research, which makes them dynamic decision-support aids for physicians. The use of an artificial intelligence algorithms that have been trained on diverse set of large-scale genomic and clinical datasets, is able to find uncommon illness quickly, that would otherwise take years to diagnose. Artificial intelligence speeds up early intervention, which in turn improves patient outcomes. It does this by spotting tiny patterns in symptoms and biomarkers. Quantum-enhanced artificial intelligence is also being investigated for its potential to process enormous volumes of medical data at speeds that have never been seen before. This might lead to significant advancements in areas such as drug development, precision medicine, and real-time diagnostics. As artificial intelligence (AI) continues to advance, it is not only enhancing human knowledge but also actively changing the process by which medical decisions are made. This is paving the way for a healthcare ecosystem that is more intelligent and adaptable (Sreedhar et al., 2025).

5.2 ML Models on Edge for Predictive Healthcare

The application of the Machine Learning (ML) models (Sun & Ansari, 2016) on an edge device is changing the mechanism of the predictive healthcare works. These models make people able to took decisions and perform analyse on data in a real time. Edge-based machine learning processing makes it possible to do healthcare analytics directly on medical devices like wearables, smart monitors, and diagnostic tools. This is different from the typical cloud computing-based AI that needed to send the data to a distant server (Wang et al., 2020). The ML models that executed on edge enabled biosensors can be able to keep track of the patient's vital signs that include the heart rate variability, oxygen levels, and glucose levels, all the time. These models can find problems that could mean the start of diseases like cardiac arrhythmia, sepsis, or diabetes-related issues. This real-time analysis that makes an early intervention possible, which helps to lowers the number of the hospitalizations and also improves patient outcomes (Yu et al., 2018). Another big benefit of using ML on edge devices is that it can help people keep track of their health. Smart implants, fitness trackers, and remote patient monitoring systems can change alarms and recommendations on the fly by tailoring their predictive analytics to each patient's data. For example, people with asthma can take steps to avoid flare-ups by wearing an ML-powered device that can predict them based on environmental factors, past events, and real-time lung function values. Federated learning and edge-based ML models work together to make security and privacy even better. A number of edge devices use this decentralized learning method to train on patient data that is stored locally, so it doesn't have to be sent to a central server. This also makes sure that the HIPAA and GDPR standards are met and this would be very helpful for the big hospital networks that want to use an AI insight, while still following strict rules for protecting patient data. Another new thing is resource-efficient machine learning optimization, which makes models smaller and faster so they can work well on low-power edge devices without losing accuracy. The strategies such as knowledge distillation, pruning, and the model quantization help the deep learning models to work better on the medical devices that run on batteries. By using the machine learning models directly on the edge devices helps the predictive healthcare become much faster and easier to get to more personalized. This does away with the need for cloud-based infrastructure and makes sure that interventions happen quickly and that patient care is better. This change is making it possible for advanced, real-time healthcare systems to protect patient data while improving effectiveness and outcomes.

5.3 Minimizing Cloud Reliance for AI in Healthcare

The amalgamation of 5G technology with AI-driven medical applications is shown in Fig. 2 which, improves real-time connectivity among edge devices. Rapid data transfer rates facilitate instantaneous AI analysis in telemedicine, robotic surgery, and remote diagnostics, hence enhancing efficiency in medical decision-making.

- *Real-Time AI Processing*: AI models integrated directly into medical devices, including advanced imaging tools and biosensors, provide immediate diagnosis and monitoring. This obviates the necessity for cloud-based inference, hence facilitating expedited treatment and diminishing reliance on external networks.

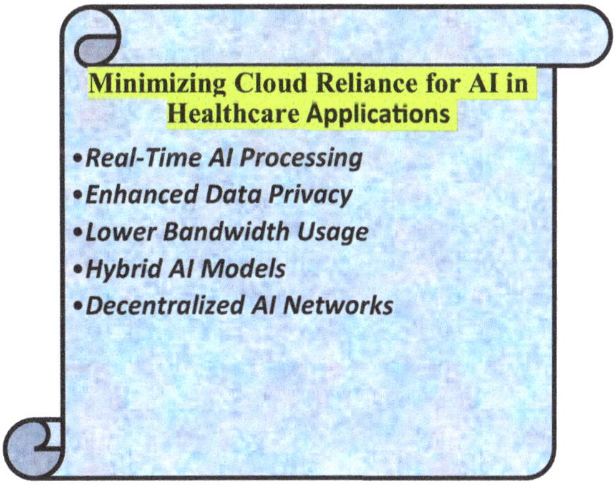

Fig. 2 Minimizing cloud reliance for AI in healthcare applications

- *Enhanced Data Privacy*: Local processing of sensitive patient information mitigates the risk of cyber threats and data breaches. Adherence to healthcare rules such as HIPAA and GDPR is reinforced, as patient data remains on-site, thereby augmenting confidentiality.
- *Lower Bandwidth Usage*: AI models functioning on edge devices markedly diminish the quantity of data required to be transmitted to the cloud. This alleviates pressure on hospital networks and facilitates uninterrupted operation in regions with restricted internet access, such as rural clinics or field hospitals.
- *Hybrid AI Models*: The integration of edge computing with cloud resources guarantees optimal AI performance. Although inference and preliminary analysis take place on local devices, intricate model retraining and extensive analytics can still utilize cloud computing. This method preserves AI efficacy without superfluous reliance on cloud resources.
- *Decentralized AI Networks*: AI-enabled devices can interact and exchange information locally without reliance on centralized cloud servers. This peer-to-peer AI methodology facilitates secure collaboration among medical institutions, preserving data sovereignty and minimizing reaction times in clinical operations.

6 Energy Efficiency and Hardware Constraints

6.1 Optimizing Computational Loads

As artificial intelligence and the data-driven technologies are added to healthcare, it is become important to optimized computing loads. So that real-time processing can be happened without giving too much strain on the medical infrastructure. The AI-driven diagnostics with predictive analytics, and remote monitoring are all considered as the examples of healthcare applications that requires a lot of the computing power. Without load optimization, hospitals and clinics may have problems with performance, waste energy, and take too long to make decisions. Sometimes, the distributed computing systems are being used to optimize the demands on the computers. Instead of using a centralized cloud server. A healthcare organization can run AI workloads on edge devices on premise servers and the hybrid cloud environments. This method does real-time tasks like monitoring patients and making emergency diagnoses on the spot, and it does computationally expensive tasks like training deep learning models in the cloud. By dynamically balancing workloads, hospitals can cut down on latency and make things run more smoothly. It's also important to have lightweight machine learning models for situations where resources are limited. Model quantization, pruning, and knowledge distillation make AI models with high accuracy use less computing power. These types of optimized models make portable medical devices to act like a wearables, diagnostic imaging systems, and point-of-care testing kits that make real-time inferences and also giving the important information without needing a lot of hardware resources. To make big hospital networks work as efficiently as possible, load balancing is needed. The AI-driven workload allocation systems are automatically assigning a processing tasks to the available the system based on the importance of the task. An AI-powered radiology system in a smart hospital might scan the most important patients first and put less urgent cases on hold until later. This makes the best use of the medical resources, that help to speeds up the system and allows for quick patient care. In addition to the software-based improvements, a better AI processor, FPGAs, and TPUs to help to optimize the computational loads. The dedicated processors is use to speed up the complicated math's and use the less energy, which makes AI work better. Such hardware makes medical AI systems to act faster for performing analysing on the data and also it is more reliable. Healthcare providers can make medical applications work better by using distributed computing, lightweight AI models, smart load balancing, and specialized hardware. By optimizing computational loads, AI-driven healthcare can stay scalable, responsive, and cost-effective, which leads to better patient outcomes and clinical workflows.

6.2 *Sustainable Infrastructure for Long-Term Deployment*

To make a healthcare system that lasts. It is needed to find a balance between efficiency, scalability, and the environmental responsibility. The AI, IoT, and edge computing are now becoming more common in hospitals. So, it is essential that they are strong and reliable. The sustainable infrastructure is able to make the most of operating efficiency, energy efficiency, system resilience, and long-term savings. The energy-efficient computers are considered as an important part of the sustainable healthcare infrastructure. Hospitals collect a lot of data from imaging, patient monitoring, and electronic health records (EHRs). It requires a lot of computing power to process this type of data, which consumes a lot of energy. To save the energy and also keep the performance up, healthcare facilities are using a low-power AI models, energy-efficient CPUs, and cooling systems that are made just for them. Solar and wind power are two examples of renewable energy sources that can also help keep medical computing systems running. Another thing to think about is system architecture that is modular and scalable. As healthcare needs change, systems need to be able to handle new technology and more data. Cloud-edge hybrid models make the computing bigger by executing a non-urgent task in the cloud and an important task on the local edge devices. This method makes better use of the available resources, that the lowers the costs of an expanding infrastructure and also makes better use of the computing resources. To deploy in a way that is good for the environment, you need to make sure that hardware lasts as long as possible and that e-waste is kept to a minimum. A lot of electronic waste collected from the healthcare comes from process of the upgrades and replacing hardware. To fight this, hospitals are using a hardware that can be upgraded and circular economy strategies like fixing and reusing old technologies. The infrastructure that is defined by using the software and can also update the systems without replacing the hardware is consider as a more sustainable. Healthcare IT systems lessen their impact on the environment by improving how they store and manage data. The smart data archiving, compression, and tiered storage able to cut down on duplicate data storage and the carbon footprint of the big cloud data centres. Decentralized storage systems have distributed computing tasks more evenly, which benefits the environment. Healthcare facilities can make their infrastructure last by using energy-efficient computers, modular design, durable hardware, and good data management. This helps make sure that digital healthcare systems stay affordable, flexible, and strong while also making sure that medical technology can last around the world.

7 Conclusion

The edge computing and the Internet of Things (IoT) have changed the healthcare sector by making it possible to process data in real time. This helps to cutting down on latency and also making medical applications work better. These technologies help to make it possible to diagnose the patients faster and also keep an eye on them. By decentralizing the data processing, a healthcare organization can make their systems more responsive and their networks faster. Less reliance on the cloud makes it easier to follow the rules and protect patient privacy. IoT devices and edge nodes have made the healthcare system smarter, bigger, and more reliable. It can now handle complicated medical data in real time. To get the most out of these technologies, people from different fields need to work together. To use edge computing and the Internet of Things (IoT) in healthcare, doctors, engineers, data scientists, and policymakers must work together. To make sure that AI models and IoT technologies meet clinical needs, medical professionals need to work with technology experts. Cybersecurity experts keep private medical records safe from hackers and other cyber threats. Governments, regulators, and leaders in the industry need to agree on ethical AI frameworks, interoperability protocols, and consistent standards. By working together across the fields. The healthcare systems can be able to get the most of the digital transformation and also solving problems with technology, ethics, and rules. The future of healthcare technology is the infrastructures that are scalable, safe, and a money on safe, low-latency, and interoperable solutions to keep digital healthcare available, useful, and flexible.

References

Ai, Y., Peng, M., & Zhang, K. (2018). Edge computing Technologies for Internet of things: A primer. *Digital Communications and Networks, 4*, 77–86.

Alahi, M. E. E., Sukkuea, A., Tina, F. W., Nag, A., Kurdthongmee, W., Suwannarat, K., & Mukhopadhyay, S. C. (2023). Integration of IoT-enabled technologies and artificial intelligence (AI) for Smart City scenario: Recent advancements and future trends. *Sensors, 23*, 5206.

Arcas, G. I., Cioara, T., & Anghel, I. (2024a). Whale optimization for cloud–edge-offloading decision-making for smart grid services. *Biomimetics, 9*, 302.

Arcas, G. I., Cioara, T., Anghel, I., Lazea, D., & Hangan, A. (2024b). Edge offloading in smart grid. *Smart Cities, 7*, 680–711.

Boopathi, S., Pandey, B. K., & Pandey, D. (2023). Advances in artificial intelligence for image processing: Techniques, applications, and optimization. In *Handbook of research on thrust technologies' effect on image processing* (pp. 73–95). IGI Global.

Chen, J., & Ran, X. (2019). Deep learning with edge computing: A review. *Proceedings of the IEEE, 107*, 1655–1674.

Cicirelli, G., Marani, R., Petitti, A., Milella, A., & D'Orazio, T. (2021). Ambient assisted living: A review of technologies, methodologies and future perspectives for healthy aging of population. *Sensors, 21*, 3549.

Deng, S., Zhao, H., Fang, W., Yin, J., Dustdar, S., & Zomaya, A.Y. 2020. Edge intelligence: The confluence of edge computing and artificial intelligence. *IEEE Internet of Things Journal, 7*, 7457–7469.

Khan, W. Z., Ahmed, E., Hakak, S., Yaqoob, I., & Ahmed, A. (2019). Edge computing: A survey. *Future Generation Computer Systems, 97*, 219–235.

Kumar Pandey, B., Pandey, D., Nassa, V. K., Ahmad, T., Singh, C., George, A. S., & Wakchaure, M. A. (2021). Encryption and steganography-based text extraction in IoT using the EWCTS optimizer. *The Imaging Science Journal, 69*(1–4), 38–56.

Ometov, A., Molua, O. L., Komarov, M., & Nurmi, J. (2022). A survey of security in cloud, edge, and fog computing. *Sensors, 22*, 927.

Pandey, B. K., & Pandey, D. (2025). Securing healthcare medical image information using advance morphological component analysis, information hiding systems, and hybrid convolutional neural networks on IoMT. *Computers in Biology and Medicine, 185*, 109499.

Premsankar, G., Di Francesco, M., & Taleb, T. (2018). Edge computing for the internet of things: A case study. *IEEE Internet of Things Journal, 5*, 1275–1284.

Shi, W., Cao, J., Zhang, Q., Li, Y., & Xu, L. (2016). Edge computing: Vision and challenges. *IEEE Internet of Things Journal, 3*, 637–646.

Sreedhar, C., Suresh Kallam, G. S., Pradeep Ghantasala, S., Anthoniraj, S., Kumarganesh, K. M., Sagayam, K. M., & Pandey, D. (2025). Enhancing healthcare data security using RFE and CRHSM for big data. *Computers in Biology and Medicine, 190*, 110063.

Sun, X., & Ansari, N. (2016). EdgeIoT: Mobile edge computing for the internet of things. *IEEE Communications Magazine, 54*, 22–29.

Wang, X., Han, Y., Leung, V. C. M., Niyato, D., Yan, X., & Chen, X. (2020). Convergence of edge computing and deep learning: A comprehensive survey. *IEEE Communications Surveys & Tutorials, 22*, 869–904.

Yu, W., Liang, F., He, X., Hatcher, W. G., Lu, C., Lin, J., & Yang, X. (2018). A survey on the edge computing for the internet of things. *IEEE Access, 6*, 6900–6919.

Deep Learning for Disease Prediction and Early Diagnosis

Prithu Sarkar, Mahadev Gawas, Mallareddy Adudhodla, Niladri Maiti, Priyanka Rajesh Patil, Hari Kumar Singh, and Ali Ihsan Alanssari

Abstract The deep learning has now become a revolutionary tool used for the predicting diseases and making an early diagnosis that makes the healthcare more accurate and effective. AI-driven models look at large amounts of medical data, like electronic health records, imaging, genomic sequences, and data from wearable sensors, to find patterns that help find diseases early and tailor treatment to each patient. The applications span multiple fields such as cancer detection, neurological disorders, cardiovascular diseases, diabetes management, and the prediction of the infectious disease outbreaks. Explainable AI (XAI) is necessary to make deep learning models more open and understandable. These healthcare professionals check the AI-generated insights and also improve their decision-making. Despite these

P. Sarkar
Amity School of Communication, Amity University Kolkata, Kolkata, India
e-mail: prithusarkar90@gmail.com

M. Gawas
State Higher Education Council, Directorate of Higher Education, Panaji, Goa, India
e-mail: gawas-dhe.goa@gov.in

M. Adudhodla (✉)
Department of IT, CVR College of Engineering, Hyderabad, India
e-mail: mallareddyadudhodla@gmail.com

N. Maiti
School of Dentistry, Central Asian University, Tashkent, Uzbekistan
e-mail: m.niladri@centralasian.uz

P. R. Patil
Department of Computer Science and Engineering, Prof Ram Meghe College of Engineering & Management, Badnera, India
e-mail: priyanka.amuc@gmail.com

H. K. Singh
Department of Electronics and Communication Engineering, M.J.P. Rohilkhand University, Bareilly, Uttar Pradesh, India
e-mail: harsdik@gmail.com

A. I. Alanssari
Al-Nisour University College, Nisour Seq Karkh, Baghdad, Iraq
e-mail: ali.ih.eng@nuc.edu.iq

D. Pandey et al. (eds.), *Smart Healthcare*, https://doi.org/10.1007/978-981-95-8828-2_5

advancements, the challenges remain in ensuring equity, reducing biases, and integrating AI into a clinical operation. To solve these problems, it is required to keep looking into the method to improve models. The deep learning could have a big impact on healthcare by making the diagnoses more accurate, making predictive medicine easier, and tailoring treatments to each patient. By improving the AI algorithms, making sure they work for different groups of people, and making sure that ethical AI is used by creating clear policy frameworks. Deep learning is getting better, and it could change how we care for patients by making it easier to intervene early and improving health outcomes around the world.

Keywords Deep learning · Disease prediction · AI · Healthcare · Machine Learning · Neural networks · Predictive analytics

1 Introduction

In modern medicine, prediction of the diseases and diagnosing them early are considered as a very important. This makes the doctors to find the diseases before it gets worse. In the past, doctors relied on patients' reported symptoms, physical exams, and lab tests to make a diagnosis. However, these technologies often identify diseases only after significant progression. The healthcare industry has changed a lot thanks to new technologies, especially deep learning. These technologies use prediction models to look at complex medical data and identify patterns that could mean a disease is starting to develop. The predictive healthcare uses information about a person's past health, their genes, and their environment to figure out how they get certain diseases. The deep learning models can perform analysis at a lot of medical imaging data such as MRIs and CT scans, to find the problems that people might miss. The wearable devices and real-time health monitoring systems have generated continuous data streams that can aid in the early identification of diseases such as diabetes, cardiovascular disorders, and neurodegenerative conditions. Timely diagnosis is crucial for the management of chronic and life-threatening diseases. Cancer, Alzheimer, and heart disease are considered examples of the conditions that often show small signs that, if caught early, can greatly improve the effectiveness of the treatment and the chances of survival for patients. Deep learning algorithms allow healthcare systems to move from reactive methods that treat diseases after symptoms appear to proactive methods that predict and stop them before they get worse. As AI and deep learning continue to improve, using these technologies in regular medical practice will make it easier to prevent, diagnose, and treat illnesses.

1.1 AI and Deep Learning in Medical Applications

The artificial intelligence (AI) and deep learning have changed the field of medicine by the making diagnoses more accurate by streamlining procedures, and allowing for the creation of personalized treatment plans. These technologies use a lot of a medical data, like imaging, electronic health records, and genomic sequences, to find patterns and accurately guess what will happen with diseases. Unlike the most rule-based algorithms, the deep learning models can automatically learn complex features from the raw data. Due to this skill, it becomes the very helpful for things like finding diseases along with finding the anomalies, and suggesting therapies. One of the most important ways that AI is used in medicine is to analyse medical images. Convolutional Neural Networks (CNNs) have shown to be very good at finding diseases like cancer, pneumonia, and retinal problems using X-rays, MRIs, and CT scans. Models based on deep learning have also done very well at finding other diseases. These AI technologies help radiologists by pointing out possible problems, making it less likely that they will make a wrong diagnosis, and speeding up the process of interpreting the data. Artificial intelligence (AI) powers natural language processing (NLP) tools that read clinical notes and research papers. This helps doctors stay up to date on the latest medical technology breakthroughs and makes it easier for them to make decisions (Ahsan et al., 2021). In addition to diagnostics, artificial intelligence is also important for personalized treatment and predictive healthcare. Machine learning algorithms can look at a patient's medical history, lifestyle, and genetic predispositions to figure out how likely it is that they will get sick and suggest personalized ways to avoid getting sick. The artificial intelligence helps a lot to speed up the process of finding potential drug candidates by predicting how molecules will interact with each other. This cuts down on the time and money needed for the pharmaceutical research by a large amount. Robots that use artificial intelligence are being used in surgeries to make them more accurate and less likely to make mistakes, which leads to better results for patients. The integration of artificial intelligence and deep learning into healthcare is expected to enhance productivity, reduce costs, and elevate the quality of patient care. However, to ensure a safe and an effective implementation in the medical applications. It has become essential to tackle the challenges, such as safeguarding data privacy, ethical concerns, and the necessity for regulatory approval (Ahsan et al., 2020a).

2 Fundamentals of Deep Learning in Healthcare

2.1 The Foundations of Deep Learning

The deep learning is a type of a machine learning that basically focusses on training an artificial neural network to find patterns and make predictions based on large sets of data. It is based on how the human brain works and how its neurons are connected to each other. Neurons analysis input to find important information. Deep learning models, on the other hand, can automatically learn complex features from raw data. This makes them very good at tasks like recognizing images, processing speech, and diagnosing medical conditions. Artificial neural networks (ANNs) are a big part of deep learning. They are made up of many layers of connected nodes (neurons). A deep neural network (DNN) is a neural network that has a lot of hidden layers. Each neuron uses math and activation functions to look at incoming data. This makes the network non-linear and lets it learn complex relationships. ReLU (Rectified Linear Unit), Sigmoid, and Tanh are some of the most common activation functions. Each one has its own job to do to help the learning process. The backpropagation is a key part of deep learning that changes the model internal parameters that weights based on the difference between predicted out come and the actual outcome. Stochastic Gradient Descent (SGD) and Adam are the two important examples of the optimizers that help make these changes better, making sure that the model makes fewer and fewer mistakes over time. The Deep learning models often require a large number of the datasets to generalize effectively and to handle a situation, when a model memorizes the training data instead of learning general patterns. To lessen this, techniques like dropout regularization and batch normalization are used to make models more general. The different types of the deep learning architectures are designed for a specific task (Ahsan et al., 2020b). In computer vision, CNNs used a lot for things such as object detection, facial recognition, and analysing medical images. They use a special parts known as convolutional layers to pull out features from the images, like edges, textures, and patterns. The Recurrent Neural Networks (RNNs) have been designed, specifically for the analysis of the sequential data (Ahsan & Siddique, 2021). Because RNN can remember things from the past. It is considered as a great option for tasks like speech recognition and text prediction. Transformers have changed deep learning in natural language processing by using self-attention mechanisms. They are now the basis for models like GPT and BERT. The deep learning is getting stronger and also more flexible as computers become more powerful and data becomes easier to obtain. It is used in fields like an autonomous driving, medical diagnosis, finance, and robotics, which encourages new ideas and changes the way businesses work. However, a significant challenge such as high computing costs, necessity of labelled datasets, and ethical concerns regarding, the AI implementation must be addressed to ensure the responsible and effective utilization of deep learning technology (Balogh et al., 2015).

2.2 *Traditional Machine Learning and Deep Learning*

In traditional machine learning, the statistical algorithms are used to train models. To make this model more accurate, the experts pick out the most relevant features. This method works well for the problems that use the structured data for finding fraud, filtering emails, and making predictions about the money. But when it comes to working with unstructured data like pictures, videos, or plain text, it doesn't work very well. With deep learning, you don't have to do feature extraction by hand. The neural networks learn to make the structured representations from simple data on their own. This is why they are so good at the difficult tasks like diagnosing medical conditions, processing speech, and recognizing images. Deep learning models, on the other hand, need a lot of labelled data and a lot of computing power, which makes them very resource-intensive. Deep learning is better at handling a lot of unstructured data, which is why it's often used for new AI projects. Traditional machine learning is easier to understand and works well for simple tasks. It really depends on how hard the problem is, what data we have, and how much computing power we have available to us. Table 1 shows how traditional machine learning and deep learning are different.

Table 1 Comparison between traditional machine learning and deep learning

Aspect	Traditional machine learning	Deep learning
Definition	A subset of AI that relies on statistical models and algorithms to make predictions	A specialized form of ML that uses artificial neural networks to automatically learn patterns from data
Feature extraction	Requires manual feature extraction, where domain experts define key attributes	Automatically learns features from raw data without manual intervention
Data dependency	Works well with small to medium-sized datasets	Requires large amounts of data to perform efficiently
Computational power	Requires moderate computational power and can run on standard CPUs	Needs high computational resources, often requiring GPUs or TPUs
Performance on complex tasks	Limited capability for highly complex tasks like image recognition or NLP	Excels at handling complex tasks, such as image processing and speech recognition.
Interpretability	More interpretable, as models like decision trees and regression provide clear reasoning	Often considered a "black box," making it difficult to interpret model decisions
Training time	Faster training due to simpler models and fewer parameters	Longer training time due to deep architectures and numerous parameters
Common algorithms	Decision trees, support vector machines (SVM), random Forest, and logistic regression	Convolutional neural networks (CNNs), recurrent neural networks (RNNs), and transformers
Applications	Fraud detection, email filtering, recommendation systems, and customer segmentation	Image classification, speech recognition, medical diagnosis, and self-driving cars

3 Data Sources for Disease Prediction

3.1 Electronic Health Records (EHRs)

Electronic Health Records (EHRs) are the computerized systems that keep track to organize all of the patient's medical information. Electronic health records (EHRs) are different from traditional paper records because they store all patient information in one digital format that healthcare providers can easily access, update, and share. These records contain an important type of the information such as medical history, diagnosis, treatment plans, lab results, prescriptions, and imaging reports. Electronic Health Records (EHRs) make it easier for the healthcare providers to work together to make more accurate diagnoses and to get better results for patients by digitizing patient information. One of the best things about the EHRs is that, it can work with other healthcare systems that making it easier for hospitals, clinics, pharmacies, and labs to work together. This constant flow of data lets healthcare providers get real-time information about their patients, which lowers the chances of mistakes and unnecessary tests. EHRs help people get more done by streamlining administrative tasks, cutting down on paperwork, and making it easier for automated reminders to be sent for follow-up appointments or drug regimens. Electronic Health Records (EHRs) make it easier to make decisions by using decision support systems (DSS) (Brownlee, 2016). These AI-powered apps look at patient data and give clinical advice, such as finding possible drug interactions, allergies, or strange test results. This feature makes patients safer and helps doctors make decisions based on facts. EHRs also help medical research by giving researchers access to anonymized datasets that they can use to look for patterns in illnesses, see how well treatments work, and find new ways to improve healthcare. Even though EHRs have benefits and they also come with problems such as data security issues, high costs, and the need for thorough training. To keep trust in a digital health system. It is considered as an important to protect patient privacy and make sure that standards like HIPAA (Health Insurance Portability and Accountability Act) are followed. As technology advances, an enhancement in artificial intelligence and the cloud computing will help to improve the effectiveness of an electronic health records to optimize their management and utilization of healthcare data.

3.2 Medical Imaging (X-Rays, MRIs, CT Scans)

Medical imaging is an important part of modern medicine because it lets doctors see inside the body to make diagnoses and treat patients. X-rays, MRIs, and CT scans are imaging tools that find problems, follow the progress of diseases, and help doctors plan treatments. These imaging techniques have revolutionized diagnostic medicine by providing non-invasive insights into organs, tissues, and bones without the need for exploratory surgery. X-rays are often used to find broken bones, infections, and lung problems. They send electromagnetic waves through the body, and different tissues absorb them at different rates. White bones and grey softer tissues. X-rays are good for looking at bones, but not soft tissues. To get a more complete picture, other tests are needed. MRI uses radio waves and strong magnetic fields to look inside organs, soft tissues, and the nervous system. MRI is safer to use often than X-rays because it doesn't use ionizing radiation. It helps find problems with the brain, the spinal cord, and the joints. MRI's high-resolution pictures help neurologists and orthopaedists plan treatments. The CT scans combine the X-rays taken from different angles to make cross-sections of the body. This method is great for finding cancers that causes internal bleeding, and vascular disorders because it makes internal structures look clearer than regular X-rays. CT scans are used in an emergency rooms to quickly and accurately find strokes occur and the serious injuries. AI makes medical imaging better. Radiologists use AI to find problems, make images clearer, and lower the number of mistakes they make when diagnosing. These technologies speed up diagnosis, which helps patients and makes interventions more effective. Combining imaging technologies with deep learning should make it easier to find and treat diseases (Chandraman et al., 2025; Chinnasamy et al., 2025).

3.3 Genomic and Biomarker Data

The genomic and biomarker data have changed precision medicine in a big way by making it is possible to customize the disease diagnosis, treatment, and the prediction. Genomics is known as the study of a person's genetic makeup that includes the changes in DNA to make them more likely to get sick. By looking at the DNA sequences, researchers and doctors can find out about the inherited problems to predict a patients' risk of getting certain diseases and tailor treatments to each person's genetic makeup. This method makes medical treatments to work better and also lowering the risk of the side effects. On the other hand, a biomarker also known as the biological markers can be measured and show normal or abnormal bodily processes. These may consist of a metabolites, proteins, hormones, or specific gene expressions that associated with a disease. Biomarkers are commonly employed for prognosis, monitoring therapeutic response, and early detection. For example, some proteins in the blood may show that cancer is getting worse, and some genetic markers may help doctors figure out if someone has an inherited disease. Early detection of disease enables swift medical intervention, significantly enhancing patient outcomes (Coon et al., 2014). Improvements in deep learning and artificial intelligence have made it possible to analysis genomic and biomarker data much faster. This has made it easier to recognize disease patterns more accurately. Machine learning algorithms analysis large datasets to identify genetic correlations with complex diseases such as cancer, cardiovascular disorders, and neurological conditions. These computational methods help create personalized medicines and improve the process of finding new drugs by predicting how patients will respond to certain treatments. Despite the potential of genetic and biomarker research, challenges such as data privacy, prohibitive costs, and ethical dilemmas remain significant obstacles. To establish the customer trust, genetic information needs to be stored safely and used in a responsible way. By combining genomic and biomarker data with the digital health technology will enhance disease prediction and treatment as research advances, facilitating more personalized and effective healthcare solutions (Houssein et al., 2021).

3.4 Wearable Sensor Data

The wearable sensor technology is now an important part of the modern healthcare because it makes the doctors keep an eye on physiological data all the time. The smartwatches, fitness trackers, and medical-grade sensors are some of the devices that can be used to collect real-time data on heart rate, oxygen saturation, body temperature, and physical activity. This information helps find the diseases early to manage a chronic disease, and also improve the overall health. Wearable sensors make it possible to monitor the people without having to touch them. This facilitates people keep an eye on their own health and enables healthcare providers draw smart decisions based on data. The people primarily employ the wearable sensors to perform monitoring on their heart health. Electrocardiogram (ECG) sensors are capable of identification heart rhythms deemed not normal, including atrial fibrillation, which is a major risk factor for strokes. Regular evaluation provides it easier to deal with problems right away, which diminishes the effects of heart disease. People with diabetes are able to control their condition with wearable glucose devices that help them maintain track of their blood sugar levels and send them quick alerts. Along with keeping an eye on vital signs, wearable technology has been employed more and more in neurological and respiratory conditions. Sensors that track how people move are making it easier to spot neurodegenerative diseases like Parkinson's disease as early as possible. Wearable respiratory monitors additionally determine how well the lungs are functioning, thus being helpful for people with asthma or chronic obstructive pulmonary disease (COPD). These applications help the patients to get better care, and they also make it easier for healthcare facilities to keep an eye on a patient's health from a distance. By adding artificial intelligence to the wearable technology helps to greatly improves its features. The machine learning algorithms can look at data that has been collected to find the patterns to predict the possible health risks, and make personalized recommendations. This proactive approach helps stop illness and makes it easier to get medical help quickly. To fully realize the potential of wearable sensor technology in healthcare, problems like data accuracy, privacy, and device reliability must be fixed. These discoveries will be important for advancing preventative medicine and improving patient outcomes as improvements continue (Ma et al., 2020).

4 Disease Prediction with Deep Learning

1. *CNNs*: CNNs are often used in medical imaging to the find trends and strange things in a X-rays, MRIs, and CT scans. These neural networks instinctively pull out the image features use to identify cancers, broken bones, and infections of the lungs. CNNs have helped make radiological diagnosis much more accurate through reducing human error and speeding up the process of finding problems promptly. Transfer learning may additionally be utilised for training CNNs on medical datasets that already have been created. This makes them better at recognizing complicated conditions despite needing labelled data.
2. *RNNs and LSTM Networks*: RNNs and LSTMs are capable of looking at time-series medical data to EHRs and wearable sensors since these devices are capable of handling medical data that comes within order. These models employ patient data to predict the manner in which diseases will progress and find health risks determined by trends. LSTMs find arrhythmias by looking at heart rate rhythms in people with heart problems. These networks keep an eye on blood sugar levels and predict problems with diabetes care. By modelling the time-based dependency of patient data, it can better predict and customise medication (McPhee et al., 2010).
3. *Autoencoders*: The set of medical data known as automatic encoders tend to be deep learning models that are capable of discovering outliers. It comprehends how to minimise and reconstruct data to find unusual health patterns that could mean someone has become sick. Autoencoders are helpful when there aren't many datasets with labels and things are strange. They help radiologists find minor flaws in medical images, which specialists might miss. They show unusual patterns in information about patients, such as sudden changes in vital signs, which could mean that a patient is getting sick early in their electronic health records.
4. *Generative Adversarial Networks*: Healthcare providers are employing Generative Adversarial Networks (GANs) to make fake medical imagery that can be used to train deep learning models. In these networks, two different neural networks a generator and a discriminator make data that appear real. This method is useful for imaging when it's challenging to get tagged datasets. GANs help AI models learn to more accurately anticipate cancer, retinal disorders, and brain problems by training them on a wide range of high-quality synthetic images. GANs also speed up the process of finding new drugs by making molecular frameworks.
5. *Healthcare Transformers*: Transformers have now transformed the manner in which natural language processing works in healthcare by allowing AI examine at and learn from huge amounts of content. These models evaluate clinical records, doctor-patient interactions, and research findings to determine patterns in diseases and help with diagnosis. Transformers are employed in chatbots for diagnosis, automated medical coding, and summarizing the medical information of a patient. Transformers are designed to cut down on medical paperwork

through utilizing cognitive mechanisms to make more accurate predictions that take context into account.

6. *Hybrid Deep Learning Models*: Hybrid models incorporate different data sources and deep learning architectures to make disease prediction more precise. CNN-LSTM amalgamations are capable of looking at healthcare imagery and health data over time. This method functions efficiently whenever it requires both radiology images and the medical information of a patient to fully assess their disease. Hybrid models incorporate deep learning methods to make predictions better, and this makes them useful for healthcare providers.
7. *Medical AI Federated Learning*: Federated learning makes AI models acquire data from numerous sources without giving confidential patient information. This plan enables hospitals and research groups relate to each other while keeping information safe. Federated learning helps researchers study rare diseases because hospitals could not possibly have enough cases to make good models. Federated learning enhances disease prediction and adheres to healthcare confidentiality standards by integrating data drawn from various sources (Nithya et al., 2020).

The deep learning algorithm continues to improve the medical decision-making in more accurate, efficient, and personalized. Particularly when it comes to predicting diseases. AI-powered models are going to grow more important for diagnosing illnesses promptly, preventing them, and treating patients in a way that puts them first through their work with real-time health monitoring systems, cloud computing, and edge devices. Deep learning makes it easier to foretell diseases, which makes healthcare more prepared, accurate, and efficient. These models are going to integrate with real-time health monitoring systems and cloud platforms to make predictive analytics and early intervention better. Figure 1 shows deep learning methods for disease forecasting.

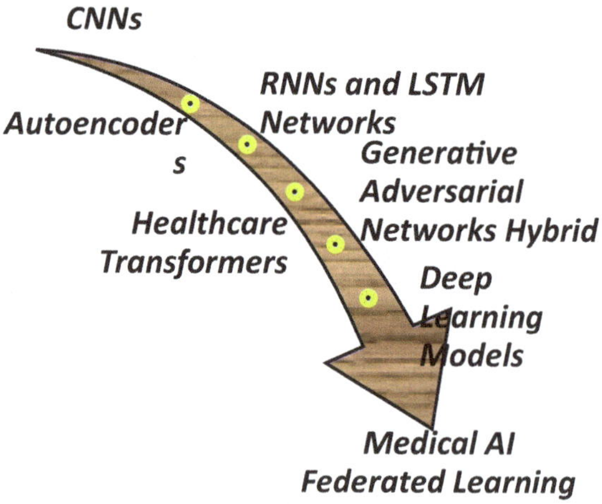

Fig. 1 Deep learning techniques for disease prediction

5 Disease Prediction and Early Diagnosis

The prediction and early diagnosis of the disease are very important in the modern healthcare because this makes it possible to treat the patients faster with a fewer complications and better outcomes. Artificial intelligence (AI), deep learning, and medical data analytics have all made it much easier to find diseases. The AI-powered models can be used to find diseases early by analysing the data obtained from medical imaging, electronic health records (EHRs), wearable sensors, and the genomic studies. This makes it is possible to give each person correct treatment and the care. One of the best ways to use deep learning in healthcare is to find out if someone has cancer. Finding the skin, breast, and lung cancer in the early stages makes treatment more effective and also increases the survival rates of the patient. The Convolutional Neural Networks (CNNs) are widely used in a medical imaging to look for the problems in the CT scans, mammograms, and the thermoscopic images. The AI-powered cancer detection helps to lowers the number of false positives, makes the diagnoses more accurate that helps doctors to find the cancers in their early stages. For example, predicting lung cancer means looking at chest X-rays and seeing dangerous nodules. For breast cancer screening, AI-driven mammography tests are used to find cancers with great accuracy. In dermatology, CNN models are also used to tell the difference between benign and malignant skin lesions, which helps find melanoma and other skin cancers early. Early diagnosis is important for treating neurological diseases like Parkinson's and Alzheimer's disease. The AI-based models use the brain scans, genetic data, and cognitive tests to find an early signs of a neurodegeneration. Using MRI scans, deep learning algorithms, it is possible to find the patterns of brain shrinkage in Alzheimer's disease. Speech and motor function analysis powered by artificial intelligence can help doctors' spot early signs of Parkinson's disease. The wearable sensors also make it easier to keep an eye on the progress of an illness of the patient. Artificial intelligence has made an early intervention of the techniques like cognitive therapy and the personalized medication. These techniques use to slow the progression of some of the neurological diseases and also improve the quality of life for those affected. Artificial intelligence also helps with early diagnosis of cardiovascular disease (CVD), which is another very important area. Artificial intelligence algorithms look at wearable sensor data, echocardiograms, and electrocardiograms to find strange things that could be linked to heart disease (Pandey & Pandey, 2025). Recurrent neural networks (RNNs) and Long Short-Term Memory (LSTM) networks process time-series heart rate data to predict possible heart problems. AI-based (Rajendran et al., 2020) risk assessment models also look at things like blood pressure, lifestyle choices, and lipid profiles to find people who are more likely to get diseases like coronary artery disease and heart failure. Finding heart problems early on lowers the risk of serious problems by taking steps to prevent them, such as changing your lifestyle, taking medicine, and getting regular checkups. Diabetes and metabolic disorders affect millions of people around the world. The AI-driven models (Samuel, 1959) can tell how likely someone is to get diabetes by just looking at their blood sugar levels, insulin resistance data, and medical history. Continuous glucose monitoring (CGM) devices that use the AI algorithms give real-time information (Sreedhar et al., 2025) about the changes occur in the blood sugar levels, which makes it possible to find out early if someone has prediabetes or diabetes. The deep learning techniques also use to analysis the lifestyle patterns and a genetic marker to predict a metabolic disorder such as obesity and the metabolic syndrome. The artificial intelligence helps doctors to find problems as early as possible that can stop long-term problems like neuropathy, kidney disease, and heart disease by changing the way people eat, giving them exercise advice, and changing their medications. This makes it easier for people to get the care they need on time. The ability of public health to respond to infectious disease outbreaks depends on how well they can predict them. Artificial intelligence and big data analytics are very important for keeping an eye on and predicting how diseases spread by looking at epidemiological data, social media trends, and travel patterns around the world. During the COVID-19 epidemic, AI-powered models (Tsao et al., 2018) used real-time health records and genomic sequencing data to keep track of changes in the virus and predict how outbreaks would spread. Machine learning methods can also help doctors figure out what diseases a person has by looking at chest X-rays and finding patterns of bacterial infection. By adding artificial intelligence to disease surveillance systems, healthcare companies can make timely interventions, run targeted vaccination campaigns, and lessen the impact of infectious disease outbreaks. Artificial intelligence and deep learning have changed the mechanism of the disease prediction and an early diagnosis in general by making them more accurate, by speeding up the process of making a diagnosis, and allowing people to take the proactive steps to protect their health. As these technologies continue to evolve alongside real-time monitoring systems, cloud computing, and medical decision-support tools, preventive medicine and patient-centred care will see significant enhancements. The future of healthcare will be fully defined by using AI-driven breakthroughs to find diseases as early, and then tailor treatments to improve health outcomes around the world.

6 Conclusion

The application of deep learning in the healthcare field has made an early diagnosis and the disease prediction much better. AI-powered models use to look at a lot of different medical data sources, such as imaging, genetic sequencing, and data from wearable sensors to find diseases as soon as possible. The deep learning and medical decision-making can help the doctors make the most of patient management strategies to improve the accuracy of diagnoses and also customize the treatments of patient. Artificial intelligence has been very helpful in finding diseases in many fields, from oncology to neurology, cardiology to infectious disease surveillance. Advanced neural networks are used to process the complicated datasets to find patterns that human experts might not be able to see and analysed. This ability to see at the high-risk people before the symptoms start not only speeds up diagnosis but also helps the preventative healthcare. Explainable artificial intelligence (XAI) makes predictions clear and easy to understand, which makes people more trusting of medical AI systems. The deep learning in healthcare could change the methodology use for the treatment of the patients. The AI-driven innovations can help to make an early intervention plans better to cut down on diagnosis errors and to further improve the therapy outcomes. To ensure ethical use, the data privacy, and compliance with laws, the widespread use of artificial intelligence in clinical settings requires a team of the engineers, doctors, and lawmakers to work together. Policy frameworks should also help to make sure that artificial intelligence is to be used safely by setting up rules for the security, validation, and integration with an existing healthcare infrastructure policy. The deep learning growing impact on predictive medicine, precision treatment, and public health campaigns will lead methodology for a more efficient and proactive healthcare system as it evolves.

References

Ahsan, M. M., Ahad, M. T., Soma, F. A., Paul, S., Chowdhury, A., Luna, S. A., Yazdan, M. M. S., Rahman, A., Siddique, Z., & Huebner, P. (2021). Detecting SARS-CoV-2 from chest X-ray using artificial intelligence. *IEEE Access, 9*, 35501–35513.

Ahsan, M. M., Gupta, K. D., Islam, M. M., Sen, S., Rahman, M., & Shakhawat Hossain, M. (2020b). COVID-19 symptoms detection based on nasnetmobile with explainable ai using various imaging modalities. *Machine Learning and Knowledge Extraction, 2*, 490–504.

Ahsan, M.M., & Siddique, Z. 2021. Machine Learning-Based Heart Disease Diagnosis: A Systematic Literature Review. *arXiv*, https://arxiv.org/abs/2112.06459.

Ahsan, M. M., T, E. A., Trafalis, T., & Huebner, P. (2020a). Deep MLP-CNN model using mixed-data to distinguish between COVID-19 and non-COVID-19 patients. *Symmetry, 12*, 1526.

Balogh, E. P., Miller, B. T., & Ball, J. R. (2015). *Improving diagnosis in health care*. National Academic Press.

Brownlee, J. (2016). Machine learning mastery with python. *Machine Learning Mastery Pty Ltd, 527*, 100–120.

Chandraman, M., Santhiyakumari, N., Shree, K. V. M., Malathi Murugesan, S., Kumarganesh, P., Rishabavarthani, S., Thiyaneswaran, B., et al. (2025). Enhancing cardiovascular disease analysis in healthcare systems with hybrid random Forest and neural network algorithm. *Engineering Reports, 7*(9), e70373.

Chinnasamy, P., Subashini, B., Ayyasamy, R. K., Kiran, A., Pandey, B. K., Pandey, D., & Lelisho, M. E. (2025). Blockchain based electronic educational document management with role-based access control using machine learning model. *Scientific Reports, 15*(1), 18828.

Coon, E. R., Quinonez, R. A., Moyer, V. A., & Schroeder, A. R. (2014). Overdiagnosis: How our compulsion for diagnosis may be harming children. *Pediatrics, 134*, 1013–1023.

Houssein, E. H., Emam, M. M., Ali, A. A., & Suganthan, P. N. (2021). Deep and machine learning techniques for medical imaging-based breast cancer: A comprehensive review. *Expert Systems with Applications, 167*, 114161.

Ma, F., Sun, T., Liu, L., & Jing, H. (2020). Detection and diagnosis of chronic kidney disease using deep learning-based heterogeneous modified artificial neural network. *Future Generation Computer Systems, 111*, 17–26.

McPhee, S. J., Papadakis, M. A., & Rabow, M. W. (Eds.). (2010). *Current Medical Diagnosis & Treatment*. McGraw-Hill Medical.

Nithya, A., Appathurai, A., Venkatadri, N., Ramji, D., & Palagan, C. A. (2020). Kidney disease detection and segmentation using artificial neural network and multi-kernel k-means clustering for ultrasound images. *Measurement, 149*, 106952.

Pandey, B. K., & Pandey, D. (2025). Securing healthcare medical image information using advance morphological component analysis, information hiding systems, and hybrid convolutional neural networks on IoMT. *Computers in Biology and Medicine, 185*, 109499.

Rajendran, K., Jayabalan, M., & Thiruchelvam, V. (2020). Predicting breast cancer via supervised machine learning methods on class imbalanced data. *International Journal of Advanced Computer Science and Applications, 11*, 54–63.

Samuel, A. L. (1959). Some studies in machine learning using the game of checkers. *IBM Journal of Research and Development, 3*, 210–229.

Sreedhar, C., Kallam, S., Ghantasala, G. P., Anthoniraj, S., Kumarganesh, S., Sagayam, K. M., & Pandey, D. (2025). Enhancing healthcare data security using RFE and CRHSM for big data. *Computers in Biology and Medicine, 190*, 110063.

Tsao, H. Y., Chan, P. Y., & Su, E. C. Y. (2018). Predicting diabetic retinopathy and identifying interpretable biomedical features using machine learning algorithms. *BMC Bioinformatics, 19*, 111–121.

Risk Assessment in Healthcare Investments: A Fuzzy Logic Approach

Naveenraj Xavier, E. Nirupama, Christabell Joseph, Sreeanandan, M. K. Sharma, A. Durai Ganesh, and Ali Ihsan Alanssari

Abstract The risk assessment constitutes a very important part of a decisions making about money. Particularly in areas that are continually challenging and ambiguous. Conventional assessment techniques frequently struggle to handle the ambiguous information that often leads to inaccurate risk categorization. This work explores the application of the fuzzy logic as an effective approach to feed risk assessment within a simpler and a more adaptable investment decision-making framework. The approach of fuzzy logic offers an increasingly nuanced perspective on risk levels by integrating linguistic factors, membership functions, and rule-centered prediction techniques. The work presents fuzzification, inference procedure, rule bases, and defuzzification as essential parts of a fuzzy logic system. It additionally demonstrates the manner in which these parts work together to cope with both quantitative and qualitative information. The investment community will benefit substantially from this method because it helps them assess risk better, lowers ambiguity, and makes decisions based on data. Policymakers might additionally employ this method to

N. Xavier (✉)
Faculty of Management, SRM Institute of Science and Technology, Chennai, Tamil Nadu, India

E. Nirupama
Saveetha School of Management, Saveetha Institute of Medical and Technical Sciences (SIMATS), Chennai, Tamil Nadu, India
e-mail: enirupama2005@gmail.com

C. Joseph
School of Law, Christ University, Bangalore, India
e-mail: christabell.joseph@christuniversity.in

Sreeanandan
PSG Institute of Management, PSG College of Technology, Coimbatore, Tamil Nadu, India

M. K. Sharma
Chaudhary Charan Singh University, Meerut, Uttar Pradesh, India

A. Durai Ganesh
Department of Mathematics, PET Engineering College, Vallioor, Tamil Nadu, India

A. I. Alanssari
Al-Nisour University College, Nisour Seq Karkh, Baghdad, Iraq
e-mail: ali.ih.eng@nuc.edu.iq

D. Pandey et al. (eds.), *Smart Healthcare*, https://doi.org/10.1007/978-981-95-8828-2_6

develop rules and financial policies that work better for the marketplace as it evolves. Instead of precise classifications, fuzzy logic allows it move smoothly between risk levels, thus making the risk evaluation better. Combining fuzzy logic alongside artificial intelligence and advanced data analytics to be financial markets change could enhance investment strategies substantially more. This makes the situation a useful tool for dealing with tough economic situations.

Keywords Fuzzy logic · Risk assessment · Healthcare investments · Uncertainty · Decision-making · Financial modeling · Artificial intelligence

1 Introduction

A lot of money is pumped into the healthcare sector throughout fields like healthcare infrastructure, medicines, biological sciences, digital health solutions, and many more. The goal for all of these investments has been to make technology, patient care, and research in medicine better. The medical field has become complicated because of issues with the economy, the law, and technology. Due to such complexity, risk assessment must be performed for healthcare investments to be financially sound as well as last. It is hard to make investments in healthcare because of worries about the marketplace and following the rules. Policies from the government, reforms in healthcare, and industry standards are all having an effect on investment decisions. In the event the rules, authorization, or reimbursement policies shift suddenly, it could hurt your finances and make it harder to succeed in the long run. To lower risk, those making investments need to diligently contemplate these uncertainties. The advancement of technology also changes the risks that come with investing in medical treatment. Recently developed medical technologies, drugs, and treatment methods can assist people improve, yet there may be additionally dangerous. It takes a lot of time, money, and research to get novel medicinal products and medical technologies approved by the government. The worries about safety or effectiveness could cause initiatives to take longer, cost more, or even make markets disappear. Prior to putting money into something, investors need to think about how likely it is to succeed and how likely it is to not succeed. Several of the risks that health care investors worry about has been managerial hazards. The manufacturing sector requires employees that understand exactly what they are doing, new tools, and distribution chains that work well. A shortage of workers, malfunctioning machinery, and problems with logistics may all impact the delivery of services and economics. For example, a healthcare facility development endeavor could be put on hold in the event that medical equipment has been late or there does not exist enough staff. These risks have to be taken into consideration in developing financial estimates and plans to reduce risk. Risks associated with markets like recessions and changes to demand make it hard to decide where to put money. Economic uncertainty may alter the amount that people spend on healthcare, and this could impact the financial standing of hospitals, insurance companies, and drug companies. The dynamics of the marketplace may additionally shift because of shifting customer preferences, competition, or other treatments. Individual investors need to do analysis of the markets to be able to forecast and adjust to modifications like these. The models of statistics and scenario analysis frequently get employed to figure out risks associated with investments since these issues are so complicated. These methods could fail to sufficiently account for ambiguity within the healthcare system and nonlinear interactions. Therefore, investigators have begun looking into fuzzy logic to help people make better decisions about healthcare investments and assess the risks involved.

1.1 Accurate Risk Evaluation in Healthcare Finance

For investment decisions for financial planning, as well as the future prosperity of the industry, the finance team in healthcare needs to be able to precisely evaluate hazards. Healthcare initiatives consume a lot of money and require an extended period to finish, therefore if you don't accurately assess potential hazards, it might forfeit money, waste time, or even lose the entire endeavor. A comprehensive risk evaluation will assist shareholders, policymakers, and healthcare officials find an appropriate compromise between making money and protecting public health. Any modifications in regulations can affect how healthcare gets accounted for, so it's important to assess the risks. A shift in government health care policies, reimbursement, and compliance could have an effect on financial security. Health care reimbursement or drug price adjustments could cause hospitals, clinics, and drug companies to incur losses in money. In the absence of a good risk assessment, investors could disregard these changes and lose money they could not expect (Amiri et al., 2017). The rising costs for healthcare and technology have become very important. It costs a lot of money to develop new therapies, digital health solutions, and medical gadgets. Several new ideas are widely accepted or approved by the government at large. A clear risk assessment method allows stakeholders to figure out if these kinds of innovations are financially sound, so they can put money into initiatives that have a good chance of continuing to grow. Hospitals spend a lot of money on their infrastructure, medical equipment, and staff. Lack of workers, problems with the supply chain, and unexpected operating costs might all hurt finances. In the event these risks have not been dealt with right away, healthcare organizations could go over budget, have had delays in service, or provide worse care to patients. A business may construct backup plans and budget their money better whenever they do a good job of assessing potential hazards. Changes in the economy, the population, and the services that patients want may all influence the demand for healthcare. As the population gets older, there will probably be a greater need for long-term care facilities. On the other hand, telemedicine could minimize the need for outpatient services. Investors must periodically look at these patterns to make sure that their financial commitments match exactly what the market shall require in the future. To account for this complexity, typical financial models have a hard time capturing the fluctuating nature of healthcare. The risk assessment makes use of fuzzy logic, AI, and predictive analytics. Including inconsistencies, expert knowledge, and real-time data makes it easier to make financial decisions and provide healthcare (Cai, 1996).

2 Healthcare Investments

2.1 Significance of Medical Spending

The investment of funds into the healthcare sector involves making expenditures on hospitals, medicines, biotechnology, medical devices, digital health solutions, and building up infrastructure. The money that is being set aside has been designated to improve the delivery of services, improve patient outcomes, encourage technological innovation, and make sure that medical systems continue to operate for a long time. The main financial donors have been governments, private investors, venture capital firms, insurance companies, and international groups that work toward enhancing and grow medical services. These investments are significant for more than merely making money since they additionally possess an immediate impact on public health and well-being. The support to feed research and development of drugs facilitates it more feasible to find new ways to manage both common and rare diseases. Making investments in the growth of hospitals, telemedicine, and digital solutions additionally helps make healthcare more accessible, making sure that people in underserved areas can get the help they need. A lack of funding could prevent essential services from accommodating rising patient requirements, leading to ineffectiveness and a deterioration in care quality. A healthcare system that is well-funded has become a big part of economic growth (Chandima Ratnayakea & Antosz, 2017). A successful sector boosts employee productivity by giving them quick and effective treatment, lowering absenteeism, and getting more people to work. This industry provides many jobs for medical professionals, researchers, technicians, and administrative staff, which helps the economy grow (Chang et al., 2018). Investing in infrastructure like hospitals, clinics, and diagnostic centers makes services much better. Contemporary medical facilities with the latest technology make sure that diagnoses have been accurate and treatments are quick. The funding that is raised toward providing medical supplies makes sure that important medicines, vaccines, and tools will always be available. It also cuts down on the requirement for imports and makes the marketplace steadier. A significant incentive to put money into this area has to do with new technologies are constantly being made. The application of AI, robots, and data analytics within diagnosis and treatment planning has revolutionized the manner in which patients receive medical treatment that facilitating to use more accurate and tailored methods. The help given to emerging tech companies and research centers accelerates the process of turning these ideas into reality, ultimately resulting in medical solutions that have become less expensive and less invasive. This is important to organize the funds carefully so that hospitals continue to grow up and get better as the world anticipates more high-quality and affordable treatments. These investments include hazards that are already there, so a full evaluation and analysis have to be done to make better use of resources. A thorough risk assessment makes sure that stakeholders benefit the most out of economic and social benefits while preventing problems. This is important for the long-term growth of this large sector (Chinnasamy et al., 2025).

2.2 Stakeholders in Healthcare Investments

The investments in the medical sector encompass a range of stakeholders, as illustrated in Fig. 1, that impact financial decisions, infrastructure development, technology integration, and policy formulation.

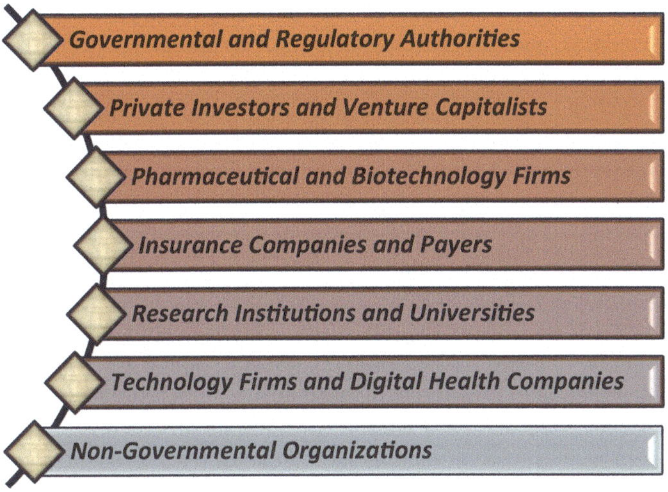

Fig. 1 Healthcare investment key stakeholders

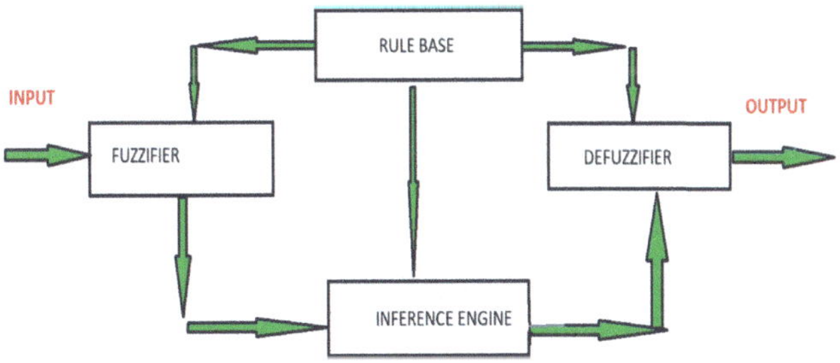

Fig. 2 Elements of fuzzy logic systems

These organizations have had unique instead related roles in promoting sustainable growth and delivering services effectively. To make smart financial choices and improve the manner in which resources are employed, it's necessary to know exactly what everyone in the group wants as well as how they will affect the situation. Each group of stakeholders plays a unique role in developing investment strategies, shaping policy decisions, and fostering innovation. Working together will contribute to making sure that these groups use their money wisely, which will lead to long-term growth and better health outcomes around the entire globe.

1. *Governmental and Regulatory Authorities*: Public institutions are essential in formulating legislation, financing public healthcare initiatives, and regulating industry standards. Health ministries, regulatory bodies, and public health organizations establish protocols for drug approvals, medical device safety, and service quality. Authorities promote investment and guarantee affordability and accessibility through programs such as subsidies, tax incentives, and public-private partnerships. Furthermore, regulatory control safeguards patient rights, upholds ethical standards, and mitigates financial risks for investors.
2. *Private Investors and Venture Capitalists*: Private equity firms and venture capitalists propel innovation by financing developing technology, pharmaceutical research, and startup enterprises. Their investments expedite the advancement of innovative therapies, digital health technologies, and medical apparatus. In exchange, they pursue financial gains via market expansion, acquisitions, or public offerings. Their participation provides proficiency in financial management and strategic growth planning, facilitating sustainable business models in the field (Duraisamy et al., 2025).
3. *Pharmaceutical and Biotechnology Firms*: Pharmaceutical manufacturers and biotechnology companies necessitate significant capital for research, clinical trials, and production. Investment in this industry propels progress in treatments, vaccines, and gene therapies. Due to the substantial expenses and protracted approval procedures, securing financial support from investors, government grants, and industry collaborations is imperative. Effective inventions generate new cash sources while tackling significant global health issues.
4. *Insurance Companies and Payers*: Health insurers and financial intermediaries affect investment trends by determining reimbursement policies and coverage programs. Their involvement in negotiating pricing frameworks, managing risk pools, and evaluating treatment expenses directly influences investment choices. Insurance companies assess market trends to evaluate the feasibility of new services, influencing financing distribution across different sector groups.
5. *Research Institutions and Universities*: Academic institutions are pivotal in medical progress through the execution of basic and applied research. Universities engage in partnerships with industry stakeholders to obtain funding and investments for clinical research, pharmaceutical development, and technical advancements. These collaborations connect theoretical research with practical applications, resulting in innovative discoveries and enhanced patient care (Gallab et al., 2019).

6. *Technology Firms and Digital Health Companies*: The emergence of artificial intelligence, telemedicine, and wearable health technologies has integrated technology businesses into the financial arena. Startups and established companies focused on software development, data analytics, and automation obtain investment to incorporate intelligent solutions into medical practices. These innovations augment productivity, diminish expenses, and refine decision-making procedures inside the sector (Grassi et al., 2009).
7. *Non-Governmental Organizations* (NGOs): International organizations and NGOs offer financial support and specialized knowledge, especially in underprivileged areas. Organizations including the World Health Organization (WHO), the World Bank, and non-profit foundations endorse programs tackling global health issues. Their contributions enhance research, infrastructure development, and disease prevention initiatives, guaranteeing fair access to high-quality care.

2.3 Major Risks in Healthcare Investments

The investment of money into the healthcare field could give rise to big financial gains and new ideas. Still, it comes with a lot of hazards because of complicated laws, changing markets, new technologies, and operational problems. Taking into account and reducing these risks has been very important for making sure that the business stays profitable and sustainable over the long term. A lack of clarity about rules and compliance has become a major risk within this area. It has strict rules for pharmaceuticals, medical equipment, insurance plans, and healthcare service activities. These rules undergo revision often that may impact investment decisions. The regulatory agencies have strict rules for approving drugs, conducting clinical trials, and making sure they are safe. This often leads to long approval times and high costs. In the event these rules are not adhered to then it could result in delays, legal problems, or even the complete denial of newly introduced items or services. This could pose a big risk for investors. The hazards related to technology and innovation have been a big problem. Healthcare technology breakthroughs are occasionally very helpful, but regularly cost a lot of money to pursue and develop. Organizations that put money into new therapies, diagnostic tools, or digital health solutions have been unsure about how well their technologies work (Ilbahar et al., 2018). Rapid technological progress potentially renders products currently under development useless before they have been sold. Those with investments in this field cannot be sure of their money because rivaling advances or unexpected failures in clinical trials may result in big losses. As soon as the market has become volatile, this makes the situation harder to make investment decisions. The shifts in population, disease rates, and the economy all affect the need of healthcare goods and services. As the population gets older, the need for long-term care might increase. However, the contrary side, improvements in telemedicine technology might ultimately render people less reliant on standard medical facilities. Economic difficulties may negatively affect consumer spending on elective surgeries and private healthcare, which causes revenue fluctuations. The investors need to do a lot of research on the market to see the manner in which trends will evolve and alter their plans to meet the necessities of a growing industry. Investment and operational problems have become a big risk factor. The high costs of building infrastructure, buying medical equipment, and managing staff are factors that make this hard to stick to an investment budget. In the absence of careful financial planning, healthcare facilities could find themselves over budget, provide lower-quality services, or even go bankrupt. By considering these challenges, the healthcare investments involve thorough risk assessment methodologies. To make smart financial decisions investors need to spend time looking at the rules, new technologies, market changes, and the operational problems. By combining predictive analytics, risk management frameworks, and flexible investment strategies, stakeholders are able to minimize potential losses while maximizing long-term profits (International Standard ISO 31000, 2018).

3 Traditional Risk Assessment Methods

- The conventional method risk assessment methods provide a structured methods to look at unpredictability to guess at financial risks, and put in place ways for minimizing them prior to choosing to invest in the medical field. The above techniques use previous information, input from experts, and mathematical modeling to help investors to make smart choices. The conventional approaches provide the structured frameworks to evaluate the financial risks. However, their bodies frequently fail to accommodate the dynamic and uncertain characteristics of healthcare investments. New developments in the law, disruptions in the market, and new technologies make things more complicated than static models could demonstrate. Also, those techniques can't be used to predict future risks very well because they depend on historical data. To address these difficulties, sophisticated risk assessment methodologies, including fuzzy logic-based models, are being increasingly investigated. These models take into account uncertainty, inaccurate data, and complicated relationships between variables, making them a more flexible and adaptable way to manage risk within the healthcare field.
- *Qualitative Risk Assessment*: This method incorporates expert opinions, knowledge of the industry, and personal analysis in order to find out precisely what the risks are for the industry. It divides risks into groups based on the probable likelihood they ought to be to happen in addition to how bad they would be if they took place. This helps stakeholders figure out which risks to worry about prior to others. Risk matrices, which rank threats from low to high risk, and scenario evaluation that examines at possible future events, are two tools that help people make informed decisions. These methods tend to be helpful as soon as don't have enough or any quantitative data. But depending on subjective judgment may bring about inconsistencies, which makes qualitative assessments less accurate for financial planning.

- *Quantitative Risk Assessment*: This method makes use of the statistical models and numbers to figure out possible financial risks. The Monte Carlo simulations and the other methods can be determining the chances of a different outcomes to create multiple risk scenarios. This gives a more thorough understanding of possible financial exposure. The use of sensitivity analysis and probability distributions examine at the way changes in costs or policies affect the performance of investments. This data-driven method helps people make better decisions by giving them measurable insights. However, its accuracy depends on exactly how good and available past data is, which may not always show how things will be in the future.
- *Financial Risk Analysis*: This method uses a well-known financial measure such as the Net Present Value (NPV), Internal Rate of Return (IRR), and Discounted Cash Flow (DCF) to calculate out the risks of investing. These methods help the investors to find out weather, the health care initiatives are worth their time and money by looking at cash inflows, funding needs, and market stability. NPV looks at the quantity that an investment will be worth in the long run, while IRR looks at the total revenue an initiative could make compared to its costs. Also, DCF analysis can guess how much money you'll make in the future by taking into account inflation and discount rates. This method gives a clear picture of the finances, but it needs accurate forecasting models to be reliable (Jaderi et al., 2019).
- *Scenario Analysis and Stress Testing*: These methods examine different market conditions, such as best-case, worst-case, and base-case scenarios, to evaluate how investments perform under varying circumstances. This approach helps investors prepare for uncertainties by simulating changes in demand, funding, or regulatory policies. Stress testing, a related approach, assesses the resilience of investments under extreme market fluctuations, such as economic recessions, pandemics, or regulatory disruptions. These techniques provide valuable risk insights but require extensive data modeling and advanced computational tools for accurate projections.
- *Sensitivity Analysis*: This method measures how fluctuations in key variables impact investment outcomes. By adjusting parameters such as interest rates, regulatory frameworks, cost structures, and patient demand, investors can identify critical risk factors affecting profitability. This technique is particularly useful for understanding financial vulnerabilities and making proactive adjustments to investment strategies. However, sensitivity analysis requires comprehensive data inputs and may not fully capture complex interdependencies between variables.

4 Fuzzy Logic in Risk Assessment

4.1 Fuzzy Logic and its Fundamental Principles

This computational method has been developed to deal with uncertainty, imprecision, as well as partial truths. These characteristics render it especially useful for making decisions that need to take plenty of different things through account. Conversely to the usual binary logic, which at first only allows outcomes to be either true (1) or false (0), this method facilitates values be present on a continuum ranging from zero to one. It has advantages for modeling real-world systems because it is able to use in instances when strict categorization could prove to be possible. The reasoning framework first introduced by Lotfi Zadeh in 1965 had the objective to replicate cognitive functions in humans. This had been done by using degrees of truth instead of simple logical choices. Over the years, this has been used throughout various fields, such as medical diagnostics, financial risk assessment, control systems, and artificial intelligence. It has contributed to helping people deal with data that has been wrong or uncertain in a way that works and has been useful. The basic ideas involve making use of linguistic variables, fuzzy sets, membership functions, and inference procedures. These variables allow it to use words that resemble a human, like low, medium, or high, instead of exact numbers to show input data. The use of fuzzy sets assists with helping it figure out how much an element fits into a group of elements. It provides a clearer indication of how ambiguous something is with their classification (Jamshidi et al., 2013). The functions of membership give a number between 0 and 1 that demonstrates how true an input value represents. After this, the inference mechanism will implement a set of rules in order to look at the inputs and give an output. Then, it is going to choose choices based on rough reasoning instead of exact reasoning. This flexible technique can be especially useful in areas at which the data has been unclear or subjective, like figuring out how risky healthcare investments are considered. It doesn't make sudden categorizing; on the contrary, it facilitates risk categories change slowly, thereby leading to a more detailed and flexible way of making decisions (Li et al., 2019).

4.2 Fuzzy Logic in Addressing Uncertainty

The main strength of this approach consists of the fact it is capable of managing uncertainty and imprecision, thus rendering it very useful to arrive at complicated decisions. This approach uses for an intermediate value that demonstrating the inherent ambiguity of real-world situations. This differentiates itself from classical binary logic, which only labels information as true or false. This flexibility has been especially useful in areas that include the healthcare investments, where it is not always possible to accurately measure financial risks, changes in regulations, and market dynamics. An additional advantage that has to do with it allows for looking at data that has been removed or unclear without needing exact numbers. When it is necessary to deal with incomplete or unclear information, traditional risk assessment models are susceptible to trouble, which might result in wrong or imprecise predictions. This method may incorporate phrases like "high risk," "moderate risk," or "low risk" to help decision-makers figure out what to do by using approximate reasoning instead of strict numerical limits. This feature makes things more flexible and gives a more precise understanding of complicated problems. The mechanism has been very adaptable to changing circumstances. In the world of investing, changes in the economy, government policy, and the market contribute to the environment consistently changing. As soon as new data comes in, conventional mathematical models sometimes need to be recalibrated on a regular basis. However, this sort of approach could potentially able to adapt to changes without major changes. The rule-based structure makes it easy to add new criteria to ensure that risk assessments are continually relevant to modify as per the change of the situations. This strategy makes it easier for people to make decisions by making the reasoning process more like a person. This technique is especially useful for looking at qualitative data because it imitates individuals use their experience and intuition to understand and organize information. This is especially necessary in areas where subjective judgment must be exercised, like figuring out if new medical technologies have been financially feasible, predicting the number of individuals who will need them, or figuring out how global health emergencies could impact investment returns. Given that it processes quickly, it is a good alternative for real-time applications. This method gives quick and reliable outcomes through fairly simple calculation (Mahdevari et al., 2014).

5 Fuzzy Logic Framework

5.1 Fuzzy Logic System Components

A fuzzy logic system has contained many parts that work together to make sense of vague data and give useful results. The parts have been fuzzification, an engine for inference, a rule base, and defuzzification, among others. Each one has significance for turning vague or linguistic information into useful decisions. The first step in the process has been fuzzification use to turns exact numbers into fuzzy values. By giving different fuzzy sets different levels in membership, this change facilitates the system deal with the uncertainties of the real world. In the context of investing in healthcare, the system might not solely say that the financial risk has been "high" or "low." Instead, this might say that the risk level is moderately high or slightly low. The roles of membership measure how closely an input relates to a certain category, which makes it easier to analysis information in a more flexible way. The Inference Engine has become the part of the system that makes decisions. It uses well-known logical rules to look at the fuzzified inputs and come to conclusions. This part relies on rules of if-then that clarify the process to understand certain situations. A rule might state, "If market stability has been low and regulatory risk has become high, then overall investment risk becomes extremely high." The inference mechanism processes many rules simultaneously, combining different inputs to come to logical conclusions (Mallik et al., 2025).

The Rule Base serves as a collection of the if-then rules that tell people the manner to make decisions. These rules are founded by the professionals to know, what has happened in the past, or what has worked in the past. The fuzzy system's accuracy (Niczyporuk, 1997) and reliability depend on the quality and completeness about the rule base. In financial risk assessment, the regulations might be considered into account the things like interest rate changes, changes in regulations, and investment returns. This enables the system adapt to changing economic conditions (Radosavljević et al., 2009). Defuzzification has become the last step, in which the inference engine's fuzzy outputs can be transformed into exact numbers. This process makes sure that the results can be understood in practical terms. There are numerous ways to get a single representative value from the fuzzy set, such as the centroid method and the mean of maximum. This method in investment decisions turns subjective assessments, like "moderate risk," into a clear risk score that stakeholders can employ to plan their strategies. By combining these parts, a fuzzy logic system provides a methodical but flexible way to make decisions, which helps make more accurate risk assessments in situations that are constantly uncertain and changeable.

5.2 *Fuzzy Rules for Risk Evaluation*

Making a list of if-then statements constitutes the way fuzzy rules for risk evaluation get created. These statements transformed qualitative assessments as numbers. These rules tend to be very important for closing the gap within expert knowledge and numerical analysis. The organization make certain that a range of unknowns in investment situations have been taken into account. The first step in the method has become to find the most important risk factors, such as changes in the market, changes in regulations, and problems with operations. Next, linguistic variables have been identified that describe these factors in a way that is similar to how people talk. Experts are a very important part of making these rules. The organization look at how different risk factors affect the overall investment profile by using their past experience in the field and historical data. As an illustration, a rule might mandate that investment risks that come from bad market conditions and big regulatory risks need to be classified as very high (Sreedhar et al., 2025). The system may additionally take into account the other level of risk, instead of just giving the two possible outcomes. Since each rule serves as the purpose of demonstrating the complex relationship exists between the different parts. After the first rules have been established, the membership functions for each linguistic phrase have been more clearly defined. The degrees of membership of these functions give to the variables that have been entered into consideration show how well a certain condition has been met. This method has been flexible enough that the system can handle a wide range of risk levels, from low to high, and give more detailed output scores. This stage of development has been iterative means that the rules have been modified and updated, which are based on the results of simulations and feedback from experts in the field. This ensure that, the model accurately represents real-world situations. The validation has become an important part of the development process and to make sure that, the results match the expected levels of risk, the rules that have been set are checked against past data or made-up situations. After this testing process, it is able to make more changes. This helps to find the differences that may have happened. The process of building rules is iterative, which means that the model will stay strong and flexible, able to handle new information and changes in the market. At the end of the day, the fuzzy rules for risk appraisal help people make better decisions by combining expert opinions with careful analysis. This strategy takes into account the unpredictable investment settings and it also gives stakeholders more information to ensure that it can make better decisions that balance the possible rewards and risks in a world that is always changing and growing.

6 Conclusion

Risk assessment becomes essential for making financial decisions, especially when it comes to investment strategies that remain continually shifting and uncertain. Traditional models have been helpful, but they have trouble with incomplete and wrong information, which makes it hard to assess risk. Fuzzy logic makes risk assessment more flexible and adaptable, which at first enables people make more nuanced decisions. This method incorporates language variables, membership functions, and rule-based inference algorithms to deal with uncertainty and give an improved understanding of financial risks. Fuzzy systems may collaborate with qualitative data and turn it into useful information because of the manner in which its components are structured, the manner in which they make inferences, the manner in which they employ rules, and how they defuzzify. Through incorporating expert knowledge and historical trends, this method eliminates the likelihood of financial mistakes and helps people understand investment threats better. This method includes an effect on both investors and policymakers. It gives investors a formal way to look at financial risks in situations where things may not always be clear, which helps them make better choices. This becomes especially helpful in fields during which changes in the market, regulations, and operations could have a big effect on finances. By applying this model, investment strategies can be modified to find a better balance between risk and reward, and this will help with long-term financial planning. This strategy helps policymakers considering it uses data to make laws and give financial advice. The regulators are able to customize risk mitigation measures to the needs of businesses when they have to deal with unclear or incomplete information. This makes sure that while making the financial decisions, more than just numbers are looked at whenever it requires to decide the stability of the economy. Fuzzy-based risk assessment embraces uncertainty, makes decisions more accurate, and gives investors an official mechanism to look at investment risk. This system smooth changes in risk levels that make it more responsive to the real-world financial situations than other models. As financial markets change, risk evaluation methods need to get smarter and stronger. The combination of qualitative and quantitative data makes this strategy helpful for making financial decisions. AI and data analytics could make it more powerful, which would make it very important for investors and politicians in times of economic uncertainty.

References

Amiri, M., Ardeshir, A., & Zarandi, M. H. F. (2017). Fuzzy probabilistic expert system for occupational hazard assessmentin construction. *Safety Science, 93*, 16–28.

Cai, K. Y. (1996). System failure engineering and fuzzy methodology. An introductory overview. *Fuzzy Sets and Systems, 83*, 113–133.

Chandima Ratnayakea, R. M., & Antosz, K. (2017). Development of a risk matrix and extending the risk-based maintenance analysis with fuzzy logic. *Procedia Engineering, 182*, 602–610.

Chang, Y., Wu, Y., Chen, G., Ye, J., Chen, B., Xu, L., Zhou, J., Yin, Z., & Ren, K. (2018). Comprehensive risk assessment of deepwater drilling riser using fuzzy Petri net model. *Process Safety and Environmental Protection, 117*, 483–497.

Chinnasamy, P., Subashini, B., Ayyasamy, R. K., Kiran, A., Pandey, B. K., Pandey, D., & Lelisho, M. E. (2025). Blockchain based electronic educational document management with role-based access control using machine learning model. *Scientific Reports, 15*(1), 18828.

Duraisamy, M., Thangavel, M., Lalitha, S., Jayaram, K., Kumarganesh, S., Martin Sagayam, K., Pandey, B. K., Pandey, D., & Sahani, S. K. (2025). Development of an ion-sensitive field-effect transistor device for high-performance diagnostic and clinical biomedical applications. *Engineering Reports, 7*(4), e70126.

Gallab, M., Bouloiz, H., Alaoui, Y. L., & Tkiouat, M. (2019). Risk assessment of maintenance activities using fuzzy logic. *Procedia Computer Science, 148*, 226–235.

Grassi, A., Gamberini, R., Mora, C., & Rimini, B. (2009). A fuzzy multi-attribute model for risk evaluation in workplaces. *Safety Science, 47*, 707–716.

Ilbahar, E., Karaşan, A., Cebi, S., & Kahraman, C. (2018). A novel approach to risk assessment for occupational health and safety using Pythagorean fuzzy AHP & fuzzy inference system. *Safety Science, 103*, 123–136.

International Standard ISO 31000. 2018*Risk Management—Guidelines*. ISO.

Jaderi, F., Ibrahim, Z. Z., & Zahiri, R. Z. (2019). Criticality analysis of petrochemical assets using risk based maintenance and the fuzzy inference system. *Process Safety and Environmental Protection, 121*, 312–325.

Jamshidi, A., Yazdani-Chamzini, A., & Yakhchali, S. H. (2013). Developing a new fuzzy inference system for pipeline risk assessment. *Journal of Loss Prevention in the Process Industries, 26*, 197–208.

Li, W., He, M., Sun, Y., & Cao, Q. (2019). A novel layered fuzzy petri nets modelling and reasoning method for process equipment failure risk assessment. *Journal of Loss Prevention in the Process Industries, 62*, 103953.

Mahdevari, S., Shahriar, K., & Esfahanipour, A. (2014). Human health and safety risks management in underground coal mines using fuzzy TOPSIS. *Science of the Total Environment, 488–489*, 85–99.

Mallik, B. B., Mukherjee, G., Kar, R., Özer, Ö., Pandey, D., & Pandey, B. K. (2025). Computational intelligence solutions for real-life problems: Theories. *Applications, and Advances*.

Niczyporuk, Z. T. (1997). Risk assessment in mining technologies. *Archives of Mining Sciences, 42*, 163–175.

Radosavljević, S., Lilić, N., Ćurčić, S., & Radosavljević, M. (2009). Risk assessment and managing technical system in case of mining industry. *Strojniški vestnik, 55*, 119–130.

Sreedhar, C., Suresh Kallam, G. S., Pradeep Ghantasala, S., Anthoniraj, S., Kumarganesh, K. M., Sagayam, B. K., & Pandey, D. (2025). Enhancing healthcare data security using RFE and CRHSM for big data. *Computers in Biology and Medicine, 190*, 110063.

AI and ML in Medical Imaging: Enhancing Diagnosis Accuracy

Suneet Gupta, Ashish Kumar, Mahadev Gawas, Bandi Rambabu, Nithin Kumar, B. Vidhya, and Ali Ihsan Alanssari

Abstract The utilization of artificial intelligence (AI) and machine learning (ML) in a medical imaging has rendered diagnosis much more accurate, faster, and more automated. The modern imaging techniques enable the identification of diseases promptly to improve the treatment planning, and cut down on human errors through the implementation of deep learning, transfer learning, and explainable AI. New advances in the computing power, like high-performance GPUs, cloud computing, and quantum algorithms have created it possible for AI to analyse complex medical scans more quickly and more accurately. The role of AI in specialized imaging fields included the oncology, neurology, cardiology, pulmonology, ophthalmology, and musculoskeletal diagnostics. The problems of an algorithmic bias, data privacy, and the need during large, well-annotated datasets that need to be fixed before widespread use in clinical settings. The growing significance of an AI in precision medicine, highlighting the capability to the customize diagnoses and a treatments based on an individual patient data. An important point involves the fact that radiologists, data scientists, engineers, and policymakers have to collaborate together to make

S. Gupta · A. Kumar
School of Computer Science and Engineering, Galgotias University, Greater Noida, India

M. Gawas
Directorate of Higher Education Goa India, State Higher Education Council, Penha de Franc, India
e-mail: gawas-dhe.goa@gov.in

B. Rambabu (✉)
Department of CSE, CVR College Of Engineering, Hyderabad, India
e-mail: rambabubandi@gmail.com

N. Kumar
School of Dentistry, Central Asian University, Tashkent, Uzbekistan
e-mail: n.kumar@centralasian.uz

B. Vidhya
Department of Computational Intelligence, SRM Institute of Science and Technology, KTR Campus, Chengalpattu District, India

A. I. Alanssari
Al-Nisour University College, Baghdad, Iraq
e-mail: ali.ih.eng@nuc.edu.iq

D. Pandey et al. (eds.), *Smart Healthcare*, https://doi.org/10.1007/978-981-95-8828-2_7

a strong, ethical, and understandable AI solutions. The future of medical imaging will be significantly shaped by the improvements in federated learning, quantum computing, and adaptive AI models. These are expected to enhance the accuracy of diagnoses, facilitate it easier to make decisions in real time, and contribute to making healthcare more accessible.

Keywords Artificial intelligence · Machine learning · Medical imaging · Deep learning · Precision medicine · Radiology

1 Introduction

Medical imaging has been going through an enormous transformation since the introduction of smart automation, leading to diagnoses more accurate, speeds up workflows, and cuts the number of mistakes made by people. The radiologists and doctors that interpret scans by hand remain able to commit mistakes and be unpredictable, even though they are experts. Innovative computational models nowadays automate image processing, thereby assisting people make decisions and making the situation easier for people in remote and underserved areas to get to. The development of a smart imaging systems has been made possible by the use of the huge datasets, powerful computers, and advanced neural networks. The latest deep learning methods, such as convolutional and transformer-based architectures, enable the identification of very precise complex anomalies. Initially, an application concentrated on recognizing patterns in radiographs, their bodies now able to encompass the detection of cancers, microcalcifications in mammograms, and vascular irregularities in angiograms the fact that might have been missed in manual evaluations. The machine-learning segmentation accurately shows that the structures of organs, tumours which greatly helps in the diagnosis and treatment planning. These new technologies have enhanced image quality and reconstruction in addition to detection. MRI and CT scans, which are common procedures used to look inside the body, have problems with noise, motion artefacts, and low resolution. Artificial intelligence models have been employed to fill in missing information, improve image clarity, and make high-resolution outputs from scans that do not look very good. These improvements reduce down on the number of times patients have to have imaging done, which saves money and lowers their dependency on radiation. Also, integrating images in real time during surgery makes things more accurate, which helps with decision-making during the operation. A further promising use is predictive analytics, which uses old imaging data and patient records to find diseases early. In neurodegenerative disorders such as Alzheimer's, early detection facilitates prompt interventions that may decelerate disease progression. Radiomics, and this gets quantitative biomarkers from scans, helps make predictions regarding the way diseases will act and how well treatments will work. The integration of imaging data with genomics and clinical records has rendered personalized medicine more possible. This means that treatment plans ought to be made for each of the patient based on their unique profile. The regulatory agencies have established frameworks to test and standardize these technologies, making sure it is safe and reliable for use in medicine. To make the most of these new technologies, while staying true to ethical standards. The data scientists, radiologists, and policymakers need to work together. In the future, more progress will speed up, the development of intelligent imaging. The quantum computing has the potential to enable an intricate image processing at unparalleled velocities, thereby facilitating, a real-time diagnostics and sophisticated disease modelling. The combination of wearable imaging devices with health applications for mobile devices will make it possible to diagnose problems outside of hospitals, giving patients easy access to health monitoring. The upcoming decades of medical imaging will be shaped by new technologies that are coming together. These will assist in making the process more efficient, accurate, and focused on the patient.

1.1 Accurate Diagnosis in Healthcare

Accurate diagnosis is important for healthcare efficiency, treatment choices, and the patient outcomes. Inaccurate or late diagnoses are susceptible to wrong treatments, worsening illnesses, and even death. Accurate medical diagnoses make healthcare systems better by cutting down on unnecessary procedures, stay at hospitals, and treatment costs. The AI and ML in medical imaging make diagnoses more accurate, cut down on mistakes made by people, and speed up treatments. For many medical conditions, getting a diagnosis beforehand and correctly makes treatment work better. In oncology, finding tumours promptly makes it possible to do surgery, chemotherapy, or radiation therapy right away, which may significantly improve survival rates. An AI-assisted imaging is capable of identifying blockages in arteries and other problems with the cardiovascular structure, and this can help prevent heart attacks early afterward. For neurological diseases like Alzheimer's and stroke, getting the right diagnosis and treatment early may impede down the illness's progress and improve the person's standard of life. For personalized medicine to work, it is essential to get the right diagnosis. In modern healthcare, patients are offered treatments that depends on their genetics, environment, and way of life. Artificial intelligence-powered imaging is capable of discovering biomarkers that show the manner in which a patient will respond to a treatment, thereby helping doctors make the best treatment choice. AI-driven radiomics are capable of looking at tumour characteristics and predicting the extent to which the tumour is going to become, which might assist doctors' choose the best treatment for cancer. This method cuts down on trial-and-error when choosing treatments and makes the outcomes for patients better. AI accuracy enhances diagnoses more accurate and makes the most of healthcare resources. Remote hospitals and poor countries usually do not have enough trained radiologists or advanced diagnostic tools. AI-powered diagnostic tools will assist healthcare workers make smart decisions by giving them automated, highly accurate evaluations. Cloud-based AI imaging systems are making it possible for specialists to look at medical images from anywhere and give advice to local healthcare providers. A correct diagnosis additionally safeguards people from getting unnecessary medical care and stay in hospitals (Avanzo et al., 2021). A lot of patients have invasive biopsies or imaging procedures because the first evaluation did not include clear. Artificial intelligence-driven precision imaging cuts down on false positives and negatives, so only people that need more tests or treatments have been tested. This makes patients safer and lessens the emotional and financial stress on patients and health care institutions.

1.2 Computational Progress on AI-Enhanced Imaging

The rapid progress of computing technology has made automated image analysis within medicine much more effective. The intelligent systems have the ability to analyse diagnostic images with incredible speed and accuracy with help of an advanced processing units, complex algorithms, and better ways to manage data. These improvements are changing the way things are done and also making it easier to find the illnesses faster, see them better, and plan treatments more effectively. The arrival of high-performance computing hardware is a big step forward. The modern architectures like GPUs (Graphics Processing Units) and TPUs (Tensor Processing Units) are able to perform the parallel processing, rather than the traditional processors that carry out tasks in order. This new idea has cut down on the time; it takes to train deep learning models and do the complicated image analysis. The deep neural networks used in the radiology can now quickly look at large datasets, which greatly help to improve the efficiency of a diagnostic facility. The integration of cloud and edge computing within the medical imaging systems represents a substantial level of the advancement. The remote computational resources allow the hospitals to use an advanced analytical method without having to buy an expensive equipment (Dembrower et al., 2023). This is especially helpful in places where resources are limited, because remote access to advanced diagnostic tools makes it easier to get quick evaluations. On the other hand, an edge computing helps to add the ability to process data in real time. So that the analysis can perform in correctly without having to rely on a centralized data centre. The quantum computing could make these advancements even better by enabling the systems to look at large datasets. In fields like high-resolution MRI imaging and 3D reconstructions. A traditional machine learning methods need a lot of data and a computing power. Quantum computing can be used to calculate many possibilities at once, which could greatly speed up and improve the accuracy of the process use for early disease diagnosis and complex anatomical modelling. Better algorithm design has also made it easier to understand pictures. The traditional deep learning techniques depended heavily on a large labelled dataset. However, a recent progress in self-supervised and transfer learning has diminished this requirement. These methods make the models to adapt with the less data, making it possible to do automated diagnostics even for rare diseases when there aren't enough annotated samples. Recent advancements in generative models and transformer-based architectures have revealed new possibilities in the processing of medical images. The Generative Adversarial Networks (GANs) and other similar methods are used to improve image quality, reduce artefacts, and create fake medical data for model training. At the same time, transformer-based architectures that were first made for language models are being used for the spatial analysis that makes it easier to understand complex image patterns. These changes together help to make diagnostic tools faster, more accurate, and easier to use. As computers get better, medical imaging technology will get better too, which will lead to better care for patients and more personalized treatment plans (Zanca et al., 2022).

2 AI and ML Techniques in Medical Imaging

2.1 Deep Learning and Neural Networks

Deep learning is transforming medical imaging by making this possible to automatically and accurately analyse complex visual data. The conventional method rule-based approaches frequently needed substantial human effort and expert oversight whereas modern neural networks can independently identify patterns in vast datasets. These models have significantly streamlined the ability to locate, sort, and cut up medical photos making diagnostic tests more accurate and faster. The progress of Convolutional Neural Networks (CNNs) has become a big step forward in the field of image analysis. In comparison with traditional algorithms the fact that rely on manually created features, CNNs are capable of recognizing spatial features like edges, textures, and structures. This ability has become particularly valuable in the field of radiotherapy where small differences in MRIs, ultrasounds, and CT scans are indicative that a disease is in its early stages. CNNs make it easier for radiologists to find problems including cancers, fractures, and organ anomalies by correctly identifying them. The automated picture segmentation has become a big step forward because it lets you accurately draw the lines around anatomical features. A precise segmentation is crucial in applications such as tumour boundary detection, organ volume measurements and surgical planning (Armato et al., 2023). The models created using deep learning may distinguish the difference between healthy and tissues that are ill which means that intrusive diagnostic methods are less likely to be needed. In order to make segmentation more accurate and better find diseased sectors techniques like U-Net and Mask R-CNN have been used frequently. The networks of neurons can help with picture improvement and reconstruction within addition to recognition and segmentation. The computational models might enhance the low-quality or noisy scans by an increasing resolution and reducing artefacts without requiring additional scans. This can be especially helpful for patients who required the imaging treatments over and over again because it reduces their exposure to radiation. The transformer-based computer architectures that were first made for language processing have since been adopted for medical imaging. This makes simpler to understand complex patterns in context. The use of deep learning is poised to further enhance the diagnostic imaging. Due to continuous advancements in processing capacity and algorithmic development that makes it more accessible and reliable. The integration of neural networks into clinical practices enhances efficiency and assists medical professionals in making prompt and informed decisions (Radanliev & de Roure, 2021).

2.2 Transfer Learning for Domain Adaptation

The transfer learning technique has come to prominence as a potent methodology for enhancing the efficacy of image analysis algorithms especially in contexts characterized by a scarcity of labelled data. As opposed to training models from scrape this method uses what was learnt from pre-trained networks on large datasets and then tweaks them for specific medical uses in order to make them work better. The application of transfer learning minimizes down on the time it takes to train a model and makes it more precise especially when working with small or specialized datasets. This is done by using the feature extraction abilities of models that have already been made. The most the best things about this approach is the fact that this can change general image recognition models to work in a wide range of medical fields. A person might employ networks that were first trained on huge databases of natural images like Image Network. To find problems in diagnostic scans like radiography, magnetic resonance imaging (MRI), and other methods. This permits the lower layers of these models to keep important image processing features like edge detection. The upper layers, on the other hand, are able to respond to characteristics that are specific to the domain, which ensures very accurate classification and segmentation. An additional significant advantage has to do with it makes it easier to generalize across different types of imaging. Medical scans often look different from each other because of differences in patient demographics, procedures and technology (Samuel, 1959). Transfer learning provides a method that helps lessen the effects of these changes through enabling models adapt well instead of having to be retrained significantly. This flexibility has become especially helpful in fields like pathology and the field of eye care where there cannot be many high-quality annotated datasets. The institutions can enhance existing models with only a small amount of data. This enables them to make custom solutions for each disorder. This means that it no longer requires thousands of medical photos that have been marked up. The combination of this method with self-supervised learning and domain-specific augmentation techniques will significantly improve its effectiveness while guaranteeing strong performance across diverse clinical contexts (Haenlein & Kaplan, 2019).

2.3 Explainable AI (XAI) for Transparent Decision-Making

According to automated image analysis has become more common in session, transparency and interpretability have grown more and more important. Explainable artificial intelligence (XAI) fixes such an issue by making it readily apparent to doctors the way to make decisions. The techniques used by XAI differentiate themselves from regular deep learning models, which may serve as black boxes that fail to clarify how they come to their conclusions. This means that radiologists and doctors can have confidence and evaluate automated findings. Many of the best things about XAI has to be that it makes it easy for practitioners to see which elements of an image have affected a diagnosis. The techniques like Grad-CAM (Gradient-weighted Class Activation Mapping) and SHAP (Shapley Additive Explanations) help find things which include tumours or lesions by showing areas of interest in scans. This makes people more likely to trust automated evaluations and especially when the stakes are high and mistakes could lead to wrong diagnoses. Another very important benefit is being able to find and reduce bias. Medical imaging databases can sometimes have a lot of problems, like differences in imaging techniques, scanner errors, or changes in the population. XAI helps find possible biases by showing patterns in how people make decisions. It also helps researchers improve models so that they always give fair and consistent results (Turing, 2004). This is especially important to make sure that everyone has equal access to the right diagnosis when using automated methods on a number of different groups of people. The radiologists are able to make better clinical decisions by combining the information they know with the information an algorithm conveys them. This becomes especially important while machine-driven pattern recognition and human judgement work together to make diagnoses more accurate in complicated situations. As XAI expands new ways are being developed to make it even easier to understand without sacrificing performance. The addition of open decision-making to diagnostic systems could quicken up the use of automated imaging remedies which will make clinical settings more trustworthy and reliable.

2.4 Generative AI for Image Enhancement

The term generative artificial intelligence has influenced picture analysis in many various manners such as by making pictures of greater quality, having reduce distortion and adding more training to the datasets through augmentation methods. These mathematical frameworks eliminate the inconvenience of data constraints and make diagnoses more accurate at the same time. The organization do this by making genuine fake images and enhancing scans that have been previously done. This can be a very useful feature whenever it is hard to obtain high-resolution medical images or datasets it has been annotated. A few the best things about such technology happens to be that it can reduce noise and improve resolution. The Generative Adversarial Networks (GANs) and diffusion models constitute two techniques used to make high-quality images via scans that are blurry or have experienced being changed in some way. This can be especially useful for MRI and CT scans, in which shortening the scan time usually means worse quality of the image. It has been shown that generative models may increase accuracy in finding small problems via bringing back fine details. This contributes to early diagnosis more reliable. The addition of data has been another important use that deals with the problem of having insufficient enough datasets for training. The class disparities where some diseases are not represented sufficiently have been a common problem in medical imaging. These models create fake images that seem real to add to training data. This makes deep learning algorithms more robust. This technique can be especially useful for finding uncommon illnesses. Considering it can be hard to get a lot of information. CycleGANs are capable of turning CT scans into images that resemble like MRI scans and vice versa. This makes the ability to train models to work with many different imaging methods. This means that the patient is not required to have as many scans as well which means they ought to be exposed to less radiation. This makes it easier for different types of imaging to work together. As generative models keep getting better, it is expected that adding them to clinical processes will contribute to both diagnoses more accurate and easier for patients to receive (Turing, 1950).

3 Emerging Innovations in Medical Imaging

Novel applications of medical imaging have influenced the way individuals do diagnostic procedures and plan treatments. A highly sophisticated computer models could assist doctors to find the diseases earlier by using automate segmentation and provide real-time advice regarding the best way to do surgery. The methods for image augmentation make scans clearer to means that patients do not have to have the same treatment as often. Predictive analysis and radiation give personalized information, and combining data from different sources makes diagnoses more reliable and facilitates patients get better. The applications shown in Fig. 1 improve accuracy, efficiency, and accessibility. These improvements render medical imaging a more powerful tool for the diagnosis and a treatment planning.

- *Proactive Disease Identifica*tion: The early diagnosis of illnesses greatly improves the effectiveness of a treatment and the patients chances of recovery also improved. The advanced imaging techniques now make it is possible to automatically find the diseases like cancer, heart disease, and neurodegenerative disorders in their early stages. The high-resolution image analysis also helps to find the small cancers, subtle changes in tissue, and early-stage problems that might be missed in manual evaluations. Incorporating deep learning models into diagnostics improves accuracy, reduces false positives, and speeds up treatments.
- *Real-Time Imaging Assistance*: The incorporation of advanced imaging technology into a surgical and the diagnostic practices helps to improve the accuracy and the decision-making. The intraoperative imaging technologies can able to

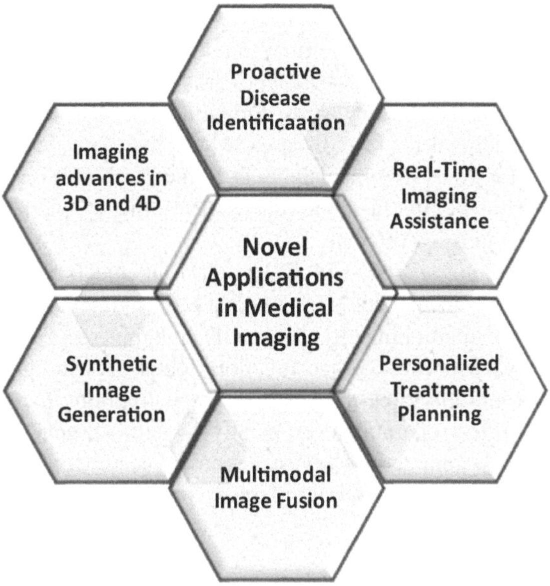

Fig. 1 Novel applications in medical imaging

offer the immediate input, aiding surgeons in a tumour excision, vascular treatments, and with minimally invasive operations. Automated anomaly detection in endoscopic and laparoscopic procedures facilitates the prompt recognition of irregularities. AI-assisted ultrasound guidance enables practitioners with minimal competence to conduct precise diagnostics, especially in emergency and remote healthcare environments.

- *Personalized Treatment Planning*: Customizing therapy according to individualized imaging data results in improved therapeutic outcomes. Imaging technologies are currently employed to forecast tumour proliferation, evaluate organ functionality, and tailor radiation therapy protocols. Through the analysis of prior scan data, prediction models enhance treatment techniques and optimize drug selection. The three-dimensional reconstruction of organs and tissues facilitates surgical planning by enabling accurate preoperative mapping and minimizing surgical risks. This method guarantees that interventions are tailored to the specific needs of each patient (Turing, 1950).
- *Multimodal Image Fusion*: Integrating imaging data from many modalities improves diagnostic precision and offers a more thorough understanding of a patient's health. Fusion techniques amalgamate data from MRI, CT, PET, and ultrasound images, facilitating enhanced visibility of soft tissues, osseous structures, and metabolic activity. This approach is especially advantageous for intricate diagnoses, such as neurological illnesses and cancer, where many imaging viewpoints enhance comprehension of disease advancement and therapeutic efficacy.

- *Synthetic Image Generation*: The creation of simulated yet realistic medical pictures have transformed model training and medical education. Methods like Generative Adversarial Networks (GANs) generate varied datasets that enhance algorithm efficacy while mitigating data scarcity. Synthetic images are especially beneficial for rare diseases, where there are few real-world instances available. Moreover, simulated datasets diminish reliance on patient data, preserving privacy while facilitating comprehensive training for medical practitioners and automated diagnostic systems.
- *Imaging advances in 3D and 4D*: Advancements in three-dimensional (3D) and four-dimensional (4D) imaging offer dynamic perspectives of organ architecture and functioning. Real-time 4D imaging records motion, rendering it essential for observing cardiac function, foetal growth, and respiratory dynamics. High-resolution three-dimensional reconstructions facilitate the planning of intricate surgical operations, especially in neurosurgery and orthopaedic interventions. These innovations boost diagnostic accuracy and improve patient outcomes by facilitating more comprehensive preoperative evaluations and minimally invasive procedures.

4 Enhancing Diagnosis Accuracy with AI

4.1 Integration of Multi-Source Data

The integration of data from different imaging modalities and diagnostic sources enhances medical analysis more accurate and complete. Thereby combining data obtained from MRI, CT, PET, ultrasound and histopathology images, doctors are able to acquire an exhaustive overview of a patient's health. Any one imaging modality provides specific insights. The MRI results indicate that the properties of soft tissues, CT shows the properties of bones, and PET scans show the manner in which the body uses energy. The combination of these different datasets also ensures a more precise diagnosis, particularly when dealing with complex conditions like neurological conditions, heart diseases, and cancer stages. A single imaging modality could not always provide a sufficient information. However, by synthesizing the various places and healthcare professionals is able to achieve a more thorough comprehension of the disease characteristics, localization, and the progression of the disease. The use of lab results, genetic information, and the electronic health records to the imaging has made it easier for healthcare providers to make decisions about the treatment of patients. The combination of radiological findings with biomarkers, pathology reports, and patient history makes it very easier to spot patterns that might not be clear from the one set of data. In the field of cancer, the combination of MRI images with genomic sequencing enables personalized treatment approaches, since several tumour subtypes exhibit unique responses to various medications. The combination of cardiac imaging with real-time electrocardiogram (ECG) data improves the assessment of cardiac output, thus making it easier to find arrhythmias and structural problems early on. The latest computational models make it easy to combine data by synchronizing, standardizing, and evaluating many inputs at once. The methods of deep learning, such as attention-based fusion networks and graph neural networks, clarify important connections between different types of data. This reduces uncertainty and makes diagnoses more reliable. Artificial intelligence programmes are capable of discovering hidden connections that human experts might miss, which makes diagnoses more accurate and cuts down on mistakes. The federated learning frameworks allow many medical institutions to work together to share and analyse data yet maintain patient privacy safe. This increases the number of diagnostic insights available. This all-encompassing approach additionally helps doctors find diseases more easily, additionally it also makes predictive modelling simpler by allowing them to more accurately predict how a disease will progress and how well a treatment will work. The ability data fusion is essential for dynamic monitoring, such as assessing tumour response to chemotherapy and evaluating recovery following a stroke. The healthcare sector is able to employ data from many sources to create a more integrated and personalized strategy that which will improve patient outcomes and make better use of resources (Garnelo & Shanahan, 2019).

4.2 Continuous Learning Models

The conventional method diagnostic systems rely on static algorithms that are incapable of adapting to new medical data, limiting their ability to respond to new diseases and changes in demographics of patients. The procedures designed for continuous improvement get around this limit by making predictions that are better with small data updates. Presently available patient data, clinical insights, and recently published research all help make diagnoses more accurate. This flexible method reduces discrimination and makes sure that tools work well for people of all ages and with different health issues. The best things about adaptive systems is the fact that their bodies can find new diseases and medical problems. During the COVID-19 pandemic an early machine learning models struggled because symptoms and imaging presentations had been different. The systems that used real-time data rapidly enhanced their ability to spot infection trends in lung CT scans. In cancer research, the diagnosis may be enhanced by integrating the most recent histopathological and radiographic data, thereby ensuring that detection techniques align with advancements in medical knowledge and treatment outcomes. A critical component of learning new systems involves performing fewer diagnostic errors. The static methodologies often encounter data drift, which is characterized by changes in patient characteristics, imaging modalities, or disease manifestations that lead to a decline in accuracy over time. The ones that constantly retrain on new data keep running at their best without needing to be completely reprogrammed (Sorantin et al., 2021). This is particularly advantageous in contexts marked by considerable diversity for example rare genetic disorders or rapidly mutating viruses, where conventional methods may struggle to manage new presentations. Feedback from doctors is very important for improving accuracy. As radiologists or pathologists fix errors in classifications. The system adds these changes to future studies. This makes the system to act as a collaborative tool that works more effectively whenever experts are involved. This feedback loop that happens over and over again and also helps to improve the accuracy of diagnoses and cultivates trust among healthcare providers by making sure that insights match clinical expertise. The medical field around the world have access to cloud-based infrastructures and federated learning to send anonymized datasets and maintain patient privacy safe. Healthcare facilities and research institutions benefit from shared knowledge, which improves the diagnosis process whilst following ethical standards for sharing data. As consequence, adaptive technology has become more robust and useful in a wider range of medical situations, which improves patient care by allowing for quick and accurate decision-making.

5 AI in Specialized Medical Imaging Fields

The use of artificial intelligence has transformed the specialised field of the medical imaging fields by making them more accurate and efficient, as shown in Fig. 2. In cancer treatments, this finds tumours early, and in neurology, this finds brain disorders. The automated heart disease analysis helps cardiology, and automated retinal disease detection enhances ophthalmology. Artificial neural network imaging also helps pulmonology and musculoskeletal diagnostics by helping doctors make accurate diagnoses and formulate treatments.

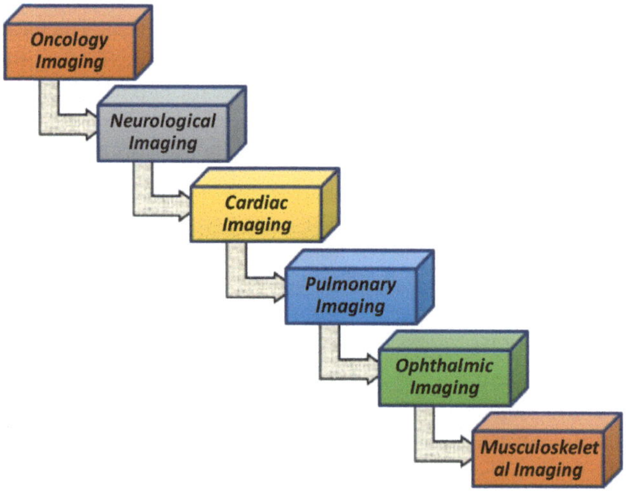

Fig. 2 AI Applications in specialized medical imaging

1. *Oncology Imaging*: The automated image analysis helps find tumours earlier in many types of cancer, such as lung, breast, and prostate cancer. Innovative algorithms can find small problems that people might not notice by looking at radiological data. Artificial intelligence radioactive substances pull out detailed information from medical images, thereby rendering it easier to classify tumours, stage them, and observe how well treatment has been working. These tools help oncologists determine the difference between benign and malignant tumours, which reduces the number of false positives and unneeded tumour biopsy. Machine learning techniques make it easier to figure out how likely it is that cancer is going to come back, thereby making it possible to make treatment plans that are specific to each patient.
2. *Neurological Imaging*: The latest image processing techniques make it easier to diagnose the neurological diseases that include the Alzheimer's, Parkinson's, and multiple sclerosis. Through looking at MRI and PET scans, the computational models are capable of discovering small changes in brain tissue that can help doctors treat patients prior to them get really sick. The AI-enhanced neuroimaging facilitates easier to diagnose a stroke by quickly finding the affected areas of the brain and measuring the extent of the damage. The automated segmentation of cerebral structures enhanced the precision of disease tracking and enabling neurologists to evaluate disease progression and treatment effectiveness.
3. *Cardiac Imaging*: In real time image analysis improves the diagnosis and treatment of heart problems. Artificial intelligence-assisted echocardiography, MRI, and CT angiography present accurate assessments of cardiac function for detecting issues such as arrhythmias, coronary artery disease, and valvar abnormalities. Artificially generated picture segmentation makes the task simpler to check blood flow to find plaque buildup, and predict the chance of heart failure. These improvements facilitate it being easier to make quick decisions in emergencies, for instance figuring out whether an individual has had a heart attack and telling them what to do, such as implanting in a stent or performing bypass surgery (Schmidhuber, 2015).
4. *Pulmonary Imaging*: The computerised techniques enable to find the lung problems like lung cancer, pneumonia, TB, and chronic obstructive pulmonary disease (COPD). The uses of the artificial neural network analysis for the chest X-rays and CT scans identifies the anomalies with a considerable precision, facilitating timely diagnosis for radiologists. In cases of lung cancer, AI (Butterworth, 2018) improves the identification and categorization of nodules, thereby rendering screening more effective and reduces the number of wrong diagnoses. Within the COVID-19 pandemic, a deep learning models had been become crucial for identifying an infection pattern in lung scans, enabling swift triage and treatment planning (Spears, 2017).
5. *Ophthalmic Imaging*: The AI-based analysis of retinal images facilitates the early detection of ocular illnesses that typically encompass diabetic retinopathy, glaucoma, and macular degeneration. The automated screening techniques are mainly used to find problems with the retina, thereby helping eye doctors' figure out what's wrong before vision loss becomes permanent. Artificial neural network

grading systems look at how bad an eye disease is to help doctors come up with the best treatment plans for each patient (Shree et al., 2025). By including portable fundus cameras, these kinds of equipment make it easier to diagnose eye problems in underserved and rural regions, thus making it easier for people to get eye care.

6. *Musculoskeletal Imaging*: The latest imaging analysis use to improve the detection and monitoring of fractures, arthritis, osteoporosis, and degenerative connective tissue diseases. The artificially intelligent models (Sreedhar et al., 2025) help radiologists check the bone density and health of joints that makes it easier to find diseases like rheumatoid arthritis early later on. In an orthopaedic surgery, a AI-driven (Chinnasamy et al., 2025) 3D reconstruction from CT and MRI scans enables the doctors to carefully plan treatments like joint replacements and the spinal surgeries. These methods speed up diagnosis and improve patient outcomes by streamlining the process of finding bone fractures in emergency situations.

6 Conclusion

The latest computational techniques used in the field of the medical imaging have been revolutionized diagnostics, enhancing accuracy, efficiency, and automation. These technologies have made it easier to find and treat the illnesses and make fewer errors, and this contributes to better health outcomes. To get widespread acceptance and confidence, the problems with data privacy for large annotated datasets, and bias in algorithms must be fixed. The balance between patient safety and innovation requires approval from regulatory bodies and ethical considerations. In addition, precision medicine gets better, computational intelligence gives doctors and patients' imaging-based diagnostic and treatment suggestions that have been specific to each patient. These tools enhance diagnoses and patient interventions through the use of the multi-modal data integration, predictive analytics, and ongoing learning. This shift from generic healthcare to patient-centred models ought to enhance the treatment efficacy and long-term outcomes. For the purpose of an AI-driven medical imaging to work effectively. The people from different fields have to work together. The r audiologists, data scientists, software developers, and healthcare policymakers must work together to come up with strong, easy-to-understand, and useful solutions. The c ross-sector partnerships may contribute new ideas by bringing together the latest research and therapeutic uses. To safely and effectively utilize these technologies in healthcare systems. There will need to be standardized model validation, ethical AI deployment, and regulatory compliance frameworks. AI, quantum computing, federated learning, and explainable models are all going to function together to make medical imaging applications more effective. By getting rid of current barriers and encouraging specialists from other fields to work together, diagnostic imaging is going to become more accurate, easier to get to, and more personalized.

References

Armato, S. G., Drukker, K., & Hadjiiski, L. (2023). AI in medical imaging grand challenges: Translation from competition to research benefit and patient care. *British Journal of Radiology, 96*, 20221152.

Avanzo, M., Porzio, M., Lorenzon, L., Milan, L., Sghedoni, R., Russo, G., Massafra, R., Fanizzi, A., Barucci, A., Ardu, V., et al. (2021). Artificial intelligence applications in medical imaging: A review of the medical physics research in Italy. *Physica Medica, 83*, 221–241.

Butterworth, M. (2018). The ICO and artificial intelligence: The role of fairness in the GDPR framework. *Computer Law and Security Review, 34*, 257–268.

Chinnasamy, P., Yarramsetti, S., Ayyasamy, R. K., Rajesh, E., Vijayasaro, V., Pandey, D., Pandey, B. K., & Lelish, M. E. (2025). AI-driven intrusion detection and prevention systems to safeguard 6G networks from cyber threats. *Scientific Reports, 15*(1), 37901.

Dembrower, K., Crippa, A., Colón, E., Eklund, M., & Strand, F. (2023). Artificial intelligence for breast cancer detection in screening mammography in Sweden: A prospective, population-based, paired-reader, non-inferiority study. *Lancet Digital Health, 5*, e703–e711.

Garnelo, M., & Shanahan, M. (2019). Reconciling deep learning with symbolic artificial intelligence: Representing objects and relations. *Current Opinion in Behavioral Sciences, 29*, 17–23.

Haenlein, M., & Kaplan, A. (2019). A brief history of artificial intelligence: On the past, present, and future of artificial intelligence. *California Management Review, 61*, 000812561986492.

Radanliev, P., & de Roure, D. (2021). Review of algorithms for artificial intelligence on low memory devices. *IEEE Access, 9*, 109986–109993.

Samuel, A. (1959). Some studies in machine learning using the game of checkers. *IBM Journal of Research and Development, 3*, 210–229.

Schmidhuber, J. (2015). Deep learning in neural networks: An overview. *Neural Networks, 61*, 85–117.

Shree, K. V. M., Pandey, B. K., & Pandey, D. (2025). Design of surface plasmon resonance (SPR) sensors for highly sensitive biomolecular detection in cancer diagnostics. *Plasmonics, 20*(2), 677–689.

Sorantin, E., Grasser, M. G., Hemmelmayr, A., Tschauner, S., Hrzic, F., Weiss, V., Lacekova, J., & Holzinger, A. (2021). The augmented radiologist: Artificial intelligence in the practice of radiology. *Pediatric Radiology, 52*, 2074–2086.

Spears, B. (2017). *Contemporary machine learning: A guide for practitioners in the physical sciences*. arXiv:1712.08523

Sreedhar, C., Kallam, S., Ghantasala, G. S. P., Anthoniraj, S., Kumarganesh, S., Sagayam, K. M., Pandey, B. K., & Pandey, D. (2025). Enhancing healthcare data security using RFE and CRHSM for big data. *Computers in Biology and Medicine, 190*, 110063.

Turing, A. (2004). *Lecture on the automatic computing engine (1947)*. Oxford University Press.

Turing, A. M. (1950) I.—Computing machinery and intelligence. *Mind, LIX*, 433–460. Accessed on 20 July 2022.

Zanca, F., Brusasco, C., Pesapane, F., Kwade, Z., Beckers, R., & Avanzo, M. (2022). Regulatory aspects of the use of artificial intelligence medical software. *Seminars in Radiation Oncology, 32*, 432–441.

Fuzzy Logic and ML in Clinical Decision Support Systems

Awanit Kumar, Nirmal Singh, and Ajay Kumar Suwalka

Abstract The integration of sophisticated computational techniques in clinical decision support systems has drastically altered modern healthcare by enhancing the accuracy of diagnostics in treatment methodologies, and management of patients. The manner in which reasoning-based and data-driven models could assist doctors make better decisions. The systems that employ human-like reasoning can deal with uncertainty well in healthcare contexts which makes it easier to understand unclear data. By employing massive datasets for building predictive models makes it feasible to speed up medical services. The suggest personalized treatments and accurately diagnose diseases. The innovations in the Internet of Things (IoT) and the big data have greatly improved the decision support systems. By allowing the real-time patient monitoring in an early disease prediction and extensive healthcare analytics, these technologies give healthcare professionals data-driven insights that make clinical workflows and patient care better. The safety of data along with ethical issues and the system interoperability are still problems that make it hard to utilize it widely. The future of clinical decision-making hinges on the amalgamation of reasoning-based methodologies alongside adaptive learning techniques, to enhance system reliability, an interpretability, and practical application. The ongoing studies in explainable artificial intelligence, federated learning, and secure data-sharing protocols will contribute to further progress in this field. As these technologies get more advanced as they will grow increasingly important for making healthcare more efficient, accurate, and focused on the patient, which will lead to better health outcomes.

Keywords Clinical decision support · ML · Fuzzy logic · Healthcare analytics · Predictive modeling · Medical diagnosis · AI

A. Kumar (✉)
Career Point University, Kota, India
e-mail: itsawanitkumar@gmail.com

N. Singh · A. K. Suwalka
Sangam University, Bhilwara, India
e-mail: nirmal.singh@sangamuniversity.ac.in

A. K. Suwalka
e-mail: ajay.suwalka@sangamuniversity.ac.in

D. Pandey et al. (eds.), *Smart Healthcare*, https://doi.org/10.1007/978-981-95-8828-2_8

1 Introduction

The clinical decisions have become a complicated process that involves a lot of uncertainty, a lot of different patient situations, and the need for solutions that are simultaneously precise and flexible. Given that it is useful for the traditional rule-based systems often have trouble with the ambiguity that is inherent in medical data. In this instance, using advanced computer methods has become very important for making intelligence-driven assistance serve better. This is a method that works well to stay dealing with information that is not readily apparent or exact. This method enables computers respond similar to people and come up with findings that are simultaneously reasonable and reliable. This technology additionally makes it possible for healthcare apps to understand symptoms that cannot be categorized into strict binary categories. This ultimately contributes to better diagnosis accuracy and therapy suggestions. A different technique brings the power of data-driven insights to the decision-making process in medicine. Through looking at huge amounts of past patient records, smart models could identify patterns, predict how a disease will progress, and suggest the best medications that have been specific to each person's needs. In contrast to traditional systems, this one remains open to learning and getting better from new information. This makes this very adaptable to changes in medical knowledge and patient demographics. Predictive analytics makes simpler to find diseases early, figure out the danger their bodies and plan care that is right for each person. The combination of these two methods creates a support system that is stronger in more flexible, and more efficient for doctors. This ultimately results to better patient outcomes and more efficient healthcare.

1.1 Clinical Decision Support Systems (CDSS)

Clinical Decision Support Systems (CDSS) have been advanced tools designed to assist healthcare professionals in analyzing medical data and providing evidence-based recommendations. Through connecting to electronic health records (EHR) and other databases. These networks are making it easier to make accurate diagnoses to plan treatments, and to assess the risks. It cut down on mistakes that stream-line workflows, and make patients safer by giving the real-time information. The h healthcare generates vast and complex datasets that making the demand for advanced decision support systems increasingly critical. There has been a lot of progress in the development of Clinical Decision Support Systems (CDSS). The earlier versions used rules that were already in place and advice from experts to send out alerts and make suggestions. They were good at making decisions that were well thought established but they had not been very good at dealing with situations that were complicated and where things were unclear. These systems have changed a lot since they added AI. They can now handle large amounts of data, spot trends and improve forecasts by learning all the time (Haleem et al., 2022). The shift from static rule-based methods to dynamic, data-driven models is rendering them much more effective in personalized medicine. The possibilities cover a wide range of medical fields. These systems help medical professionals find possible combinations, allergies, and contraindications in pharmacological management. This helps them avoid bad reactions. The organization help keep an eye on vital signs, guess what might go incorrectly and suggest quick actions in critical care settings. Application of predictive analytics makes it easier to find diseases at an early stage, which makes it easier to use proactive treatment methods. By using these characteristics, medical professionals might provide better care and achieve better results for their patients. There are issues with the accuracy of the data and the compatibility of the system with the present physical setup as well as ethical issues related to privacy and liability that need to be fixed. Subsequently is important for doctors to use their own judgment instead of relying too much on automated suggestions. These technologies tend to be set to play a bigger and bigger role in modern healthcare as they ought to keep getting better. New developments in artificial intelligence, big data analytics and cloud computing are going to make them more accurate and easier to find. As more people use them, their respective position's role in improving efficiency, lowering costs, and encouraging evidence-based medicine will continue to shape the future of patient care (DeTore, 1988).

1.2 Artificial Intelligence in Modern Healthcare

Artificial intelligence has influenced modern healthcare by making it easier to diagnose, treat, and manage patients. AI-powered systems that can analyze large amounts of medical data give healthcare professionals accurate, real-time information that helps them make better decisions. These technological advances make operations run more smoothly, reduce human mistakes and to help find diseases earlier, all of which led to better patient outcomes. The artificial intelligences most impressive work has been in medical imaging and diagnostics. The machine learning algorithms carefully look at X-rays, MRIs, and CT scans that helping the radiologists to find problems that people might not find. The artificial intelligence algorithms also have applications in pathology to look at tissue specimens that makes it easier to quickly and accurately find the cancerous cells. In personalized medicine, artificially intelligent technology helps create personalized treatment plans based on a patient's genetic makeup, medical history, and current health status. The use of predictive analytics helps doctors predict how an illness will progress and suggest the best treatments. This leads to higher recovery rates and fewer hospital readmissions. Artificially intelligent drug discovery speeds up the development of new drugs by finding potential molecules and predicting how well they will work. This cuts down on research time by a lot (Paik & Kim, 2019). AI makes healthcare management better by streamlining workflows, getting rid of unnecessary jobs, and making better use of resources. Artificially intelligence health assistants and chatbots facilitate it being easier for patients to get in touch with healthcare workers, help them figure out their symptoms, and remind them to take their medications that makes the work of healthcare workers easier (Yu et al., 2021). The artificial intelligence (AI) and robotics work together to make the surgery, rehabilitation, and elder care be better by making sure they are accurate and dependable. The use of technology can change things in a big way, by adding AI to healthcare is not without its problems. To ensure safe and reliable implementation the problems like data privacy, ethics, and the need to follow the law must be addressed. Also, this is important to find a way to combine AI-driven automation with human expertise in order to keep trust and responsibility in patient care. As technology gets better, artificial intelligence (AI) is going to have a bigger role in healthcare, leading to improvements in telemedicine, illness prevention, and remote monitoring. Given the ongoing changes, it will change the way medicine is carried out, making healthcare more efficient, accessible, and personalized (Mosavi & Santos, 2020).

2 Clinical Decision Support Systems

2.1 Fundamental Elements of CDSS

A system based on technology that assists healthcare workers make smart choices by looking at medical data and providing them with suggestions based on evidence. Through combining useful information from many sources. It makes diagnoses more accurate, treatment plans better, patients as well safer. This improves healthcare operations and reduces human errors by sending real-time alerts, protocols, and predictive analytics. These technologies are designed to work as smart assistants to make sure that medical professionals get important information quickly that help to improves patient outcomes. The entire system has to exist to improve medical decision-making, make things run more smoothly and keep patients safer. Figure 1 shows the main parts of CDSS. As these systems get better and they keep healthcare innovation going to make the medical practice more data-driven, efficient, and patient-centered.

1. *Inference Engine*: The central processing unit looks at patient data using rules to the algorithms, and a decision trees. This then makes suggestions based on the medical knowledge. This looks at different factors, weighs the possible outcomes, and suggests the best solutions. This component makes sure that complicated medical situations are looked at in a methodical way, which helps doctors make smart choices regardless of whether things are not clear. The inference engine gets better over time by taking in new examples and results, which makes it more accurate.
2. *Data Administration*: A systematic module that collects, stores, and organises patient records from electronic health systems. This combines data from numerous sources such as laboratory findings, imaging reports, and old medical records, in order to give a complete picture of a patient's health. The best rules for managing data keep patients' information private while making it easy to find

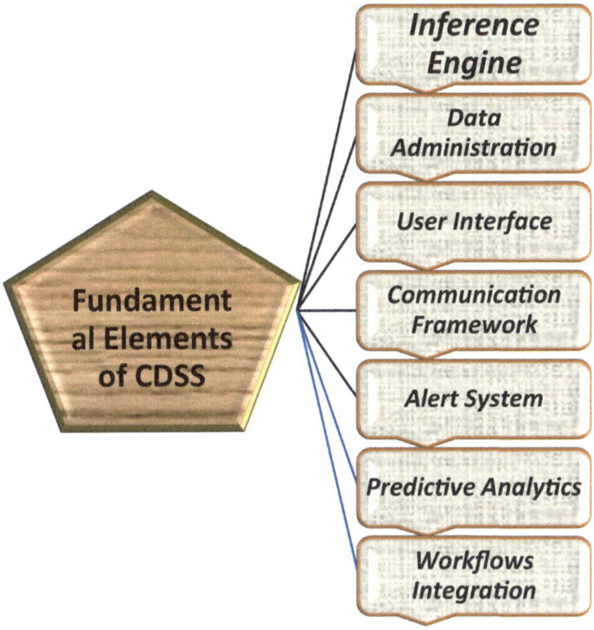

Fig. 1 Fundamental components of CDSS

important information quickly. Data management that is thorough makes sure that decisions are consistent and trustworthy (Kalra & Ingram, 2006).

3. *User Interface*: This part helps healthcare providers understand the system. The designed for ease of usage sends organized recommendations alerts, and patient data to users. The medical staff has been able to learn how to use the system more quickly because of the user-friendly interface. This means they have access to the information they need quickly and without wasting time. The system is easier to use and improves clinical workflows overall owing to a well-designed interface, customizable settings, and smooth navigation.
4. *Communication Framework*: It connects to hospital networks, the medical devices, and outside healthcare databases to make sure that data transfer continues to be possible. This connection enables the healthcare workers see real-time patient information, speak to specialists, and make decisions based on data. Effective communication between different medical departments makes things run more smoothly and cuts down on delays in patient care. Being compatible with different healthcare systems makes it easier to share information completely, which helps with treatment planning.
5. *Alert System*: The system sends out instant alerts and notification messages about potential dangers such as drug interactions, allergic reactions. Despite not following the prescribed treatment strategies. These alerts stop mistakes from happening in the healthcare facility and also make sure safety rules are observed and make it easier for quick actions to be performed. The automatic notifications

for the subsequent appointments lab tests, and prescription refills help patients stick to their treatment plans and lower the chance of bad outcomes. A properly calibrated alert system balances sensitivity and specificity to cut down on false alarms while making sure that important warnings are not missed (Delen, 2020).

6. *Predictive Analytics:* The most advanced algorithms look at the past patient data to find patterns, guess how the disease will get worse, and suggest personalized treatment plans. The rest of the system uses big datasets to help find diseases before symptoms show up. This helps figure out how dangerous they have become and lets people take action before they get worse. Doctors can quickly change treatment plans for people with chronic diseases thanks to predictive analytics. This makes it much easier to manage these diseases. This feature gets better over time because it learns more, which helps you make decisions.
7. *Workflows Integration*: The solution works well with the healthcare facility current systems to make clinical decision making better without getting in the way of normal operations. It is easy to get set up because it works with hospital management software, diagnostic equipment, and patient monitoring systems. Following established medical protocols makes things run more smoothly, lightens the load for administrators, and lets doctors focus on taking care of patients. If this part is done correctly, decision support will become a normal part of everyday practice instead of an extra job.

2.2 Rule-Based to AI-Driven Systems

The decision support technology in healthcare has undergone a significant transformation that evolve from traditional rule-based systems to advanced AI-based models. This advancement has contributed to the accuracy, adaptability and effectiveness of clinical decision-making by enabling systems to process vast amounts of complex medical data and evolve continuously. The initial decision support technologies were based on rules and reasoning that experts had already set up. These systems worked by using if–then statements to encode medical guidelines and protocols that would then make suggestions. A rule-based system might inform a clinician in the event a suggested medication had a negative effect on patients with known allergies. These models had been clear and useful for problems that were well defined and involved structured data. It needed to be updated by hand as medical knowledge grew, which made maintenance hard and costly. They had trouble dealing with medical information that was confusing, incomplete or contradictory. Their rigid personalities made it hard for them to adapt to new situations that made it harder for them to work in complex and changing healthcare settings. To solve these problems the modern systems started using machine learning techniques. These advanced models' analysis of the comprehensive patient records, research data, and clinical case studies to discern patterns, predict the development of the disease and customize treatment recommendations. In contrast to traditional rule-based systems. They constantly improve their accuracy by learning from real-world examples. A deep learning and natural language processing have substantially improved decision support systems by enabling the automated analysis of unstructured medical information such as physician notes, medical literature, and imaging reports. The use of predictive analytics has improved the early detection of diseases and the assessment of risk by making it easier to take proactive medical action. The switch to AI-driven methods has made adaptability, decision making preciseness and operational efficiency much better. These systems are changing as technology improves. They now include real-time patient monitoring, cloud computing, and personalized treatment methods to improve health outcomes (Mao et al., 2021).

2.3 Integration with Electronic Health Records (EHR)

The combination of decision support systems with electronic health records has made clinical decision making faster and more accurate. By making use of patient data and real-time analytical tools to give accurate data-driven treatment can help healthcare professionals make fewer mistakes and get more done. The transition from regulated frameworks to artificial intelligent-based models makes it easier to adapt and make predictions. The initial decision support technologies used conditional statements to write down medical rules and guidelines and make suggestions. These technologies might let a doctor know if a medicine made someone allergic. These models were easy to understand and simple to comprehend but it took a lot of time and money to keep them up to date by hand. In complicated healthcare settings. They had to deal with medical data that was hard to understand, missing, or contradictory. The process of machine learning is used by modern systems to get past static rules and solve these problems. These models look at huge amounts of patient records, research data, and clinical case studies to find trends to predict how an illness will progress, and make personalized treatment suggestions. A deep learning and natural language processing make it easier to look at unstructured medical data like doctor's notes, medical literature, and imaging reports. This helps with decision-making. The use of predictive analytics makes it possible to take the proactive steps to find diseases early and assess risks. The decision support systems and digital patient records interact seamlessly to provide complete medical histories. The connection cuts down on wrong diagnoses and unnecessary tests and makes it possible to make decisions right away. Adding analytical models to digital health systems sends clinicians quick alerts and risk assessments like when drugs interact or health gets worse, so they can start treatments right away. The automation of medication reconciliation and clinical reporting helps healthcare providers spend more time caring for patients. The safety of digital recordkeeping makes healthcare data more reliable and private for patients. By employing past data and the application of predictive analytics treatment methods can be changed to get better results and get patients more involved. As AI-driven decision support gets more sophisticated, cloud computing, interoperability standards, and real-time monitoring enable precision medicine and healthcare work better.

3 Fuzzy Logic in Clinical Decision Support

3.1 Fuzzy Logic Concept and Principles

These decisions in many everyday circumstances especially in health care involves uncertainty, fuzzy lines, and situations that overlap. Simple binary mathematical reasoning that only uses true or false values that are is unable to handle this kind of complexity. A new way to process partial truths makes it possible to reason more flexibly and like a person in situations where things cannot be clear. This method assumes that variables might possess a truth value between 0 and 1, not in fixed categories. This helps medical systems get a better idea of how symptoms and diseases really work. This is possible to assess states that are in between typical and high, for instance "borderline high" or "moderately elevated." This helps doctors make better clinical decisions. This strategy is based on membership functions, which sort data points into groups. These functions make it easy to switch between categories without making big changes to the input. This can stop doctors from changing treatment plans because of small test results. A further fundamental principle is to use words instead of numbers. Mathematical processing of "mild pain," "moderate fever," and severe fatigue might be helpful in medical guidance. The method becomes easier to understand and fits into the way doctors naturally assess patients. The reasoning process employs if–then rules to figure out what the right answer signifies. The medical guidelines are capable of being customized for individual individuals as these criteria permit varying levels of confidence, in contrast to rigid logical frameworks. Final results must be clear for clinical use. Defuzzification changes membership degrees into useful information, such as changes in dose and health risks. This step makes sure that abstract math operations give useful health care advice. These principles help medical systems deal with complicated that uncertain and constantly changing situations, which makes healthcare decisions more accurate and reliable (Verma et al., 2021).

3.2 Management of Medical Diagnosis Uncertainty

Medical diagnosis can be difficult because indicators, patient physiology, and data restrictions can all be different. It can be hard to classify diseases because numerous them have similar signs and symptoms. This vagueness causes it to be hard to use traditional computational methods, which need exact inputs that might not be available in healthcare settings. Highly sophisticated reasoning methods allow it make more flexible decisions by putting medical illnesses into groups. This makes sure that diagnoses take into account the complicated and unclear symptoms of patients. A method that determines if a patient has an underlying disease based on a number of things instead of just saying they possess it. The functions of membership assign different levels of confidence to symptoms. A high temperature of 100.4°F, along with other symptoms like tiredness and body aches, could indicate the presence of an infection. This strategy prevents misdiagnosis by considering multiple alternatives rather than imposing a binary choice. It is important to process data which is not clear or complete. Patients' descriptions of their pain are often subjective, like "mild" or "intense." Even though it's hard to put a number on these words, they can be used in diagnostic models by linking them to severity. This means that medical decision support systems can work even if the numbers aren't right. This type of reasoning additionally assists in helping healthcare systems look at many symptoms and risk factors at once. The average person can look at previous patient records, lab results, and environmental factors to get a better picture of the situation. This reduces false positives and negatives, which makes the diagnosis accurate and specific to the case. The latest medical decision-making technologies help the healthcare providers make more successful data-driven choices, which leads to better patient outcomes by handling uncertainty (Yu et al., 2019).

4 Machine Learning in Clinical Decision Support

4.1 ML Techniques Used in CDSS

- *Supervised Learning*: This method involves training models in an annotated medical dataset that possesses known for the inputs and outputs that match. The system may anticipate diagnoses for the suggest treatments and identify diseases early by looking at past medical records. For instance, image-based models trained on annotated scans can accurately identify malignancies while classification algorithms help predict disease risks based on a patient's medical history.
- *Unsupervised Learning*: This strategy reveals hidden patterns in medical data without needing pre-existing categorizations unlike supervised methods. It is widely used to group patients with symptoms that are alike, find unusual patterns in medical pictures and find new subgroups of diseases that were not known before. By grouping cases based on shared characteristics, healthcare providers can create personalized treatment plans and improve patient segmentation for targeted interventions (Chakraborty et al., 2022).
- *Reinforcement Learning*: This method allows models learn the best ways to make decisions by interacting with their surroundings and getting feedback. In healthcare it is used to improve robotic-assisted surgical procedures, change the dosages of drugs and make treatment protocols better. Constant improvement based on past actions and patient feedback helps to make personalized healthcare recommendations better and improve clinical workflows.
- *Deep Learning*: Advanced neural networks analyze complex medical data such as genomic sequences, the radiological snapshots and an electronic health record. These models are great in extracting features because they can find patterns that

regular algorithms might miss. For finding anomalies in medical images, convolutional neural networks (CNNs) are widely used. For predictive modeling, recurrent neural networks (RNNs) look at sequential patient data.
- *Natural Language Processing* (NLP): This method allows systems look at and get useful information from unstructured medical texts like doctor observations, clinical reports, and the research papers. It makes it easier to keep records automatically to assess symptoms, and to summarize medical information in real time. It also improves decision-making by turning text data into useful information.
- *Collective Learning*: By combining many models, the predictions become more accurate and cuts down on mistakes. The system can give more reliable medical advice by combining results from the different methods, such as decision trees, neural networks, and logistic regression. This methodology is particularly beneficial for identifying the complex disorders when a single model may be insufficient (Doğan et al., 2019).

By combining these sophisticated techniques, the decision support systems might enhance accuracy of diagnostics used in the treatment strategies, and patient outcomes, thereby contributing to more efficient and data-driven healthcare solutions. Figure 2 shows the methods that uses the ML in the CDSS. These methods enhance clinical decision making by analyzing complex medical data and enhancing diagnostic accuracy. The supervised training uses a labeled patient records to train models that can be able to predict diseases. The technique of unsupervised learning helps find patterns and clusters in patients which can help create personalized treatment plans. The reinforcement learning method learns from how patients respond to treatment all the time to make it better. The use of deep learning is very good at medical imaging, because it can find problems in images with great accuracy. The use of a natural languages makes documentation and decision support better by figuring out what unstructured clinical notes represent. The ensemble learning method combines several models to make them more reliable, make fewer mistakes, and give better medical advice.

5 Fuzzy Logic and Machine Learning

The use of fuzzy reasoning and machine learning play a big role in clinical decision support systems through dealing with uncertainty, improving diagnostics, and adding to treatment suggestions. However, they differ in their way of work to know how flexible these individuals and how they are complicated. The use of fuzzy logic has its foundation on how people think, which allows for smooth changes between many states instead of strict categories. It is very helpful when medical data is unclear or missing. The use of linguistic variables and membership functions makes it possible to work with imprecise inputs which is especially useful for rating symptoms and figuring out how bad a disease is in reality. Its rule-based framework is easy to understand, which makes it useful in situations where it is essential to be able to see how

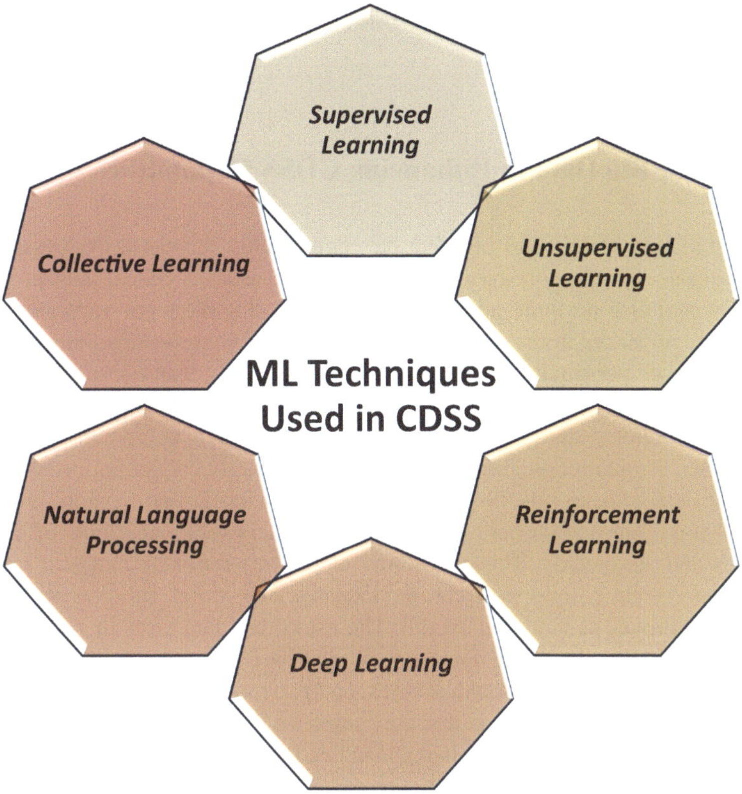

Fig. 2 Methods used by ML in CDSS

decisions are made. However, creating and changing rules requires specific expertise, which limits its ability to learn from new data in an adaptive way (Nguyen et al., 2019). On the reverse side, a machine learning finds patterns in the large datasets, which makes it easier to create predictive models and keep improving. The algorithms used for supervised learning use past records to group diseases (Du et al., 2018), while unsupervised methods find hidden patterns and groups in patient data. The use of deep learning makes image-based diagnostics better by finding problems with great accuracy (Tai et al., 2019). The use of machine learning is more scalable for large applications than fuzzy logic because it doesn't rely on preset rules. On the contrary, it adapts to real-world data. However, its decision-making process may be complicated and hard to understand, and it often requires a lot of computing power. A hybrid methodology that combines both techniques can use to take advantage of their strengths (Basha et al., 2025). The use of fuzzy logic offers an interpretability and expert-driven reasoning, whereas machine learning provides flexibility and automation. The combination of these strategies makes clinical decision support systems more accurate, more reliable, and more trusted by healthcare providers, which leads to better care for patients.

6 IoT and Big Data in Enhancing CDSS Capabilities

The combination of IoT and big data has significantly increased the possibilities of clinical decision support systems by making it easier to collect data in instantaneously, and also do more advanced analytics, and make more accurate predictions. These advances in the technology make it possible to make a more accurate, faster, and more personalized clinical choices, ultimately leading to better patient outcomes and better management of healthcare (Sreedhar et al., 2025). The wireless health monitors, smart sensors, and a connected medical equipment are actually all examples of Internet of Things devices that constantly collect important patient data comprised of heart rate, blood pressure, glucose levels, and oxygen saturation. This real-time information permits healthcare workers spot early signs of medical problems and act quickly. The monitoring of patients remotely makes it possible to keep an eye on people with chronic diseases over time. This lowers hospital stays and improves patient care overall. The use of big data takes in a lot of structured and unstructured medical data from many different sources, like genomic data, medical imaging, electronic health records, and patient-reported outcomes. The use of big data helps find patterns in diseases, improve the accuracy of diagnoses, and find the best treatment options by using machine learning algorithms and predictive modeling (Pandey & Pandey, 2025). Through looking at patterns in large groups of patients, it helps with population health management by improving early detection and prevention strategies. The Internet of Things and big data work together to make clinical decision support systems better by giving patients personalized therapies, automating data-driven insights, and making recommendations more accurate (Praveenkumar et al., 2025). However, problems with data security, interoperability, and working with current systems must be fixed before they can reach their full potential. As these technologies get better, they are going to become more and more important. They are expected to make healthcare a more proactive, effective, and patient-centered system.

7 Conclusion

The analysis points out the significance of a computational methods in the clinical decision-making. An artificially intelligent reasoning systems effectively used to the handle ambiguous health information to enhancing the interpretation of an uncertainty. Machine learning techniques that learn from big datasets make it easier to diagnose, treat, and manage patients. These approaches have made healthcare more efficient, improved the accuracy of diagnoses, and better patient care. The IoT and big data make it possible to monitor the things in a real time and use analytics to predict the future events, which makes it easier to make decisions. The latest decision support systems could assist healthcare providers in making better diagnoses, handling more work, and improving patient outcomes. These tools give you data-driven insights, advanced case evaluations, and ways to make your clinical workflow more efficient. It may be hard to keep things clear understandable and easy to use in the medical settings. The researchers need to improve these systems by using a hybrid model that can be used to combine expert knowledge with adaptive learning. For widespread use, data security, ethics, and interoperability must also be taken care of. The models based on reasoning and data will help people make better decisions about their health care. Together, these methods will make the system more reliable, adaptable to real-world situations, and trustworthy for medical professionals. Investigations into explainable AI, federated learning, and better security is going to contribute to new ideas. These technologies are going to become more and more important for making healthcare more accurate, efficient, and focused on the patient.

References

Basha, A., Jameer, R., Maheshwari, U., Pandey, B. K., & Pandey, D. (2025). Ultra-sensitive photonic crystal fiber–based SPR sensor for cancer detection utilizing hybrid nanocomposite layers. *Plasmonics, 20*(7), 4943–4957.

Chakraborty, S., Mallick, B., & Chakraborty, S. (2022). Mining of association rules for treatment of dental diseases. *Journal of Decision Analytics and Intelligent Computing, 2*, 1–11.

Delen, D. (2020). *Prescriptive analytics the final frontier for evidence-based management and optimal decision*. Pearson Education Inc.

DeTore, A. W. (1988). Medical informatics: An introduction to computer technology in medicine. *American Journal of Medicine, 85*, 399–403.

Doğan, R. I., Kim, S., Chatr-Aryamontri, A., Wei, C.-H., Comeau, D. C., Antunes, R., Matos, S., Chen, Q., Elangovan, A., Panyam, N. C., et al. (2019). Overview of the bioCreative VI precision medicine track: Mining protein interactions and mutations for precision medicine. *Database*, bay147.

Du, Y., Pan, Y., Wang, C., & Ji, J. (2018). Biomedical semantic indexing by deep neural network with multi-task learning. *BMC Bioinform., 19*, 502.

Haleem, A., Javaid, M., Singh, R. P., & Suman, R. (2022). Medical 4.0 technologies for healthcare: Features, capabilities, and applications. *Internet of Things and Cyber-Physical System, 2*, 12–30.

Kalra, D., & Ingram, D. (2006). Electronic health records. In K. Zieliński, M. Duplaga, & D. Ingram (Eds.), *Information technology solutions for healthcare. Health informatics*. Springer.

Mao, R. Q., Lan, L., Kay, J., Lohre, R., Ayeni, O. R., Goel, D. P., & de Sa, D. (2021). Immersive virtual reality for surgical training: A systematic review. *Journal of Surgical Research, 268*, 40–58.

Mosavi, N. S., & Santos, M. F. (2020). How Prescriptive analytics influences decision making in precision medicine. *Procedia Computer Science, 177*, 528–533.

Nguyen, D., Long, T., Jia, X., Lu, W., Gu, X., Iqbal, Z., & Jiang, S. (2019). A feasibility study for predicting optimal radiation therapy dose distributions of prostate cancer patients from patient anatomy using deep learning. *Science and Reports, 9*, 1076.

Paik, S.-H., & Kim, D.-J. (2019). Smart healthcare Systems and Precision Medicine. *Advances in Experimental Medicine and Biology, 1192*, 263–279.

Pandey, B. K., & Pandey, D. (2025). Securing healthcare medical image information using advance morphological component analysis, information hiding systems, and hybrid convolutional neural networks on IoMT. *Computers in Biology and Medicine, 185*, 109499.

Praveenkumar, T., Anthoniraj, S., Kumarganesh, M., Somaskandan, K., Sagayam, M., Pandey, B. K., Pandey, D., & Sahani, S. K. (2025). Enhanced circuit board analysis: Infrared image segmentation utilizing Markov random field (MRF) and level set techniques. *Engineering Reports, 7*(3), e70029.

Sreedhar, C., Kallam, S., Ghantasala, G. S. P., Anthoniraj, S., Kumarganesh, S., Sagayam, K. M., Pandey, B. K., & Pandey, D. (2025). Enhancing healthcare data security using RFE and CRHSM for big data. *Computers in Biology and Medicine, 190*, 110063.

Tai, A. M., Albuquerque, A., Carmona, N. E., Subramanieapillai, M., Cha, D. S., Sheko, M., Lee, Y., Mansur, R., & McIntyre, R. S. (2019). Machine learning and big data: Implications for disease modeling and therapeutic discovery in psychiatry. *Artificial Intelligence in Medicine, 99*, Article 101704.

Verma, D., Bach, K., & Mork, P. J. (2021). Application of machine learning methods on patient reported outcome measurements for predicting outcomes: A literature review. *Informatics, 8*, 56.

Yu, G., Chen, Z., Wu, J., & Tan, Y. (2021). Medical decision support system for cancer treatment in precision medicine in developing countries. *Expert Systems with Applications, 186*, Article 115725.

Yu, Y., Li, M., Liu, L., Li, Y., & Wang, J. (2019). Clinical big data and deep learning: Applications, challenges, and future outlooks. *Big Data Mining and Analytics, 2*, 288–305.

Explainable AI in Healthcare in Enhancing Trust in ML Models

Niladri Maiti, Babacar Toure, Neha Bharani, Nithin Kumar, Jyoti Jayesh Chavhan, Aradhana Sahu, and Hassan Khalid Abozibid

Abstract Artificial intelligence has transformed the way to the medical professionals make assessments to plan treatments and also keep an eye on patients. The lack of transparency in complex machine learning models creates significant obstacles, undermining trust and hindering implementation in clinical settings. An explicable artificial intelligence (XAI) seeks to rectify this discrepancy by making model's conclusions understandable, thereby empowering medical professionals to understand and verify, and confidently employ AI-generated information. The importance of explainability in AI-driven healthcare and the differences between accuracy and various strategies for enhancing the interpretability. It also looks at real-world uses the rules, and the importance of the human oversight in making sure that decisions are made to reliably. The standardizing explainability frameworks, encouraging collaboration between different fields, and teaching healthcare workers about AI interpretability are all important for building trust and improving patient outcomes. Finding solutions to these challenges facilitates the seamless integration of AI-driven medical advancements into clinical workflows, enhancing both efficiency and safety in modern healthcare.

N. Maiti (✉) · B. Toure
Faculty of Dental Medicine, College of Health Sciences, International University of Rabat, Rabat, Morocco
e-mail: cthakar12@gmail.com

N. Bharani
School of Computers, IPS Academy, Indore, India
e-mail: neha4bharani@gmail.com

N. Kumar
School of Dentistry, Central Asian University, Tashkent, Uzbekistan

J. J. Chavhan
CSE-DS, MGM College of Engineering Kamothe, Mumbai, India

A. Sahu
Department of Computer Science and Engineering, Rungta College of Engineering and Technology, Bhilai, India

H. K. Abozibid
Al-Zahrawi University College, Karbala, Iraq

D. Pandey et al. (eds.), *Smart Healthcare*, https://doi.org/10.1007/978-981-95-8828-2_9

Keywords Explainable AI · Healthcare · Machine learning · Clinical decision support · Model validation

1 Introduction

The artificial intelligence has significantly impacted the medical field by making, it possible to make the decisions based on data, improving medical diagnoses and making treatment plans better. The artificial intelligence is currently employed in a lot of different applications such as finding diseases, personalized medicine, robotic surgeries, and predictive analytics. These improvements help cut down on mistakes made by individuals to make better use of resources, and improve the patient outcomes. Perhaps the most important uses are in medical imaging and diagnosis. Machine learning algorithms have the ability to look at X-rays, MRIs, and CT scans with amazing accuracy, which helps radiologists find things like cancer, broken bones, and neurological disorders. A computerized diagnostic tool has also been helpful in finding diseases in their early stages, which allows for quicker treatment and better outcomes. The use of predictive analytics is important for more than just diagnostics. It is also important for predicting how a disease will progress, anticipating complications, and suggesting personalized plans for treatment. Machine learning models help doctors make better decisions by looking at a lot of patient data. This improves care and lowers costs in the long run. The development and discovery of drugs is another very important area. Conventional approaches take a lot of time and money, but computational models are capable of looking at complicated biological data to find possible drug candidates to improve the design of clinical trials. This speeds up the process of coming up with new treatments while lowering the costs and the risks. As technology keeps getting better, it will be used more and more in the healthcare. To make sure that medical decisions are made responsibly and need to deal with problems like data privacy, ethical issues, and model transparency. Explainable systems are becoming an important way to solve these problems, building trust and dependability in automated healthcare solutions.

1.1 Transparency in AI-Driven Medical Decisions

In healthcare sector, trust, safety, and accountability have been very important. Additionally, the openness has become a vital requirement. Whenever AI makes medical decisions, the doctors, patients, and regulatory bodies might not believe the models because they have no understanding how they make predictions. To make certain that automated recommendations are in line with clinical knowledge and best practices, medical professionals need to know the reason these recommendations were generated. In the event these systems are unclear, there will be a chance of wrong diagnoses, bad treatments, and less trust in them. A further significant argument for explainability is due to the fact patients need to trust the information provided. The public have been more likely to accept and follow AI-assisted recommendations if they know how the decisions were made. The healthcare professionals and patients must be able to understand the reason of the AI-driven suggestions that are made in the important situations like diagnosing cancer or planning treatment. Individuals may be hesitant to use these technologies if they have no idea how they work, which can slow down their use. Regulatory compliance is also a big reason why transparency is needed. The FDA and the European Medicines Agency are two examples of healthcare authorities that require AI-powered tools to follow strict safety and ethical rules (Bonkra & Dhiman, 2021). Transparent models help with verifying decision-making processes to make sure they follow the law and are free of biases that could lead to unfair or dangerous results. Scientists as well as developers are able to identify the mistakes, improve algorithms, and make things work better, when they ought to explain their decisions. This process of making things better over time and makes sure that AI-powered tools get better results, while still being very accurate and dependable. Artificial intelligence with an explanation builds trust by promoting the openness. It also improves patient care and makes sure that medical professionals can confidently use smart systems in their work. Without it, these new ideas can't reach their full potential, and people may worry about how reliable and fair they are (Barredo Arrieta et al., 2020).

2 The Necessity of Explainability in Healthcare AI

2.1 The Black-Box Problem in AI Models

The black-box problem has become a major concern in medical AI, since it means that people do not understand how it works. The numerous machine learning techniques especially deep learning systems, examine large datasets and make predictions, but they don't explain why they came to those conclusions. The lack of interpretability makes it hard for healthcare professionals to trust or confirm results that especially when it comes to diagnoses and treatments that could save a life. The practitioners in healthcare may struggle to pinpoint inaccuracies or biases. If they do not comprehend how a model generates its outcomes. As an example, in the event an AI system wrongly diagnoses a problem or suggests the wrong treatment, it is hard to fix the mistakes since humans can't see how it came to that conclusion. This lack of clarity could make patients feel less secure, which could make them less likely to follow medical advice from a system that is not clear. The black-box problem also raises moral and legal concerns. The laws governing healthcare require accountability in making choices, but AI models that are not explainable make it harder to follow these rules. It becomes difficult to figure out who is responsible if a patient gets hurt because of a mistake made by an AI. Inadequate openness, models may unintentionally reinforce biases present in the training evidence, leading to unfair treatment outcomes. To deal with this problem, we need to improve explainable AI methods that make decision-making processes clear. The use of AI easier to understand may help build trust, make sure that rules are followed, and make it easier to create safer, more reliable healthcare solutions (Adadi & Berrada, 2018).

2.2 Explainability's Role in Patient Safety

Making sure that patients have been safe remains the most important thing in healthcare. The AI-driven systems that are easy to understand are a big part of making this a reality. Whenever doctors use AI to figure out what's wrong with a patient to plan their treatment or assess their risk. They need to know why the system provides those suggestions. In addition, being open about things might give rise to wrong decisions, which could put patients in danger. Explainable artificial intelligence (X AI) helps keep these kinds of problems from happening by letting healthcare professionals use their clinical knowledge to check and confirm automated suggestions. The ability to understand is very important in high-stakes situations like emergency care, where decisions need to be made quickly and correctly. In the event, an AI system tells a healthcare provider to do a certain thing, comprehension of why it made that choice can help the doctor feel sure about what they ought to do. Without this, depending on black-box models could lead people to be hesitant to make mistakes, or even make medical mistakes (Gilpin et al., 2018). When AI-generated medical decisions are readily apparent, patients are more likely to trust and work with their doctors. The public are more likely to agree with a diagnosis or treatment plan if they understand how the system came to that conclusion. This is especially important when dealing with chronic illnesses or complicated conditions that require long-term treatment strategies. The patients feel better about their care. As they know that both the human knowledge and reliable technology assist with it. The ability to explain also helps find mistakes and make AI models better over time. The healthcare professionals are able to identify the discrepancies to point out possible mistakes and improve models for better accuracy when they can understand system outputs. This feedback loop makes sure that AI solutions can grow in a way that puts, the health of patients at the forefront. Healthcare providers are able to render decisions safer, build trust, and create a collaborative environment where technology supports, instead of replaces, human expertise by using explainable AI (Ahmad et al., 2019).

3 Applications of XAI in Healthcare

Explainable AI (XAI) plays a crucial role in making AI-driven healthcare solutions more transparent and trustworthy. By providing clear reasoning behind decisions, XAI helps medical professionals and patients better understand AI-based recommendations. Below are key applications of XAI in healthcare are shown in Fig. 1.

- *Disease Diagnosis & Prognosis*: XAI improves diagnostic accuracy by highlighting the specific factors that contribute to AI-driven disease detection. In conditions like cancer, diabetes, and cardiovascular diseases, explainable models show which symptoms, biomarkers, or medical history elements influenced the diagnosis. This allows doctors to validate AI predictions and make more informed clinical decisions. Additionally, AI can forecast disease progression, but without transparency, doctors may not trust these predictions. XAI ensures that physicians can see the reasoning behind risk assessments, enabling early intervention and personalized treatment strategies.
- *Medical Imaging & Radiology*: Medical imaging relies heavily on AI for detecting abnormalities in X-rays, MRIs, and CT scans. However, a lack of interpretability can make radiologists hesitant to trust AI outputs. XAI techniques like heatmaps and feature attribution methods highlight the regions in medical scans that contributed to a diagnosis. For example, if an AI model detects a tumour, XAI can indicate which part of the scan led to that conclusion. This improves diagnostic confidence, reduces false positives and negatives, and allows radiologists to verify AI findings before making final assessments (Dieber & Kirrane, 2012).
- *AI-Assisted Surgery*: Robotic surgery is becoming more advanced, with AI assisting in precision tasks. However, for surgeons to trust these systems, they need to understand how AI makes decisions during procedures. XAI ensures that robotic systems provide real-time feedback on their actions, explaining why specific movements or adjustments are made. This improves surgical precision, minimizes risks, and ensures that surgeons remain in control. Transparent decision-making also helps in post-surgical analysis, allowing medical teams to evaluate AI-assisted procedures and refine techniques for future surgeries.

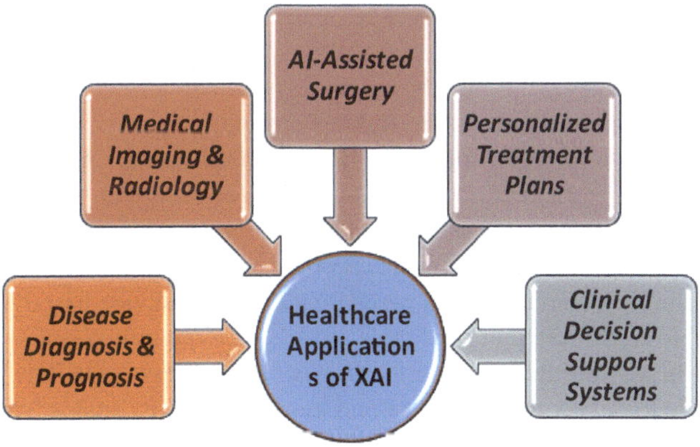

Fig. 1 Healthcare applications of XAI

- *Personalized Treatment Plans*: Treatment plans often vary based on a patient's medical history, genetics, and lifestyle factors. AI can analyse the vast datasets to recommend personalized treatments, but without explainability, doctors and patients may be unsure why a particular plan is suggested. XAI clarifies the reasoning behind recommendations, whether it's a specific medication, dosage, or therapy. This transparency increases patient adherence to prescribed treatments and helps healthcare providers modify plans when necessary, ensuring better health outcomes (Bach et al., 2015).
- *Clinical Decision Support Systems* (CDSS): Clinical decision support systems assist healthcare providers in making informed choices by analysing patient data and offering recommendations. However, without explainability, doctors may not fully trust AI-generated suggestions. XAI provides clear justifications for recommendations, showing how different variables such as lab results, symptoms, and medical history contributed to a decision. This helps reduce diagnostic errors, supports second opinions, and enhances the overall reliability of AI-powered clinical tools. Additionally, in prescribing medications, XAI can detect potential drug interactions and provide understandable warnings, improving patient safety.

4 The Human Factor in Explainable AI

4.1 Physicians' Trust in AI-Generated Explanations

As an AI-driven systems in healthcare to function properly, healthcare providers need to trust the suggestions they provide. This trust is established since the reasons behind predictions seem straightforward, reliable, and in line with exactly what is known about medicine. In the event, the decision-making process cannot be understood; healthcare providers might not want to use those instruments, which would make them less useful in clinical settings. A few of the main issues that comes up has become whether or not automated insights correspond to line with accepted clinical thinking. This is hard for healthcare professionals to check if models that give outputs without explaining them are right. There are ways to close this gap with clear methods like rule-based logic and feature identification, which show which factors have the biggest effect on predictions. This feature gives medical staff more faith in the system because it permits them check automated ideas against their own knowledge. Maintaining consistency has become a further significant issue to think about. The confidence is hurt when people get different advice based on the same information. To make sure that predictive models give the same results continually, they ought to be put through very strict testing (Chattopadhay et al., 2018). They also need to be able to deal with uncertainty and know their limits, instead of just giving the results as final answers. Healthcare providers can make smart choices without relying too much on automation in the event they are given confidence levels along with recommendations. The familiarity and training are also important factors that affect adoption. In the event healthcare providers know more about how these tools work and how to read the results they provide it is more likely to use them in their work. To make things easier to accept, learning institutions should focus on education and case studies that are based on real life. Some of the most important things have to be done to build trust are being open, consistent, and in line with clinical competence. As soon as these conditions are met, healthcare providers will be able to reliably use smart decision support technologies in providing medical treatment, which will both serve patients better and save time (Selvaraju et al., 2020).

4.2 AI-Enhanced Training for Healthcare Practitioners

Artificial intelligence has transformed the medical education by offering personalized, flexible training methods that make a learning better. These technologies provide healthcare workers interactive, data-driven tools that make it easier to make decisions, improve diagnostic accuracy, and improve procedural skills in clinical settings. T hereby adding artificial learning systems to training software medical professionals may acquire information more effectively and make fewer mistakes in real-life situations. A few the best things about AI-driven training have to be that it permits people learn in their own way. Artificial intelligence services, on the other hand, look at how a person is doing and tailor information to them. This is different from traditional methods that use a one size fits all the approach. These technologies find gaps in the understanding of a learn change the difficulty of the course, and recommend specific study materials to make sure that each student gets the right and most effective training. This approach improves skill acquisition and lowers cognitive load. Virtual simulations and advanced case studies are changing the way doctors are trained. AI-powered simulations mimic real-life patient interactions, allowing doctors to diagnose and treat illnesses in a safe, controlled setting. These fake patients show different symptoms and respond to treatments in a way that makes the experience more realistic and helps professionals make better decisions. By practicing complex situations repeatedly, thereby students improve their skills without putting real patients at risk. Artificial neural networks have additionally influenced how surgeons learn. The highly precise simulators use motion tracking and real time input to rate the performance. This helps surgeons improve their skills before performing any live procedures. These platforms check hand movements, find error and give feedback that is helpful greatly to improve accuracy. The surgery performed with robotic assistance training helps doctors get used to the advanced technology used in the minimally invasive procedures that helps to the boosts their confidence and skills. AI helps people make better decisions by giving them advanced clinical reasoning modules in addition to real-world experience. These case-based training tools help doctors evaluate patients by giving them information about possible diagnoses, treatment options, and problems that may arise. These platforms improve critical thinking and problem-solving skills by giving users a lot of different situations for consideration and explaining the reasons behind different medical choices.

Healthcare workers need to keep learning all throughout their careers, and AI helps them stay up to date on new medical knowledge (Alsharif et al., 2021). These systems look at a lot of research, guidelines, and real patient data to give you the most up-to-date advice. Healthcare providers get personalized alerts about new treatment options, drug interactions, and best practices, which helps them maintain high standards of care. AI makes it easier for people to work together by connecting people all over the world. The healthcare providers can improve the way they do their jobs by the sharing ideas, case studies, and new methods through a smart network. By employing AI-driven technologies into training gives medical staff the skills, they need to provide high-quality care, which leads to better patient outcomes and a better performing healthcare system (Antoniadi et al., 2021).

5 Strategies for Improving Trust Through XAI

5.1 Hybrid Models Combining Interpretability and Accuracy

In healthcare, it is very important for AI models to be both easy to understand and accurate. The structures of deep learning that are very complicated can make very accurate predictions, but because they are extremely hard to understand, that they also hard to trust. From the other hand, simpler models are easier to understand, but they don't always have the accuracy needed for making clinical decisions. The hybrid mathematical models solve this problem by combining the best parts of both methodologies that makes sure that predictions are both accurate and understandable. Building multiple models is one way to make them easier to understand without losing accuracy. A hybrid method might first use a deep learning model to look for patterns in medical data that are hard to understand. Then, a simpler decision tree or rule-based system could explain why the prediction was made. This makes sure that the final output can be shown to doctors and other medical staff in a way that is easy to understand, even though the underlying calculations are still complex. Another method uses attention mechanisms to show which parts of a model's decision-making process are the most important. For instance, deep learning networks can make heatmaps in medical imaging that show the areas that are responsible for a diagnosis. This makes it easier for radiologists to check the results. In predictive models for diseases, attention layers can also find important biomarkers or symptoms that helped with a risk assessment. This permits the doctors compare the AI generated insights with their own clinical knowledge. The ensemble learning is consider as another common method used in hybrid modelling. Models can able to get both high accuracy and better interpretability by using more than one algorithm, like neural networks, gradient boosting, and logistic regression. Some ensemble methods such as stacking or boosting that allow the transparent models to improve or check the results of more complicated systems, which makes them even more trustworthy. SHAP (Shapley Additive Explanations) and LIME (Local

Interpretable Model-agnostic Explanations) are two examples to turn the AI outputs into insights that people can able to understand. These methods help the medical professional and the nurses understand why a certain choice was made, which makes them less sceptical and more likely to use them in clinical settings. The hybrid models make sure that AI driven solutions stay clear, reliable, and clinically relevant by combining accuracy with interpretability. This method not only improves decision-making in healthcare, but it also improves cooperation between medical professionals and technology, which leads to safer and more effective patient care (Kaur et al., 2021).

5.2 Human-In-The-Loop Approaches

The incorporation of the human expertise to AI-driven healthcare systems makes sure the results are accurate, and in line with clinical standards. The human in the loop (HITL) methods use the machine intelligence and the knowledge of the medical professionals to keep predictive models precisely modern and better. This process of doing things over and over again builds trust and makes patient care more effective. In real time validation strengthens AI-generated concepts stronger. In advance of predictions are implemented in medical procedures, healthcare providers and other medical staff check and confirm them. This prevents mistakes in important areas like diagnosing conditions preparing treatments, and suggesting medications. Expert oversight makes sure that AI can handle complicated medical cases that are inconsistent with the training data. Regular input improves how well the model works. When doctors use AI tools, they make corrections, add notes, and suggest other options. The above method of learning lets systems change based on expert choice which makes predictions more accurate over time. In medical imaging, radiologists can use AI-generated heatmaps to mark false positives or draw attention to missed anomalies. This makes future analyses more accurate and also make it possible to reduce bias. Artificial intelligence models that use old data, may show differences that already exist in medical records. An expert review helps find and fix these biases and also making sure that different groups of patients get fair and equal treatment. Artificial intelligence (AI) models could make healthcare inequalities worse as long as they are not watched over by people. When medical professionals work with artificial intelligence systems, it's easier to understand what they are supposed to perform. When people know how decisions happen, they trust technology more and are more likely to use it. The transparent workflows in which experts can see, how a model came to a certain recommendation to build trust and make it easier to use responsibly. HITL makes sure that AI has been a helpful tool and not a decision-maker on its own by combining computational efficiency with human judgement. This partnership makes patients safer and lets AI-driven solutions get better through input from qualified professionals, which leads to more accurate and ethical uses of AI in healthcare (Naik et al., 2021).

5.3 Standardization of Explainability Frameworks

In recognition of AI models to be useful in healthcare it is important that every one of them give the same explanations (Dash & Agarwal, 2006). Without the clearly established norms, various technologies may have different levels of openly making it harder for healthcare professionals to judge and trust AI-generated insights (Refat et al., 2021). Establishment of protocols for comprehension helps create artificial intelligence in clinical settings that are trustworthy and straightforward to comprehend, and ethically responsible. For standardization to work, it is important to follow the rules. The FDA, EMA, and WHO all have been working to set clear standards for AI transparency in healthcare (Praveenkumar et al., 2025). These standards stipulate that models have to explain why they give certain outputs. This makes decisions less risky when they are not clear. The standardized frameworks allow individuals to follow the law and do the right thing which keeps patients safe and holds people accountable. When comprehension follows a systematic framework and the AI systems that can work together better (Kumarganesh et al., 2025). Hospitals and other medical facilities and practitioners employ diverse AI technologies for diagnosis, treatment planning, and patient monitoring. The cohesive explainability framework makes sure that different models explain their logic in the same manner which makes it easier to use them in clinical settings. The medical community can make better decisions with more confidence when provided with clear and comparable explanations across platforms. A comparison strategy to enhance the reliability by providing a measurable criterion for explainability (Sreedhar et al., 2025). The use of Shapley Additive Explanations and Local Interpretable Model Explanations along with the attention-based visualizations all serve as systematic ways to make AI decision-making clearer. The establishment of a clear evaluation standards for these procedures makes sure that the explanations are straightforward more accurate and applicable to clinical practice. The openness builds trust between doctors and patients. As soon as AI systems consistently offer clear explanations for their recommendations, physicians can validate decisions and corroborate predictions with their expertise (Chinnasamy et al., 2025). The patients benefit from clearer clarifications which help them understand their diagnosis and treatment options better. It is necessary for academics, business leaders, and regulatory bodies to work together to come up with universal recommendations. The international organization for standardization and IEEE is the two groups that are working together to set standards for AI explainability in healthcare. A clearly defined standard ensures that the AI technologies remain secure and in line with medical needs. The utilizing standardized explainability frameworks makes healthcare AI more trustworthy, easier to understand, and more ethical (Chandraman et al., 2025).

5.4 Educating Medical Professionals on AI Interpretability

To identify AI to be increasingly prevalent. The medical professionals need to trust and understand its results. Medical professionals might have a hard time understanding AI-generated recommendations since they do not have prior experience that would limit its ability to help them make clinical decisions. Healthcare providers become acquainted with how to use AI to understand forecasts implement what they have learnt in the course of their duties and make smart choices to maintain patients secure. Integrated training programs connect medical and AI knowledge. A person can learn about models based on artificial their advantages and disadvantages, along with how to make predictions through demonstrations, online courses, and certification programs. These training programs make AI concepts easier for medical professionals to understand by using real-life examples. Being present in the real world makes things easier to understand. Medical professionals can test AI models and figure out why they work on interactive platforms and which helps them understand better. Through simulations, case studies, and AI-assisted decision-support tools help doctors and nurses understand the manner in which algorithms functions, which makes learning more enjoyable and useful. The healthcare sector and AI developers work together to make things easier to understand. The creators of systems must give explanations that are easy for doctors to understand. Observing clear, structured reasoning behind model outputs helps doctors trust AI-assisted suggestions further. The input from medical professionals helps make explainability frameworks work in everyday circumstances. Healthcare professionals may acquire knowledge about regulatory and ethical issues to help them judge AI models against industry standards. Through knowing these facts, clinicians can push for AI applications that are open and responsible at their workplaces. Acquisition of knowledge from many different fields helps you understand AI better. Healthcare institutions, AI researchers, and technological specialists should work together to demonstrate to future doctors the manner in which to use smart technologies. AI education in medical school assists doctors get ready for how technology will change how they care for patients. Healthcare workers can utilize AI-driven insights while preserving clinical autonomy by emphasizing AI interpretability education. Through the right training, these technologies can help make decisions that are transparent, open, and ethical, which improves patient outcomes (Refat et al., 2021).

6 Conclusion

Medical professionals must have transparency in order to understand to validate, and have confidence in AI-driven solutions. Transparent models enhance security for patients, regulatory adherence, and ethical decision making by mitigating automated output blindness. As soon as AI predictions give straightforward explanations, clinicians can trust them in plans for treatment, and which leads to better results. It is hard to find a balance between accuracy while maintaining how easy it is to understand. In general, more complicated algorithms do a better job of making predictions than simpler ones. Nevertheless, their lack of transparency might make them less likely to be used. For the clinical acceptance there must be hybrid methods that keep accuracy and also give the clear explanations. Attention tasks, rule-based overlays, and post-hoc explanations assist in bridging this gap. To foster trust in AI-driven medical advances. The explainability framework needs to be improved all the time. The standardized model transparency, regulatory alignment, and human-in-the-loop assessment enhance the confidence in automated decision support systems. Healthcare providers, researchers, and regulators working together makes sure that AI advances meet the needs of the medical field. To move forward with transparent artificial intelligence. It is necessary to work together across fields. The integrating skills in medicine along with data science, ethics, and law makes frameworks that are more useful and reliable. The healthcare professionals get practical instruction on how to critically evaluate AI assisted direction. This makes sure that these technologies help people make decisions instead of taking their place. By making interpretability a top concern, healthcare AI can make patient care, uptake, and regulatory acceptance more effective. In healthcare, artificial intelligence needs to be accurate, clear, ethical, and work well with human knowledge.

References

Adadi, A., & Berrada, M. (2018). Peeking inside the black-box: A survey on Explainable Artificial Intelligence (XAI). *IEEE Access, 6*, 52138–52160.

Ahmad, M. A., Eckert, C., & Teredesai, A. (2019). Explainable AI in healthcare. *SSRN Electronic Journal.*

Alsharif, A. H., Md Salleh, N. Z., Baharun, R., & Hashem, E. R. (2021). Neuromarketing research in the last five years: A bibliometric analysis. *Cogent Business & Management, 8*, 1978620.

Antoniadi, A. M., Du, Y., Guendouz, Y., Wei, L., Mazo, C., Becker, B. A., & Mooney, C. (2021). Current challenges and future opportunities for XAI in machine learning-based clinical decision support systems: A systematic review. *Applied Sciences, 11*, 5088.

Bach, S., Binder, A., Montavon, G., Klauschen, F., Müller, K. R., & Samek, W. (2015). On pixel-wise explanations for non-linear classifier decisions by layer-wise relevance propagation. *PLoS ONE, 10*, Article e0130140.

Barredo Arrieta, A., Díaz-Rodríguez, N., Del Ser, J., Bennetot, A., Tabik, S., Barbado, A., Garcia, S., Gil-Lopez, S., Molina, D., Benjamins, R., et al. (2020). Explainable Artificial Intelligence (XAI): Concepts, taxonomies, opportunities and challenges toward responsible AI. *Inf. Fusion, 58*, 82–115.

Bonkra, A., & Dhiman, P. (2021, December 17–18). *IoT security challenges in cloud environment.* Proceedings of the 2021 2nd International Conference on Computational Methods in Science & Technology, Mohali, India, pp. 30–34.

Chandraman, M., Santhiyakumari, N., Shree, K.V. M., Murugesan, M., Kumarganesh, S., Rishabavarthani, P., Thiyaneswaran, B., et al. (2025). Enhancing cardiovascular disease analysis in healthcare systems with hybrid random forest and neural network algorithm. *Engineering Reports, 7*(9), e70373.

Chattopadhay, A., Sarkar, A., Howlader, P., & Balasubramanian, V. N. (2018, March 12–15). *Grad-CAM++: Generalized gradient-based visual explanations for deep convolutional networks.*

Proceedings of the 2018 IEEE Winter Conference on Applications of Computer Vision, WACV 2018, Lake Tahoe, NV, USA, pp. 839–847.
Chinnasamy, P., Subashini, B., Ayyasamy, R. K., Kiran, A., Pandey, B. K., Pandey, D., & Lelisho, M. E. (2025). Blockchain based electronic educational document management with role-based access control using machine learning model. *Scientific Reports, 15*(1), 18828.
Dash, S. C., & Agarwal, S. K. (2006). Incidence of chronic kidney disease in India. *Nephrology, Dialysis, Transplantation, 21*, 232–233.
Dieber, J., & Kirrane, S. (2012). *Why model why? Assessing the strengths and limitations of LIME*. arXiv:2012.00093.
Gilpin, L. H., Bau, D., Yuan, B. Z., Bajwa, A., Specter, M., & Kagal, L. (2018, October 1–3). *Explaining explanations: An overview of interpretability of machine learning*. Proceedings of the 5th IEEE International Conference on Data Science and Advanced Analytics, DSAA 2018, Turin, Italy, pp. 80–89.
Kaur, H., Koundal, D., & Kadyan, V. (2021). Image fusion techniques: A survey. *Archives of Computational Methods in Enginerring, 28*, 4425–4447.
Kumarganesh, S., Murugesan, M., Ganesh, C., Santhiyakumari, N., Thangavel, M., Jayaram, K., Sagayam, K. M., Pandey, B. K., & Pandey, D. (2025). Hybrid plasmonic biosensors with deep learning for colorectal cancer detection. *Plasmonics, 20*(7), 4895–4909.
Naik, H., Goradia, P., Desai, V., Desai, Y., & Iyyanki, M. (2021). Explainable Artificial Intelligence (XAI) for population health management—An appraisal. *European Journal of Electrical Engineering and Computer Science, 5*, 64–76.
Praveenkumar, T., Anthoniraj, S., Kumarganesh, S., Somaskandan, M., Sagayam, K. M., Pandey, B. K., Pandey, D., & Sahani, S. K. (2025). Enhanced circuit board analysis: Infrared image segmentation utilizing Markov Random Field (MRF) and level set techniques. *Engineering Reports, 7*(3), e70029.
Refat, M. A. R., Al Amin, M., Kaushal, C., Yeasmin, M. N., & Islam, M. K. (2021, October 7–9). *A comparative analysis of early-stage diabetes prediction using machine learning and deep learning approach*. Proceedings of the 2021 6th International Conference on Signal Processing, Computing and Control (ISPCC), Solan, India, pp. 654–659.
Selvaraju, R. R., Cogswell, M., Das, A., Vedantam, R., Parikh, D., & Batra, D. (2020). Grad-CAM: Visual explanations from deep networks via gradient-based localization. *International Journal of Computer Vision, 128*, 36–359.
Sreedhar, C., Kallam, S., Ghantasala, G. S. P., Anthoniraj, S., Kumarganesh, S., Sagayam, K. M., Pandey, B. K., & Pandey, D. (2025). Enhancing healthcare data security using RFE and CRHSM for big data. *Computers in Biology and Medicine, 190*, 110063.

IoT-Enabled Wearable Health Devices for Real-Time Diagnosis

N. Krishna Kumar, Bandi Rambabu, Niladri Maiti, Prabhakara Rao Kapula, M. V. S. V. Kiranmai, Sakthitharan Subramanian, and Maki Mahdi Abdulhasan

Abstract The wearable health devices compatible with the Internet of Things (IoT) contribute to the modern healthcare by allowing for a continuous monitoring of health for real-time data analysis and better patient management. These devices incorporate an artificial intelligence-based analytics, detectors, and internet connection modules to keep track of important things comprising heart rate, blood pressure, glucose levels, and oxygen saturation. It can be used for everything from managing chronic diseases and keeping an eye on a patient from finding emergencies and providing the care within hospitals. The use of mobile devices makes healthcare more efficient and improves patient outcomes by making it easier to diagnose problems early and cutting down on the number of times patients need to go to the medical professional.

N. K. Kumar
Department of CSA, University Institute of Computer Science and Applications, Guru Nanak University, Hyderabad, Telangana, India

B. Rambabu (✉)
Department of CSE, CVR College of Engineering, Hyderabad, India
e-mail: rambabubandi@gmail.com

N. Maiti
School of Dentistry, Central Asian University, Tashkent, Uzbekistan
e-mail: m.niladri@centralasian.uz

P. R. Kapula
ECE, B V Raju Institute of Technology, Vishnupur, Narsapur, Medak, Telangana, India
e-mail: prabhakar.kapula@bvrit.ac.in

M. V. S. V. Kiranmai
Department of CSE, University College of Engineering Kakinada, JNTUK, Kakinada, Andhra Pradesh, India

S. Subramanian
Department of Computational Intelligence, School of Computing, Faculty of Engineering and Technology, SRM Institute of Science and Technology, Kattankulathur, Chennai, Tamil Nadu, India

M. M. Abdulhasan
Al-Nisour University College, Nisour Seq. Karkh, Baghdad, Iraq
e-mail: maki.a.eng@nuc.edu.iq

D. Pandey et al. (eds.), *Smart Healthcare*,
https://doi.org/10.1007/978-981-95-8828-2_10

These mobile health devices work perfectly with a medical record that is stored electronically, which makes it easier for healthcare providers to work together and make sure that patients receive the right care at the right time. Artificial intelligence-based predictive analytics help prevent diseases from occurring prior to occur which lowers the number of people who need to go to the hospital and makes it easier to manage their health over time. These technologies have many benefits that are but more research is needed on issues like confidentiality of information, sensor accuracy, and interoperability. The next enhancements should concentrate on boosting consistency, security, and cost-effectiveness to facilitate broader acceptance. The smartphone and tablet used in the health technology will continue to transform healthcare for the better by encouraging proactive health management and moving medical precision forward to help patients all over the world.

Keywords IOT · Wearable health devices · Real-time monitoring · AI in healthcare · Predictive analytics · Healthcare technology

1 Introduction

The Internet of Things (IoT) has revolutionized the healthcare industry by making it possible to use intelligent, interconnected solutions that improve the treatment of patients, accelerate up treatments, and assist in making everything run more smoothly. In addition to the Internet of Things can use to keep an eye on vital signs all the time for find diseases early and get medical help when needed it. The following is made possible by combining technological advances such as cloud computing, and data analytics that happen in real time. The public can keep an eye on their heart rate, oxygen saturation, glucose levels, and body temperature with wearable health devices that constitute a part of the Internet of Things (IOE). This real-time monitoring promotes tailored treatment strategies and assists in reducing down on visits to the hospital that ultimately leads to better outcomes for patients. Practitioners in healthcare can also access patient data from distant locations, thereby making telemedicine and remote diagnostics possible. The Internet of Things-based technologies help hospitals run more effectively, keep track of their assets, and predict when medical equipment will need maintenance. It also helps keep an eye on the wellness of individuals. These improvements make healthcare better and easier to get by reducing the number of mistakes that have to be made by hand and by making the best use of resources. The Internet of Things (IoT) is making more technologies readily accessible, which will change the way medical care is delivered by making decisions based on more data and smarter choices.

1.1 Wearable Devices in Real-Time Health Monitoring

Wearable gadgets along with health technologies have transformed the way that track our health in real time by continuously and privately monitoring physiological data. These intelligent gadgets include sophisticated biosensors that collect and send important health data to connected platforms. This enables users and healthcare professionals check on their health in real time. These devices enable patients and healthcare professionals communicate to each other without any breaks by using wireless technologies like Bluetooth, Wi-Fi, or cellular networks. A few of the best things about wearable technology is that it can quickly find problems. The smartwatches, fitness bands, and bio-patches are examples of devices which monitor things comprising blood pressure, ECG signals, oxygen saturation, and stress levels. As soon as irregularities occur, careers receive notification shortly thereafter, which makes it easier for doctors to respond quickly. This feature can be particularly helpful for people with long-term illnesses like diabetes, heart disease, or respiratory problems, whenever quick answers could prevent problems (Pandian, 2016). These devices help people stay healthy by keeping track of their exercise habits, sleep quality, and metabolic rates. The company also helps people with chronic illnesses. These tools give specific input that helps people live healthier lives that helps prevent illness and improve overall fitness. Wearable ECG monitors and continuous glucose monitors provide it data in real time, helping you make better healthcare decisions based on facts. The addition of artificial intelligence to these devices makes them more effective in analysing data, thereby rendering it easier to use predictive modelling to stop diseases from happening. Wearable technology can make it easier for medical professionals and patients to talk to each other in telehealth by letting them have virtual consultations and tests from a distance. In hospitals, mobile devices improve patient care by reducing the need for manual surveillance, which allows medical staff to focus on more urgent cases. These devices are having a bigger and bigger impact on the future of healthcare as technology improves. It makes healthcare more accessible, efficient, and personalized.

2 IoT Technology in Wearable Health Devices

2.1 Architecture in Wearable Healthcare

The wearable healthcare uses IoT architecture to create a structured system. It makes easier to send data in the real time to perform analyses intelligently and keep an eye on patients all the time. Each layer of this design is important for keeping communication between healthcare systems and wearable technology running smoothly. The main layers included the sensory layer, the network layer, the processing layer, and the application layer. The IoT system is used to build on the perception layer. The biosensors use in the wearable technology collect the physiological data like heart rate, temperature, oxygen saturation, glucose levels, and electrocardiogram (ECG) readings. These sensors can help to turn biological impulses into digital data that makes it possible to analyses health conditions in a real time. Flexible electronics and tiny sensors have made wearable technologies much more accurate and comfortable, making sure that health monitoring is reliable. The network layer is responsible for sending the data that the wearable device collects to medical providers or cloud computing platforms. Bluetooth, Wi-Fi, cellular networks (4G/5G), and low-power wide-area networks (LPWAN) are just a few of the communication technologies that make data transport possible (Takizawa et al., 1998). To make real-time health monitoring easier, this layer cuts down on latency and makes sure that transmission is safe, fast, and uses less energy. The processing layer is necessary to look at and understand the data that has been sent. The cloud computing, edge computing, and artificial intelligence (AI) all work together in this layer to handle a huge amount of health data. The AI-powered algorithms help to find problems to predict possible health risks and give the personalized advice based on past patterns. The edge computing makes real-time decision even better by processing data closer to the source and getting rid of the need for constant access to the cloud. The people and healthcare providers interact with the processed data at the application layer through the use mobile applications, web dashboards, or the medical software. This layer has tools for visualizing the data, perform predictive analytics, and remote patient management that make it easier for both people and a medical professional to keep an eye on a health problem and make smart choices. The integration with electronic health records (EHR) makes sure that patient data is stored safely and can be accessed for possible future medical visits. The wearable healthcare's IoT architecture creates a smart and connected ecosystem that can improve patient monitoring, make it easier to find diseases early, and make healthcare as a whole more efficient by combining these layers. As technology gets better, wearable health devices will be able to do more things because of better connections, more accurate sensors, and AI-driven insights (Song et al., 2015).

2.2 Sensors, Processors, and Connectivity Modules

Wearable health devices must have a combination of advanced parts to make sure it can accurately monitor in immediate succession, send data without disturbance, and process this quickly. The sensors, processors, as well as communication modules have been the three main parts that make these devices operate well. This is important to have each piece in order to turn raw physiological data into useful health information. These wearable healthcare technologies rely on sensors to find and measure a number of physiological data. These types of biosensors gather information such as heart rate, blood pressure, oxygen saturation, glucose levels, and body temperature. The optical sensors employ light to check vital signs, and electrochemical sensors check glucose levels and the chemical composition of sweat. Accelerometers along with and gyroscopes are examples of motion sensors that keep track of physical activity, find falls, and look at movements over time. The biological impedance sensors monitor the level of hydration and the rate of respiration, whereas temperature sensors keep track of fluctuations in body heat. These sensors keep collecting accurate information about the body, and this allows them monitor health in real time and find diseases before they become serious. These mobile health devices have processors that act as the central processing unit. It reads and analyses the raw data which sensors collect (Atmojo et al., 2020). These microcontrollers or AI-powered circuits lower down on noise in order to make signals more precise as well as enable individuals to make decisions right away. A few processors that use the machine learning algorithms to find health problems and give a predicted insight. The modern central processing units are designed to use as little power as possible, while still keeping performance up. This helps batteries last longer. The edge computing features accelerate up processing by looking at data on the device first before sending important information to cloud storage. This reduces lower on latency and the need for a constant internet connection. The connectivity modules make it possible for healthcare professionals, wearable devices, and cloud storage to send and receive data without interruption. The Bluetooth Low Energy, Wi-Fi, and cellular networks are among the few of the many wireless communication technologies that can send data in real time. Bluetooth Low Energy is usually used for short-range, low-power connections, while Wi-Fi is used for high-speed data transfer for ongoing monitoring. Mobile communications networks, especially 5G, enhance remote healthcare applications better by giving them wide, high-bandwidth access. The use of near-field and Low-Power Wide-Area Networks are two examples of alternative communication technologies that can be used for remote patient monitoring. Near-Field Communication allows to send data securely over short distances, and Low-Power Wide-Area Networks allow it to connect over long distances with low bandwidth. Wearable health devices that use the Internet of Things (IoT) have sensors, processors, and networking modules, that work together to give real-time, data-driven insights, which makes healthcare more efficient. These parts work together to make sure that patients are always being watched, that they get medical help quickly, and that their health improves, which helps create smarter and more accessible healthcare solutions (Yetisen et al., 2018).

2.3 Data Collection, Transmission, and Cloud Integration

The wearable health devices that use the Internet of Things (IoT) must be able to move data from collection to secure transmission and cloud-based analysis with barely any problems. This interconnected system keeps watch on, analyses, and retains health data in order to medical professionals can get immediate information and give better care. Wearable sensors are capable of monitoring your heart rate, blood pressure, oxygen saturation, glucose levels, and body temperature. Highly sophisticated biosensors turn biological signals into digital data to make them more accurate and less probable to be affected by other signals. Through a lot of sensors, modern wearables may provide an exhaustive overview of a health. This level utilizes AI to get rid of noise and find significant trends in data. The information is sent to processing units or cloud platforms so that it can be evaluated. The Bluetooth Low Energy, Wi-Fi, and cellular networks all enable to send and receive data safely and quickly. The Bluetooth protocol is a good choice for short-range transmission because it uses less battery power. Wi-Fi, on the other alternative, permits this transfer data quickly to ensure a keep an eye on things all the time. The 4G as well as 5G cellular wireless network ability to connect over long distances is good for remote healthcare applications. The edge of computing allows for processing important health data on-site before sending it to the cloud. This reduces down the latency time and speeds up response time. The device uses in the healthcare needs cloud integration for more storage, better analytics, and remote access. The information is sent to secure cloud servers, in which AI and machine learning algorithms examine health threats. The cloud-based mobile applications and web dashboards enable users and healthcare professionals to observe health trends taking place. These systems work with electronic health records, which allows medical professionals get to patient information so they can perform accurate diagnoses and start treatment right away. The wearable health devices work better, since they can collect data quickly and send it reliably to the cloud. This unified approach enhances the patient outcomes and also proactive medical management via continual surveillance, early disease detection, and the personalized healthcare solutions (Park & Jayaraman, 2021).

3 Real-Time Diagnosis and Health Monitoring

3.1 Continuous Monitoring for Early Diagnosis

Continuous monitoring has become very important for early diagnosis. Since it gives the real-time information about a person's health. The wearable health devices using IoT technology allow it to keep an eye on patient's vital signs all the time. Unlike the regular check-ups, that only give you periodic assessments. This continuous data collection enables to find the minor variations in physiological parameters that could mean the beginning of a disease long before any of the noticeable symptoms develop up. Through identifying these warning signs in time, healthcare practitioners may intervene quickly, which leads to better treatment outcomes and a lower chance of serious side effects. The constant surveillance can keep an eye on long-term conditions including diabetes, high blood pressure, and heart disease. Patients with these conditions need to be watched closely all the time to keep their health from getting worse quickly. These devices keep track of important things like blood pressure, glucose levels, and heart rate fluctuations in real time. The result allows users and healthcare professionals know about potential hazards (Kekade et al., 2018). This proactive approach helps change medications, lifestyle choices, and treatment strategies based on real health trends instead of simply going to medical professional every now and occasionally. The importance of constant monitoring in finding serious medical problems includes heart attacks, strokes, and breathing problems. The wearable technology with electrocardiogram (ECG) sensors and pulse oximeters can able to find the heart rhythms which are not normal, drops in oxygen levels, or breathing patterns which are not normal. In a situation of emergency, these devices are capable of sending alerts to healthcare providers or emergency contacts, ensure that help is on the way right away. This feature is especially helpful for senior citizens and the patients who have a high risk of complications, along with those who live in remote areas where medical facilities are hardly accessible. The continuous monitoring not only helps find illness, but it also encourages users to live a healthy lifestyle, which improves preventive healthcare. The wearable health devices give a personalized information and an advice based on data collected in real time that can help maintain in better shape, sleep better, and deal with stress better. This self-awareness pushes people to make smart choices that will help them stay healthy in the long run. The use of IoT-enabled continuous monitoring in healthcare has transformed early diagnosis by moving the focus from treating problems after they happen to preventing them from happening in the first place. A wearable device uses real-time data analytics to help people and healthcare providers find, stop, and manage health problems more effectively. This improves patient care as a whole and makes healthcare systems less stressed (Escobar-Linero et al., 2022).

3.2 Health Parameters Monitored

- *Heart Rate* (HR): The wearable health devices must have heart rate monitoring as a basic feature. These devices can use photoplethysmography (PPG) sensors to accurately measure the heart rate by detecting changes in the blood flow. Tracking the pace of the heart all the time can assist to find the problems like arrhythmias, tachycardia, and bradycardia, which could be signs of heart problems. HRV analysis also gives information about stress levels, fitness recovery, along with the way the autonomic nervous system works, which makes it a useful tool for both medical diagnosis and wellness tracking.
- *Electrocardiogram* (ECG): Wearable devices with electrocardiogram (ECG) sensors keep track of the cardiac electrical activity. ECG readings are better than just checking the heart rate as they can find irregular heart rhythms like atrial fibrillation that can cause stroke or heart failure whenever not treated. Long-term ECG monitoring means that users are not required to travel to the hospital every so frequently, which makes it easier for them to keep track of their heart health.
- *Oxygen Saturation* (SpO_2): As an optimal breathing habits, it's important to understand how much oxygen is in the blood. Wearable technology can do this with integrated pulse oximeters. The aforementioned sensors utilize light to figure out the quantity of oxygen is in the blood. Constantly keeping an eye on SpO_2 can be particularly helpful for people with respiratory conditions such as COPD, asthma, and insomnia since it helps them keep track of their oxygen levels whilst they are

awake and asleep. For the sake of people who have recuperated from respiratory infections or who are living in high-altitude areas, detection of hypoxia beforehand can save their lives.

- *Glucose Levels*: individuals with diabetes can keep an eye on their blood sugar levels without the need to prick their fingers all the time, through use of the continuous glucose monitoring (CGM) systems built into gadgets that are worn. These systems have had small sensors that go under the skin and monitor glucose levels in interstitial fluid. Continuous glucose monitoring helps people with diabetes manage their condition better due to helping them change their diet, medicine, and way of life based on accurate readings. A number innovative wearable devices even use artificial intelligence to guess when glucose levels might increase or decrease, which helps users take action before things get bad (Luna-Perejón et al., 2020).
- *Additional Parameters*: Wearable health devices track several other vital signs essential for comprehensive health management, ensuring a holistic approach to monitoring and preventive care.

  i *Blood Pressure*: Blood pressure monitoring in wearable devices helps detect hypertension and related cardiovascular risks. Smartwatches and wearable cuffs use optical sensors and inflatable air pockets to measure systolic and diastolic pressure. Continuous blood pressure tracking allows early detection of hypertension, reducing the risk of heart attacks, strokes, and kidney disease.

  ii *Respiratory Rate*: Monitoring the rate of breathing helps in the early detection of respiratory disorders such as chronic obstructive pulmonary disease (COPD) and asthma. Wearable sensors track breathing patterns and detect irregularities like apnea, shallow breathing, or rapid breathing, allowing timely medical intervention. This is especially beneficial for individuals recovering from respiratory illnesses or those involved in high-altitude training.

  iii *Body Temperature*: Wearable temperature sensors provide continuous monitoring of body heat levels, enabling early detection of fever, infections, or inflammatory conditions. Body temperature fluctuations can also indicate metabolic disorders or hormonal imbalances, helping healthcare professionals diagnose underlying health issues.

  iv *Hydration Levels*: Proper hydration is essential for maintaining bodily functions, and some wearables use bioimpedance analysis to assess hydration status. Dehydration can lead to fatigue, dizziness, and kidney complications. Real-time hydration tracking helps athletes, outdoor workers, and elderly individuals maintain optimal fluid balance.

By continuously monitoring these key health parameters, which are shown in the Fig. 1, wearable devices contribute to proactive healthcare, early disease detection, and improved chronic disease management. The integration of IoT technology enhances real-time data analysis, empowering individuals and healthcare providers to make informed health decisions, ultimately improving patient outcomes.

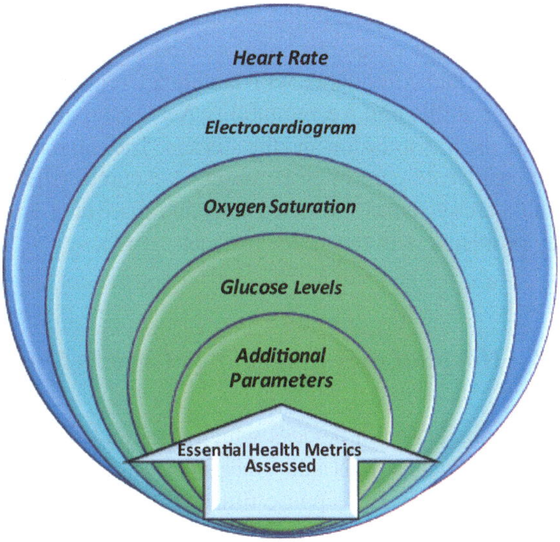

Fig. 1 Essential health metrics assessed

4 Integration with Healthcare Systems

4.1 Interoperability with Electronic Health Records

It is very important for IoT-enabled wearable health devices and a electronic health records (EHRs) to work together in order to create the cohesive healthcare environment. Through adding a real-time health data from the wearables to electronic health records. A healthcare professionals can able to obtain an exhaustive overview of the medical history of a patient. This helps to improve the process of the making choices, that perform diagnoses more precise, and allows for customized treatment plans that incorporate ongoing health monitoring instead of just periodic visits to the physician. Perhaps the most important benefits of this connection is that data can be sent in and out between wearable devices and healthcare systems without any breaks. These devices collect a lot of important health information that includes the heart rate, blood pressure, glucose levels, and oxygen saturation. This data can be sent right away to an EHR platform. This eliminates the need for data entry by hand, thereby decreasing any mistakes and makes sure that medical professionals have access to accurate and current data to improve the patient care. The ability to communicate makes it much easier to monitor patients from a distance, particularly individuals with chronic conditions like diabetes, high blood pressure, or heart disease (Guk et al., 2019). The medical professionals can keep an eye on patients' health patterns in real time, quickly spot any problems, and change treatments as needed without having to make patients go to the hospital all the time. This makes things easier for patients and takes some of the stress off of healthcare facilities through cutting down on unnecessary hospital stays and emergency procedures. To achieve seamless integration, a data security with privacy have been considered as very important parameters. An advanced encryption technique, secure storage in the cloud, and compliance with healthcare regulations such as HIPAA (Health Insurance Portability and Accountability Act) ensure the protection of patient information during the transmission and the storage. The standardized communication protocols, like Fast Healthcare Interoperability Resources (FHIR), make it easier for different healthcare systems to work together and share data across different platforms without any problems with technology (Çiçek, 2015).

4.2 Hospital and Emergency Care Settings

The wearable health devices which can connect to the Internet of Things are very important in hospitals and emergency rooms as they help make the best use of resources, boost up response times, as well as maintain an eye on patients. These devices provide healthcare providers immediate information about important health factors, and this can help them to make quick, well-informed decisions, especially in situations of emergency. The use of mobile devices allows hospitals keep an eye on patients all the time without having someone at their bedside all the time. Those receiving treatment in intensive care units (ICUs) or recovering from surgery can wear gadgets that keep track of their heart rate, blood pressure, breathing rate, and oxygen saturation. Transferring this information to centralized monitoring systems allows medical staff spot problems immediately and take action beforehand that get worse. This type of ongoing observation lowers the chance of adverse effects, reduces hospital stays, and helps patients get better faster. The wearable device is very helpful in emergency rooms because it assists doctors quickly check out and sort new patients. Emergency medical personnel can use wearable sensors to collect and send real-time patient data to healthcare facilities while they are on their way to the hospital. This gives emergency medical professionals an early idea of the patient's condition. This speeds up treatment decisions while patients arrive, which leads to better results for conditions like heart attacks, strokes, and injuries caused by trauma. For instance, wearable ECG monitors may identify heart pain or arrhythmias in patients prior to get to the hospital, so medical professionals can plan the treatments that are necessary to give them ahead of time. The wearable medical devices are additionally helpful for keeping an eye on patients after they leave the hospital. A patients may wear connected devices that give a healthcare providers the current information on their health, while they recover from surgery or deal with long-term illnesses. By taking steps to set off alarms for quick medical help when there are any worrying changes, like a sudden drop in oxygen levels or high blood pressure, it can lower the chances of readmission. Through adding wearable technology with Internet of Things capabilities to hospitals and emergency rooms, healthcare systems could greatly improve patient safety, quicken up medical procedures, and provide care that is faster and more effective. Eventually, this will raise the chances of patients living and improve the quality of care overall (Iqbal et al., 2021).

5 IoT-Enabled Wearable Health Devices

The wearable health devices that connect to the Internet of Things (IoT) improve healthcare by helping doctors keep an eye on vital signs in the present moment, finding diseases sooner, and cutting down on hospital visits. These devices help keep an eye on patients all of the time and send out alerts for medical emergencies right away that support personalized healthcare solutions. In the end, it improves overall health and make the best use of medical resources. Wearable health devices that use the Internet of Things (IoT) make healthcare better through the ability for continuous surveillance, early diagnosis, and customized treatment. The sophisticated sensors in these devices keep track of glucose, oxygen, blood pressure, and heart rate. Medical professionals can find health risks before they become serious and patients are not required to go to the hospital as often as they are monitored all the time. The control of chronic diseases is one of the most common uses for these devices. These individuals with diabetes and high blood pressure can keep track of their health indicators in real time so that they can get medical help right away. Healthcare professionals can keep an eye on those who are recovering from surgery or dealing with long-term illnesses without getting to see them in person.

Fall detection, ECG monitoring, and real-time notifications detect strokes, heart attacks, and accidents for fast medical action. Wearable sensors optimize ICU monitoring and staff efficiency in hospitals (Yang & Rhee, 2000). Wearable gadgets are also used to track fitness and mental health, helping users live an active and balanced lifestyle. Figure 2 illustrates the uses of wearable health devices with Internet of Things capabilities (Amitrano et al., 2020).

- *Chronic Disease Care*: Wearable devices play a crucial role in managing chronic conditions such as diabetes, hypertension, and cardiovascular diseases (Wang et al., 2022). By continuously monitoring vital parameters like blood pressure, glucose levels, and heart rate, these devices help patients and healthcare providers

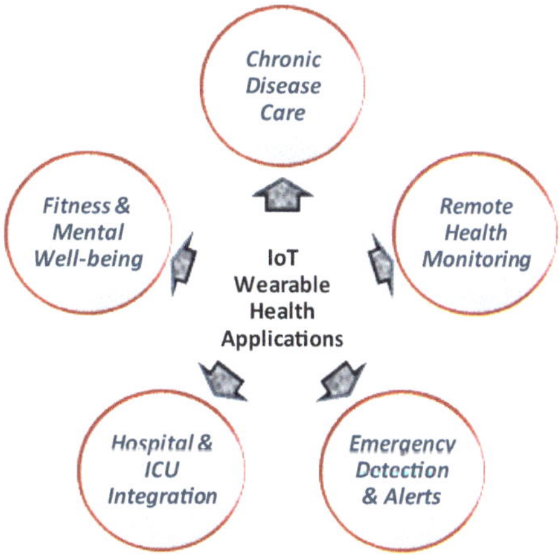

Fig. 2 IoT wearable health applications

detect early warning signs and adjust treatments accordingly. Automated (Chinnasamy et al., 2025) alerts notify users of abnormal readings, reducing the risk of complications and hospitalizations. AI-driven analytics further personalize treatment plans, enhancing long-term disease management.

- *Remote Health Monitoring*: IoT-enabled wearables allow healthcare professionals to track patients outside hospital settings, reducing the need for frequent check-ups. These devices collect and transmit real-time health data, enabling doctors to detect health issues before they escalate. Remote monitoring is particularly beneficial for elderly individuals and patients recovering from surgery, as it minimizes hospital visits while ensuring continuous medical supervision. This approach also optimizes healthcare resources, allowing doctors to focus on critical cases (Sreedhar et al., 2025).
- *Emergency Detection & Alerts*: Wearable health devices improve emergency response by detecting sudden health events such as heart attacks, strokes, or falls. Equipped with motion sensors, ECG monitors, and GPS tracking, these devices automatically send alerts to emergency contacts or healthcare providers when abnormal conditions are detected. Paramedics can receive real-time patient data before arrival, allowing for faster and more accurate treatment decisions. Such technology is especially valuable for high-risk individuals and those living alone (Pandey & Pandey, 2025).
- *Hospital & ICU Integration*: In hospital settings, wearable devices enhance patient monitoring and workflow efficiency. Patients in intensive care units (ICUs) or post-surgical recovery can be continuously monitored without constant bedside supervision. Wearable biosensors transmit real-time health data to centralized hospital systems, alerting medical staff of any sudden changes. This technology reduces manual monitoring efforts, minimizes errors, and improves overall hospital efficiency by optimizing resource allocation and staff coordination (Maheshwari et al., 2025).
- *Fitness & Mental Well-being*: Beyond medical applications, wearable devices support general health and wellness by tracking physical activity, sleep patterns, and stress levels. Advanced sensors analyse biometric data to provide personalized fitness recommendations and mental health insights. Features such as heart rate variability (HRV) analysis, guided breathing exercises, and sleep tracking help users maintain a balanced lifestyle. These devices are widely used by athletes, fitness enthusiasts, and individuals seeking better stress management.

6 Conclusion

The device health devices that use the Internet of Things (IoT) have changed healthcare by allowing for ongoing surveillance, collection of real-time information, and easy accessibility to electronic health records. These devices are important for the treating chronic medical conditions that help in reducing down on hospital visits by permitting doctors monitor patients from a far, and making emergency response procedures better by finding important health events including strokes and heart attacks. Wearable technology enhances ICU surveillance and efficiency of operations in healthcare facilities, which helps doctors get to patients faster. The fitness and mental health applications can help people to feel better by keeping track of their sleep, stress, and the activity levels. By implementing these gadgets to healthcare systems encompasses big effects on patients as well as healthcare providers. The healthcare professionals can make better decisions by minimize the need for manual monitoring, and make the better use of resources when they possess real-time access to the patient data. The devices give patients more freedom, help them find health problems promptly and make treating chronic illnesses better. Integration with electronic health records makes sure that medical histories are accurate and up recent, which makes it easier for different healthcare providers to work alongside one another. Wearable devices that use less energy, have been easier to use, and are cheaper will become more accessible and popular. The lasting effects of wearable technologies on patient outcomes will ultimately render it easier for them to become a part of regular healthcare. Internet of Things (IoT)-equipped wearables are expected to be an important part of changing healthcare, improving patient care, and encouraging personalized medicine as technological advances continue.

References

Amitrano, F., Coccia, A., Ricciardi, C., Donisi, L., Cesarelli, G., Capodaglio, E. M., & D'Addio, G. (2020). Design and validation of an e-textile-based wearable sock for remote gait and postural assessment. *Sensors, 20*, 6691.

Atmojo, J., Sudaryanto, W., Widiyanto, A., Ernawati, E., & Arradini, D. (2020). Telemedicine, cost effectiveness, and patients satisfaction: A systematic review. *Journal of Health Policy & Management, 5*, 103–107.

Chinnasamy, P., Subashini, B., Ayyasamy, R. K., Kiran, A., Pandey, B. K., Pandey, D., & Lelisho, M. E. (2025). Blockchain based electronic educational document management with role-based access control using machine learning model. *Scientific Reports, 15*(1), 18828.

Çiçek, M. (2015). Wearable technologies and its future applications. *International Journal of Electrical, Electronics and Data Communication, 3*, 45–50.

Escobar-Linero, E., Domínguez-Morales, M., & Sevillano, J. L. (2022). Worker's physical fatigue classification using neural networks. *Expert Systems with Applications, 198*, Article 116784.

Guk, K., Han, G., Lim, J., Jeong, K., Kang, T., Lim, E. K., & Jung, J. (2019). Evolution of wearable devices with real-time disease monitoring for personalized healthcare. *Nanomaterials, 9*, 813.

Iqbal, S. M., Mahgoub, I., Du, S., Leavitt, M. A., & Asghar, W. (2021). Advances in healthcare wearable devices. *NPJ Flexible Electronics, 5*, 9.

Kekade, S., Hseieh, C. H., Islam, M. M., Atique, S., Mohammed Khalfan, A., Li, Y. C., & Abdul, S. S. (2018). The usefulness and actual use of wearable devices among the elderly population. *Computer Methods and Programs in Biomedicine, 153*, 137–159.

Luna-Perejón, F., Domínguez-Morales, M., Gutiérrez-Galán, D., & Civit-Balcells, A. (2020). Low-power embedded system for gait classification using neural networks. *Journal of Low Power Electronics and Applications, 10*, 14.

Maheshwari, R. U., Paulchamy, B., Pandey, B. K., & Pandey, D. (2025). Enhancing sensing and imaging capabilities through surface plasmon resonance for deepfake image detection. *Plasmonics, 20*(5), 2945–2964.

Pandey, B. K., & Pandey, D. (2025). Securing healthcare medical image information using advance morphological component analysis, information hiding systems, and hybrid convolutional neural networks on IoMT. *Computers in Biology and Medicine, 185*, 109499.

Pandian, P. (2016). An overview of telemedicine technologies for healthcare applications. *International Journal of Biomedical and Clinical Engineering, 5*, 29–52.

Park, S., & Jayaraman, S. (2021). Wearables: Fundamentals, advancements, and a roadmap for the future. In Sazonov, E. (Ed.), *Wearable sensors* (2nd ed, pp. 3–27). Academic Press.

Song, F. X., Zhang, Z. J., Gao, F., Zhang, W. Y. (2015). An evolutionary approach to detecting elderly fall in telemedicine. In *Proceedings of the 2015 First International Conference on Computational Intelligence Theory, Systems and Applications (CCITSA), Ilan, Taiwan, 10–12 December 2015* (pp. 110–114).

Sreedhar, C., Kallam, S., Ghantasala, G. P., Anthoniraj, S., Kumarganesh, S., Sagayam, K. M., Pandey, B. K., & Pandey, D. (2025). Enhancing healthcare data security using RFE and CRHSM for big data. *Computers in Biology and Medicine, 190*, 110063.

Takizawa, M., Sone, S., Takashima, S., Feng, L., Maruyama, Y., Hasegawa, M., Hanamura, K., & Asakura, K. (1998). The mobile hospital-an experimental telemedicine system for the early detection of disease. *Journal of Telemedicine and Telecare, 4*, 146–151.

Wang, H., Wang, J., Chen, D., Ge, S., Liu, Y., Wang, Z., Zhang, X., Guo, Q., & Yang, J. (2022). Robust tattoo electrode prepared by paper-assisted water transfer printing for wearable health monitoring. *IEEE Sensors Journal, 22*, 3817–3827.

Yang, B. H., & Rhee, S. (2000). Development of the ring sensor for healthcare automation. *Robotics and Autonomous Systems, 30*, 273–281.

Yetisen, A. K., Martinez-Hurtado, J. L., Ünal, B., Khademhosseini, A., & Butt, H. (2018). Wearables in medicine. *Advanced Materials, 30*, 1706910.

Natural Language Processing for AI-Enabled Medical Documentation

Rachana Ravindra Mudholkar, Kondapakala Indumathi, M. L. M. Prasad, Mukesh Mohan More, Amit Baban Kasar, B. Vidhya, and Maki Mahdi Abdulhasan

Abstract The addition of natural language processing (NLP) to the documentation of healthcare delivery is changing the way medical records are put together, maintained and examined in a big way. Healthcare staff members might minimize the stress of administrative work whereas also improving their precision and effectiveness by using computerized speech transcription, computerized clinical note production, and medical coding automation. A further method that decision support and predictive analytics contribute to making clinical decisions better is by finding useful information in huge medical datasets. Nonetheless, there remains problems that need to be ameliorated, that include interoperability, contextual accuracy, and data privacy. In the near future, advancements will have to be made to improve models for deep learning to make them easier to understand, and make sure that systems work well

R. R. Mudholkar (✉)
PCET's Pimpri Chinchwad College of Engineering & Research, Ravet, India
e-mail: mudholkar.rrm@gmail.com

K. Indumathi
Department of CSE (Cyber Security), Siddhartha Institute of Technology and Sciences, Narapally, Ghatkesar, India
e-mail: kondapakalaindumathi.cse@siddhartha.co.in

M. L. M. Prasad
CSE(AI&ML), Joginpally BR Engineering College, Yenkapally (V), Moinabad(Md), Hyderabad, Telangana, India

M. M. More
Department of Computer Engineering, International Institute of Information Technology, Hinjawadi, Pune, India

A. B. Kasar
Department of Engineering Sciences, International Institute of Information Technology, Hinjawadi, Pune, India

B. Vidhya
Department of Computational Intelligence, SRM Institute of Science and Technology, KTR Campus, Tamil Nadu Chengalpattu District, India

M. M. Abdulhasan
Al-Nisour University College, Nisour Seq. Karkh, Baghdad, Iraq
e-mail: maki.a.eng@nuc.edu.iq

D. Pandey et al. (eds.), *Smart Healthcare*,
https://doi.org/10.1007/978-981-95-8828-2_11

together so that people can use them without any problems. The ongoing progress of smart automation might influence the way healthcare professionals' document things by cutting down on unused time and accelerating up workflows, and ultimately improving the care that patients receive, which natural language processing (NLP) and artificial intelligence (AI) do to make documentation easier, including the main benefits, problems, and possible new directions.

Keywords NLP · Medical documentation · Medical coding · Predictive analytics · Decision support · Deep learning · Healthcare automation

1 Introduction

The recording process, maintaining, and storing patient records is an important part of healthcare. It is an important tool for communication between providers that ensures continuity of hospital treatment to help in the making clinical decisions, and makes sure that legal and regulatory rules are adhered to. This practice helps to include a wide range of information, such as observations from medical professionals, reports from nurses, lab results, diagnostic imaging data, prescriptions, and summary of discharge. In the past, patient records were maintained on the paper, which made it hard to keep, find, and share information. The electronic health records also known as EHRs are now the standard because of the improvements in digital technology. It makes easier to access the medical data to reduce the mistakes and streamline workflows. By bringing together patient information, treatment plans, and test outcome data into one place. For the sake of the safety and quality of care of patients, records must be accurate and well-organized. It makes sure that symptoms, diagnoses, and treatments have been recorded correctly that lowers the chance of medical mistakes and malpractice. Standardized reports make billing and coding easier that ensures that healthcare professionals get paid fairly for their work. The developments in artificial intelligence (AI) and natural language processing (NLP) have changed the way clinical documentation is done in the last few years. AI-driven applications make it easier to take observations, pull useful information out of messy clinical documents, and help with coding and decision-making. These new technologies make things easier for the doctors and nurses, allowing them to focus more on caring for patients. Despite progress in technology, difficulties remain, such as maintaining confidentiality, addressing interoperability issues among diverse EHR systems, and ensuring data accuracy. To enhance efficiency and also to maintain compliance to improve healthcare outcomes. The record keeping needs to be optimized with standardized methods and AI-augmented solutions.

1.1 NLP in Medical Documentation

The natural language processing (NLP) has transformed the way healthcare providers keep track of the patient records by making them more accurate, efficient, and easy to get to. As the amount of unstructured clinical data grows, the automated processing methods help extract and make sense of text that greatly cuts down on the amount of work performed by the medical professionals. With speech recognition technology, doctors can dictate notes about patients, which turns spoken words into structured digital text. This cuts down on the amount of work that needs to be performed by hand and also speeds up the required process of documentation. It is also giving doctors more time to care for patients. The advanced text processing techniques need to find and pull-out important information from the clinical notes, lab reports, and the discharge summaries. This makes sure that important information is always available for diagnosis and treatment planning. Another big benefit is that the medical coding and billing will get better (Rajpurkar et al., 2022). The automated classification of diagnoses and the procedures ensure that the coding is correct, which helps to cuts down on the mistakes and stops claims from being denied. This helps healthcare organizations manage their money in a better way while still following the rules. The AI-driven text analysis also helps the decision support systems by finding patterns in a patient record that pointing out possible risks, and giving predictive insights. This helps with early diagnosis, personalized treatment suggestions, and better results for patients. The advanced language models to use in a clinical setting is not an easy work. It involves making sure that the data is to kept private, reducing bias, and making sure that they work with an existing electronic health record (EHR) system. To get the most out of intelligent documentation solutions and improve healthcare delivery, it's important to get past these problems.

2 Natural Language Processing (NLP)

2.1 NLP Techniques

- *Tokenization*: Tokenization has been a method of breaking text into smaller pieces, for instance sentences or words, so that it can be easier to perform understand. A word tokenization can be useful in medical records to identify specific words that have to do with medical conditions, medications, and procedures. A sentence tokenization has become helpful for organizing long clinical reports. For instance, it can break up a patient's progress note into useful parts to make it easier to process. Tokenization is very important for afterwards NLP tasks involving entity recognition and sentiment analysis. This makes sure that medical records persist as nicely organized and simple to understand.

- *Named Entity Recognition* (NER): The NER serves as a sophisticated method for finding and sorting important words in medical documents that include the patient names, diagnoses, drug names, lab test results, and procedures for medicine. By mapping an obtained entities to standardized a healthcare database that consisting of SNOMED CT, ICD-10, and RxNorm. This technique assists in organizing large amounts of unstructured data. NER is going to identify "metformin" as a drug and "type 2 diabetes" as a disease in a clinical note, which says, "Patient had been given metformin for type 2 diabetes." This makes it easier to automate the medical coding process, manage patient information, and systems to support clinical decisions.
- *Lemmatization and Stemming*: Both methods help text analysis work better through making sure that different forms of the same word remain the same. The lemmatization employs rules from language to change words to their dictionary form. For example, "diagnosed", "diagnosing", and "diagnosis" have all been changed to the "diagnose". The stemming on the other hand reduces words down to their roots by taking off their endings. In medical records, lemmatization makes sure that clinical records are consistent, which makes it easier to search and cuts down on duplicate information in databases. This is especially helpful in decision support systems and predictive analytics, where using the right words is very important.
- *Speech Recognition*: This method changes spoken language through written material that enable doctors and other medical staff dictate records for patients instead of writing them down by hand. To make speech recognition techniques more accurate, advanced AI-driven models have been developed on large datasets that include medical terms. These systems are able to accurately transcribe complex medical phrases, accents and changes in speech patterns. For instance, voice sensitive EHRs permit doctors record diagnoses, symptoms, and treatment plans without having to type them down, which makes the workflow more efficient. Furthermore, the integration with natural language understanding (NLU) allows for processing in real time, which makes sure that transcribed records are formatted adequately and that relevant information has become automatically sorted (McCorduck & Cfe, 2004).
- *Text Summarization*: Given that there is so much paperwork associated with healthcare, summarization methods have become essential for making short versions of long medical records, patient histories, or research articles. There are basically two main types of summarizations that are extractive summarization, which picks out significant words from the original text, and abstractive summarization that generates new, shorter sentences that keep the same meaning. For instance, a medical professional looking over the medical history of a patient might get a short summary that lists the main diagnoses, treatments, and recent laboratory findings that would help them make a quick decision. This method has become especially helpful for clinical research, discharge summaries, and literature reviews because it makes things more efficient and reduces the mental load on healthcare workers.

- *Medical Coding Automation:* Automating the assignment of standardized medical codes contributes to making sure that billing rules have been followed, minimises down on mistakes, and speeds up the procedure of receiving reimbursement back. In order to employ this method, it looks at clinical text and match terms to coding systems like ICD-10 which stands for diseases and conditions, CPT for medical procedures, and HCPCS (for healthcare services). By way of example, in the event the healthcare provider writes that a patient enjoyed "laparoscopic cholecystectomy", NLP-driven coding systems determine the correct ICD-10 code (K80.20) and CPT code (47,562). This makes sure that billing is correct. This method greatly improves financial management and compliance with rules in healthcare facilities by getting rid of coding mistakes made by hand and making the process more efficient (Alpaydin, 2020).

Figure 1 demonstrates the way natural language processing (NLP) methods that turn unstructured clinical writing into structured. Thereby keeping medical records more accurate and efficient. The techniques, including the speech recognition, named entity recognition, and tokenization to make it easier to organize and find patient records. The automated medical coding, lemmatization, and text summarization enhanced data consistency, reduce mistakes, and speed up procedure. These methods help with continuous collection and make clinical decision support better by drawing smart conclusions from huge amounts of medical data. By using these novel techniques, healthcare providers can more closely adhere to the rules, make their jobs easier, and give their patients the best care attainable.

Fig. 1 NLP techniques

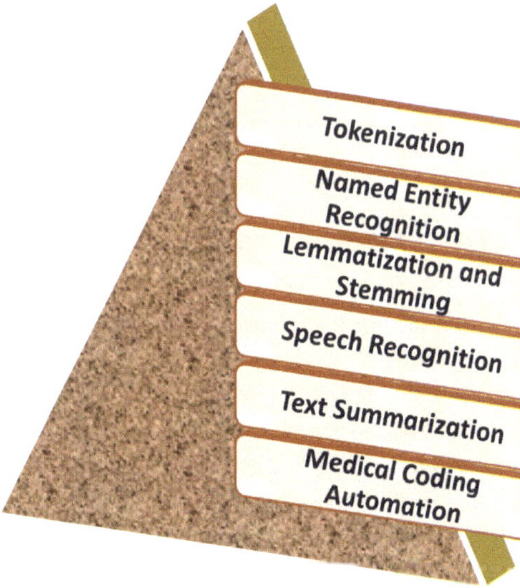

2.2 Machine Learning-Based NLP

The natural languages processing, which employs machine learning uses data driven models to comprehend, read, and compose medical text with a lot of the accuracy and the speed. These models differentiate themselves from traditional rule-based approaches given that they learn from a lot of healthcare data and become better at processing complex terms from medicine and unstructured content over time. This has made it possible for a machine learning to work in many areas of the healthcare, such as clinical record keeping, decision support systems, and medical coding. Supervised learning is an established technique in a medical NLP that used to train the algorithms on datasets with labels which connect input text to the right outputs. This method works really well for things that include the medical coding to classifying diseases and recognizing the speech. For instance, a simulation trained on annotated patient records will autonomously identify the diagnoses and assign the right ICD-10 codes. This makes billing simpler and cuts down on mistakes. An unsupervised machine learning, on the other hand, finds patterns in clinical text which is not structured without needing labelled data. Techniques including clustering and topic modelling help sort through a lot of patient notes, lab reports, and prescriptions. These techniques have been especially helpful for finding patterns in patient information, spotting emerging illnesses, and making medical research better by looking at large healthcare datasets. Models developed using deep learning, especially transformer-based architectures like BERT and GPT, have transformed NLP in healthcare even more revolutionary. These advanced models have been very good at summarizing clinical notes, answering requests from patients, and helping doctors make decisions due to their ability retain the context, figure out meaning, and write text that sounds corresponding to a person. Healthcare facilities are able to significantly enhance the efficiency of documentation, the accuracy of diagnoses, and the quality of overall patient care through the integration of machine learning-based NLP techniques to electronic health records (EHRs) systems (LeCun et al., 2015).

2.3 Deep Learning and Transformer Models

The deep learning has changed natural language processing through rendering the medical records more accurate while offering them in a more context. Deep learning employs neural networks with many layers to process huge amounts of unstructured text to recognize complicated connections between words and terminology in medicine. These models have been great at recognizing medical phenomena, transforming speech onto text, and interpreting clinical documents. The BERT and GPT transformer models have enhanced medical NLP applications more efficient. These architectures comprehend words through context as opposed to through keywords. The BERT-based models may accurately retrieve patient symptoms, test data, and prescribed therapies from EHRs, helping with clinical decision-making. The GPT-based models make it easier for healthcare providers to write clinical notes and summaries patient histories by automating the creation of reports. Models developed on Transformers make medical documents available in many various languages, making healthcare more accessible around the world. These algorithms find patterns in patient records to make predictive analytics more proficient to find diseases earlier in time and suggest customized treatments. Whenever using deep learning in medical applications, there can be problems with data privacy, interpretability, and large annotated datasets. Through the utilization of deep learning and transformer models, medical systems may improve documentation faster, more accurate, and more automated. These improvements facilitate easier for administrators and doctors to do their jobs and give patients improved treatment by giving them more reliable and organized healthcare data.

3 AI-Enabled Medical Documentation

3.1 AI-Driven Medical Documentation Systems

The artificial intelligence powered healthcare helps the record keeping systems that are composed up of many parts that function together to make clinical records more accurate, productive, and simple to gain access. These components use AI techniques like natural language processing (NLP), machine learning, and deep learning in order to look at unstructured medical data and generate organized documents. Speech recognition serves as the key part that permits healthcare workers record patient notes instead of typing them in by hand. Highly sophisticated models that know medical terms ensure that spoken language has become accurately transcribed into organized text. This makes the situation easier for administrators to keep records in real time. These systems also work with electronic health records (EHRs) making it easier to enter data without stopping. The Natural Language Understanding (NLU) has become another important part that helps the algorithm to comprehend the meaning and context of a clinical content. The NLU makes certain that the medical records have been accurate and complete by getting the information about symptoms, diagnoses, drugs, and treatments. This element has become very useful for connecting patient data to uniform coding systems like ICD-10 and SNOMED CT. The artificial intelligence does automated coding in medical purposes, and this is a very important job that uses the medical data which has been collected to assign the right billing and diagnosis codes. This element helps a medical professional to follow the rules, speed up the billing procedure, and cut down on claim denials by making the coding more accurate and consistent. The support of clinical decisions is use to improves documentation by using patient records, historical data, and prediction analytics to give the insights. The artificial intelligence generated alerts could assist healthcare professionals make smart decisions by pointing out possible risks, suggesting treatments, or permitting them know when data has gone missing (DuBois, 2019). The information security and compliance rules make sure that patient records continue to remain private and that healthcare laws like HIPAA and GDPR are observed. Encryption, access controls, and audit trails have been used to keep private medical information safe from people who shouldn't have it and who might misuse it. AI-driven medical documentation solutions put these parts together to make things work better, cut down on mistakes in paperwork, and let healthcare workers focus more on taking care of patients than on paperwork (Davenport, 2018).

3.2 *AI in Medical Documentation*

AI makes the medical records less inaccurate, speeds up processing, and also makes sure that records are all identical, and gives decision support in real time. It makes administrative tasks easier by automating the entered information, report writing, and coding. Figure 2 shows how artificial intelligence could assist with medical documentation. The use of AI makes security and compliance more effective, lowering the chance of data breaches while also making sure that healthcare standards are met. This ultimately contributes to better patient care and more efficient work.

- *Higher Accuracy*: AI-powered documentation systems minimize human errors by intelligently interpreting medical terminology and context. Advanced NLP models can recognize abbreviations, correct misspellings, and understand variations in medical language, ensuring that patient records are precise and comprehensive. AI also cross-references patient histories and physician notes to detect

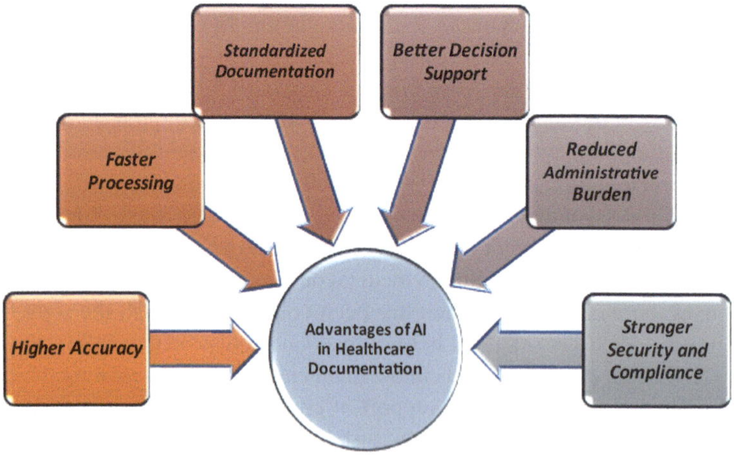

Fig. 2 Advantages of AI in healthcare documentation

inconsistencies, flagging potential discrepancies that may require verification. Additionally, automated quality checks ensure that records meet documentation standards before being finalized, reducing the likelihood of medical errors and misdiagnoses.

- *Faster Processing*: AI significantly accelerates the documentation workflow by automating repetitive tasks such as voice-to-text conversion, form filling, and report summarization. Doctors can dictate notes directly into an AI system, which transcribes and organizes them in real time, eliminating the need for manual entry. AI-powered tools can also extract key insights from complex medical texts, quickly summarizing patient histories, lab results, and prescriptions. This reduces the time required for physicians to review extensive records, allowing them to make faster clinical decisions and improve overall patient throughput.
- *Standardized Documentation*: AI enforces uniformity in medical records by ensuring adherence to standardized coding systems and clinical documentation guidelines. By analysing historical data and institutional best practices, AI can suggest optimal phrasing and terminology to maintain consistency across different healthcare providers. Automated coding assistants assign accurate procedural and diagnostic codes, minimizing discrepancies between medical notes and billing claims. AI-driven documentation systems also facilitate interoperability, ensuring that patient records are structured in a way that allows seamless data exchange between hospitals, insurance providers, and regulatory bodies (Hosny et al., 2018).
- *Better Decision Support*: AI-integrated documentation systems enhance clinical decision-making by providing real-time data insights and predictive analytics. These systems analyse vast amounts of patient data, identifying trends and correlations that may not be immediately apparent to healthcare providers. AI can detect early warning signs of disease progression, recommend alternative treatment options, and highlight potential drug interactions based on a patient's medical history. Additionally, AI-powered decision support tools integrate with electronic health records (EHRs), ensuring that clinicians have access to up-to-date information that aids in precise diagnosis and treatment planning.
- *Reduced Administrative Burden*: AI automates labour-intensive documentation tasks, reducing the workload for healthcare professionals and administrative staff. Intelligent document management systems categorize and index patient records, making retrieval and updates faster and more efficient. AI-powered chatbots and virtual assistants help clinicians quickly retrieve relevant information without manually searching through extensive records. Additionally, AI reduces redundant paperwork by auto-generating discharge summaries, progress notes, and follow-up recommendations based on existing patient data, allowing medical staff to focus more on patient care rather than clerical duties.
- *Stronger Security and Compliance*: AI enhances data security by implementing advanced encryption techniques, real-time threat detection, and automated access control mechanisms. Machine learning models can detect unusual activity, such as unauthorized access to patient records or inconsistencies in data entry, preventing potential breaches. AI also ensures compliance with regulatory standards such as HIPAA and GDPR by continuously monitoring documentation practices and

identifying areas where security policies need reinforcement. Furthermore, AI-driven compliance tools help healthcare organizations keep up with evolving legal requirements by automatically updating documentation protocols in response to new regulations (Kagiyama et al., 2019).

4 NLP Applications in Medical Documentation

4.1 Speech-To-Text Transcription for Medical Notes

Employing the speech-to-text technology, it is able to write down medical observations. The use of speech transcription technology has transformed the way medical professionals keep records of patient data by making it possible to write down in real time and effortlessly using their hands. The AI-driven transcription systems may transform spoken words into text that is organized since they comprehend the way individuals communicate. This means that doctors don't have to write or type prescriptions by hand. In light of this, healthcare providers are able to devote less time on administrative tasks, which not only makes them more effective but also enables them focus more on treating patients. Highly sophisticated speech recognition models, which have been tuned in on medical terminology are able to accurately transcribe complex terms, drug names, and diagnoses. These systems continue to acquire knowledge from modifications and keep adapting to different speech patterns, accents, and ways of pronouncing words. The integration with electronic health records (EHR) additionally allows you enter data without stopping that cuts down on the number of errors committed whenever someone enters it by hand and makes sure that patient records continue to be complete and up to date. One of the best things about speech-to-text transcription is the fact that it allows for work flow more smoothly. Medical professionals can write notes during or right after seeing someone being treated, which cuts down on the time they spend on record-keeping (Huang et al., 2020). In high-pressure situations including emergency rooms, timely documentation has become even more important. The artificial intelligence powered transcription systems that may identify and highlight the important patient information including symptoms, allergies, and prescribed drugs. This makes it this easier for healthcare teams to quickly go through records. There are a lot of benefits to transcribing speech to text in a medical file, but there are also a lot of problems exist with it. These problems include the background noise that makes it hard to hear and the need for strict data security measures. The latest transcription systems use the noise reduction algorithms, contextual understanding skills, and standards like HIPAA to deal with these problems and also keep the patient information private. Speech-to-text transcription has emerged as an important tool as artificial intelligence (AI) continues to make progress. This can help make healthcare more efficient and speed up medical paperwork.

4.2 *Automated Clinical Note Generation*

Automated clinical note creation has transformed the way healthcare records are kept by using AI to make organized, accurate, and complete patient records without any help coming from people. The use of NLP and machine learning by these systems to transform healthcare provider patient conversations, medical histories, and test results to structured clinical notes. The reason for this greatly reduces the stress on health care providers, allowing them to focus more on caring for patients and less on administrative tasks. A few of the main benefits of automated taking notes is that it makes record keeping more consistent. Artificial intelligence-driven solutions keep things consistent by following established frameworks and clinical requirements. The result reduces down on differences in how data gets recorded (Binhowemel et al., 2023). This makes it easier for different healthcare facilities to work alongside one another and allows medical professionals to communicate to each other. These systems reduce mistakes and missed information by checking patient data against past records, which makes sure that the information is complete and accurate. The integration with electronic health records (EHRs) has made it much easier to automatically create clinical notes. These systems automatically update the records of patients, which cuts down on the need to enter the same information over and over again and makes sure that healthcare workers always have access to the most up-to-date medical information. Several AI-powered systems could assist with therapy by looking at past data, finding important patterns, and suggesting possible diagnoses (Guan et al., 2023).

4.3 *Medical Coding and Billing Automation*

The medical coding and the billing automation employ an AI to make it easier to assign the conventional codes to the operations, diagnoses, and the procedures. In the past, competent workers possessed to peruse through patient records by hand and then transform clinical data into standardized codes like SNOMED CT, CPT, and ICD-10. Automation powered by artificial intelligence accelerates this process by looking at electronic health records (EHRs) and making precise codes (Waring et al., 2020). This reduces human error and boosts worker efficiency. Some of the best things about automated medical coding is the fact that it is capable of making things more accurate and compliant. Through natural language processing (NLP), AI systems ensure sure that the right codes have been employed by looking at lab results, clinical documentation, and healthcare provider notes (Nezamabadi et al., 2022). The result lessens the differences that may give rise to audits or insurance claims being denied. Automatic systems additionally update coding systems in real time so that their bodies can keep up with changes to medical coding standards and rules (Coronato et al., 2020). The use of automation makes revenue cycle management more efficient by cutting the delays in making claims and getting paid. Artificially intelligent billing systems identify any incorrect or incomplete information before claims are sent out in. This cuts down on denied claims and helps medical providers get paid faster. Furthermore, by foreseeing potential claims issues, these technologies aid companies in implementing proactive corrective measures (Sarvamangala & Kulkarni, 2022).

4.4 Decision Support and Predictive Analytics

Decision support and predictive analytics (Maheshwari et al., 2025) have begun healthcare by using artificial intelligence to help healthcare providers to make the smart medical decisions and predict the manner in which patients will respond to treatment (Chinnasamy et al., 2025). Artificial intelligence-based decision support systems examine a lot of clinical data and identify the patterns, trends, and possible dangers that healthcare professionals might not have been able to see at that moment. These systems give healthcare providers real time suggestions that are informed by the person's health history, lab results, and current medical literature (Sreedhar et al., 2025). This helps these individuals make treatment decisions based on evidence. To identify and prevent diseases promptly. The predictive analytics seems very important. Although severe symptoms appear, machine learning algorithms examine medical records to find those individuals who are at a higher risk for diseases like heart disease, diabetes, or sepsis. This makes simpler to act quickly and create customized treatment plans, which improves patient outcomes while lowering hospital readmissions and healthcare costs. A significant advantage of AI-driven decision support is the fact that it can help make diagnoses more accurate. AI can offer potential illnesses, propose more tests, and identify possible drug interactions by comparing patient data with large medical knowledge databases. This helps doctors deal with challenging circumstances and makes it less likely that they will make mistakes when diagnosing patients. AI may be able to forecast the number of patients that will be admitted, improve how staff is split up, and figure out which supplies will be needed, all of which will lead to better use of resources. This also helps find mistakes in billing and claims handling, which helps stop fraud and save money.

5 Conclusion

The natural language processing (NLP) has transformed healthcare documentation much more accurate and the efficient. The automation of clinical note generation that uses the text to speech transcription, and medical coding have each made workflows easier, and this has made it easier for healthcare professionals to do their jobs. The support of decisions and the predictive analytics make healthcare decisions even better by giving a real time information and tailored made suggestions. Notwithstanding with these improvements, there are still problems like making sure that the data is accurate in context, which maintaining it private, and making sure it works well with existing systems. In the future, the focus will be on making it easier to understand the context, reducing bias, and making it easier for institutions to work together. Deep learning models, which include transformers and large-scale language processing frameworks, are expected to enhance the process of getting information out of documents, thereby rendering documentation systems easier to use as well as more accurate. To earn the trust of healthcare professionals and make sure that technology that makes decisions is open and honest, models that can be explained will be very important. The artificially intelligent automation has transformed the way medical records are kept by making them more efficient, standardized, and better for the patients. By getting rid of boring tasks, doctors and nurses will have more time caring for patients instead of doing paperwork. As these technologies become better, the focus will be ensuring that they follow the rules that are used in a way that is ethical and keep data safe. The next generation of documentation systems will continue to be driven by ongoing innovation and collaboration between industries. These systems will assist in making healthcare safer, more accessible, and smarter while still protecting patient safety and trust.

References

Alpaydin, E. (2020). *Introduction to machine learning*. MIT Press.

Binhowemel, S., Alfakhri, M., AlReshaid, K., & Alyani, A. (2023). Role of artificial intelligence in diabetes research diagnosis and prognosis: A narrative review. *Journal of Health Informatics Developing Countries, 17*, 1–12.

Chinnasamy, P., Subashini, B., Ayyasamy, R. K., Kiran, A., Pandey, B. K., Pandey, D., & Lelisho, M. E. (2025). Blockchain based electronic educational document management with role-based access control using machine learning model. *Scientific Reports, 15*(1), 18828.

Coronato, A., Naeem, M., De Pietro, G., & Paragliola, G. (2020). Reinforcement learning for intelligent healthcare applications: A survey. *Artificial Intelligence in Medicine, 109*, Article 101964.

Davenport, T. H. (2018). *The AI advantage: How to put the artificial intelligence revolution to work*. MIT Press.

DuBois, K. N. (2019). Deep medicine: How artificial intelligence can make healthcare human again. *Perspectives on Science and Christian Faith, 71*, 199–201.

Guan, Z., Li, H., Liu, R., Cai, C., Liu, Y., Li, J., Wang, X., Huang, S., Wu, L., & Liu, D. (2023). Artificial intelligence in diabetes management: Advancements, opportunities, and challenges. *Cell Reports Medicine, 4*, Article 101213.

Hosny, A., Parmar, C., Quackenbush, J., Schwartz, L. H., & Aerts, H. J. (2018). Artificial intelligence in radiology. *Nature Reviews Cancer, 18*, 500–510.

Huang, S., Yang, J., Fong, S., & Zhao, Q. (2020). Artificial intelligence in cancer diagnosis and prognosis: Opportunities and challenges. *Cancer Letters, 471*, 61–71.

Kagiyama, N., Shrestha, S., Farjo, P. D., & Sengupta, P. P. (2019). Artificial intelligence: Practical primer for clinical research in cardiovascular disease. *Journal of the American Heart Association, 8*, Article e012788.

LeCun, Y., Bengio, Y., & Hinton, G. (2015). Deep learning. *Nature, 521*, 436–444.

Maheshwari, R. U., Paulchamy, B., Pandey, B. K., & Pandey, D. (2025). Enhancing sensing and imaging capabilities through surface plasmon resonance for deepfake image detection. *Plasmonics, 20*(5), 2945–2964.

McCorduck, P., Cfe, C. (2004). *Machines who think: A personal inquiry into the history and prospects of artificial intelligence.* CRC Press.

Nezamabadi, K., Sardaripour, N., Haghi, B., & Forouzanfar, M. (2022). Unsupervised ECG analysis: A review. *IEEE Reviews in Biomedical Engineering, 16*, 208–224.

Rajpurkar, P., Chen, E., Banerjee, O., & Topol, E. J. (2022). AI in health and medicine. *Nature Medicine, 28*, 31–38.

Sarvamangala, D., & Kulkarni, R. V. (2022). Convolutional neural networks in medical image understanding: A survey. *Evolutionary Intelligence, 15*, 1–22.

Sreedhar, C., Kallam, S., Ghantasala, G. P., Anthoniraj, S., Kumarganesh, S., Sagayam, K. M., Pandey, B. K., & Pandey, D. (2025). Enhancing healthcare data security using RFE and CRHSM for big data. *Computers in Biology and Medicine, 190*, 110063.

Waring, J., Lindvall, C., & Umeton, R. (2020). Automated machine learning: Review of the state-of-the-art and opportunities for healthcare. *Artificial Intelligence in Medicine, 104*, Article 101822.

Fuzzy Logic for Risk Assessment and Early Disease Prediction in Healthcare

Deepali Virmani, Savneet Kaur, Sonakshi Vij, and Vidisha Khetarpal

Abstract Initially, the medical diagnosis and illness forecasting gets more complicated. Thus, it is necessary to have advanced systems for making decisions that can handle uncertainty and lack of information. The role of expert-driven models in the healthcare sector, highlighting their ability to enhance risk assessment and promote early disease detection. In opposition to traditional statistical and machine learning techniques, these mathematical models blend expert knowledge with computational reasoning, facilitating making decisions that are adaptable, interpretable, and adaptable. The main benefits are that these experts are capable of looking at ambiguous or unreliable medical data, facilitate approximate thinking, and make diagnoses more accurate. A comparative analysis indicates that while machine learning models achieve high accuracy, they ought to often lack transparency, which makes them difficult to interpret in clinical settings. On the other however, expert systems provide a more straightforward framework. Therefore, being suitable for medical professionals seeking reliable and comprehensible support for decision tools. The findings demonstrate that the integration of these technologies into healthcare could significantly improve disease prevention and patient outcomes via early detection and timely interventions. Incorporating real-time processes for learning, strengthening rule-based frameworks, and addressing ethical concerns to enable widespread adoption in medical practice.

Keywords Fuzzy logic · Disease prediction · Healthcare AI · Medical diagnosis · Uncertain data · Decision support · Machine learning

---

D. Virmani (✉) · S. Kaur
Department of Information Technology, Guru Tegh Bahadur Institute of Technology, GGSIPU, New Delhi, India
e-mail: Deepalivirmani@gmail.com

S. Vij
VSET, VIPS-TC, New Delhi, India

V. Khetarpal
Department of ECE, Guru Tegh Bahadur Institute of Technology, GGSIPU, New Delhi, India

D. Pandey et al. (eds.), *Smart Healthcare*,
https://doi.org/10.1007/978-981-95-8828-2_12

1 Introduction

In the field of healthcare, the risk assessment has become an important step in figuring out the reason that endanger the wellness of a patient, clinical results, and the overall efficiency of the system of healthcare. It entails the proper identification, analysis, and the mitigation of risks related to the medical conditions, treatments, and an operational procedure. The medical community can estimate the likelihood of a disease onset and then further take necessary steps towards avoiding it. By carefully and systematically examining things like the individual's past health status, lifestyle, and genetic predisposition. Thorough risk assessment makes patients safer, cuts down on readmissions to the hospital, and enables medical facilities use their resources better. The statistical models, expert judgement, and rule-based frameworks have been employed in traditional risk assessment to figure which health risks might happen. These methods provide us valuable knowledge, but they often have trouble with inconsistencies, insufficient information, and personal bias. The medical conditions tend not to adhere to strict trends, which makes it hard to use traditional methods to make accurate conclusions. In these situations, novel computational models like fuzzy logic, artificial intelligence, and machine learning provide greater flexible and precise ways to assess risk. These innovations facilitate sophisticated the choice making, permitting healthcare practitioners to look into ambiguous or overlapping symptoms. As diseases get more complicated and the population ages, along with changing environmental factors, the world requires more advanced risk assessment models. In order to prevent serious problems, conditions such as heart disease, diabetes, and cancer need to be found early. Particularly, the risk assessment tools along with the tailor preventive measures, ensure that medical responses have been quick. By employing real-time data from electronic health records, wearable devices, and genetic testing makes risk prediction even more accurate. The healthcare risk assessment also includes the systemic risks like hospital infections, medication errors, and ineffectiveness in treatment, in addition to risks that exist for an individual patient. A thorough assessment of these factors facilitates to improve the policymaking and healthcare administration. As medical science develops, risk assessment methodologies evolve, including emerging technologies that improve predictive capabilities and enhance patient outcomes.

1.1 Early Disease Prediction in Preventive Medicine

The proactive illness forecasting has become essential in preventive medicine. It enables the timely treatments, reduces the price of healthcare, and enhances patient outcomes. Through identifying risk factors and diagnosing diseases from their inception. A healthcare providers may undertake preventive measures, modifications to lifestyles, as well as early interventions to mitigate disease progression. This preventative strategy shifts the focus from reactive medical care to prevention, and these eases the burden on healthcare systems. Advances in healthcare technology, computational intelligence, and data analytics have made significant improvements in the accuracy of predicting diseases. These models examine the medical history of an individual, predisposition to genes, influences from the environment, and current health data in order to determine out how susceptible they have been to get certain diseases (Chen et al., 2022). This makes more straightforward to find individuals who are at high risk, which allows for targeted tests and personalized preventive treatments. In chronic diseases such as diabetes and cardiovascular disease, being able to predict them beforehand enables it easier to make changes to diet, exercise, and medications, which lowers the risk of serious complications. Initial detection supports efforts to improve public health by giving policymakers the information required to make decisions based on data regarding the best way to stop diseases from spreading. By looking at patterns within the population as a whole, healthcare professionals are able to come up with campaigns to raise awareness, vaccination programmes, as well as early screening strategies to stop outbreaks of disease and lower death rates. This becomes especially important for determining the illnesses that are infectious, in which a quick detection and control measures may prevent the further spread of the disease. Beginning illness prediction faces challenges such as concerns about data confidentiality, the need for high-quality information, and ensuring the reliability of model accuracy across diverse populations. The right data management, continual model improvements, and connections to healthcare infrastructure might assist in making predictive systems work better by reducing these issues. In conclusion, using early disease prediction improves the practice of preventive medicine that leads to healthier people and better healthcare delivery (Sun & Zhang, 2021).

1.2 Fuzzy Logic and Its Relevance in Healthcare

Fuzzy reasoning has become a complex computing tool designed to assist people make decisions by dealing with ambiguity and vagueness. This method enables present different levels of truthfulness, that lets believe more freely. The aforementioned differentiates itself from standard binary platforms, which allow it to determine whether something is true or false. It is very helpful while attempting to deal with information that is ambiguous, has insufficient details, or has been inconsistent (ISO & SAE, 2021). In the field of healthcare, it is an extremely significant position to deal with the complicated nature of medical evaluation and therapy. As soon as healthcare providers make choices about medical treatment, they ought to often have to deal with ambiguous facts because symptoms cannot always be matched up with a set list of diseases. It can be hard to classify and predict illnesses because the symptoms are able to be very different from one patient to the subsequent one. This method could make diagnoses more reliable since it enables medical professionals look at the information the patient provides them in more detail. This application helps bring together numerous kinds of information like clinical findings, medical history, and laboratory outcomes that may not always be clear or consistent. It enhances the ability to model complex interactions between various health determinants, which include lifestyle choices, genetic predispositions, and environmental influences. Given that this method can be used in many different ways, medical professionals can create customized treatment plans for their patients. This is especially helpful for people with chronic illnesses or conditions that have multiple risk factors. This strategy assists in identifying diseases early and keeps an eye on risk by processing unclear data and providing more flexible explanations. This leads to better outcomes for patients in the long run. By incorporating this technology into clinical decision support systems facilitates timely implementation of treatments and enhances preventative care efforts (Macher et al., 2015).

2 Fundamentals of Fuzzy Logic

2.1 Principles of Fuzzy Logic

Fuzzy logic is a type of mathematical procedure that helps people function in situations in which the information does not appear to be accurate, as well as has no clear boundaries. This method enables statements to have different levels of truth, opposed to classical Boolean logic that permits statements be true or false. This is based on the idea of partial association, which means that an element could belong to more than one set with different levels of certainty. Given that it is so flexible, it functions well for modelling actual circumstances, which are unclear and subjective. The membership functions, linguistic variables, and a rule-based inference mechanism have been the main parts of this reasoning system. The member functions demonstrate the extent that an input fits into a specific group, with 0 meaning "utterly untrue" and 1 meaning "fully true". The values in between indicate the manner in which much of the truth is present. Words such as "high temperature" or "moderate risk" facilitate the transformation of numbers into human-like logical thinking. If–then rules are utilized for processing all of these variables. These constraints have been exactly, what this system employs to make decisions. There are actually three main steps in the inductive process: fuzziness, rules evaluation, and defuzzification of information. This process transforms clear numbers into fuzzy values that work alongside the reasoning model. The rule assessments stage uses established standards in order to figure out the way inputs and outputs are related. This procedure changes the resulting fuzzy values back into a clear result that can be acted upon. This structured method makes simpler to make decisions that are additionally adaptable and malleable, which can be especially helpful in fields where this is hard to make exact classifications. This method is frequently employed in control systems, artificial intelligence, medical diagnosis, and risk assessment due to it makes it easier to solve problems like an individual would have to do. It is an important tool in complex, information-driven environments (Gennarelli & Wodzin, 2005) since it can handle unpredictability well.

2.2 Classical and Fuzzy Logic Systems

One of the most important differences between fuzzy logic and classical logic is the way each system handles uncertainty and imprecision. Fuzzy logic is better for solving real-world problems that are unclear since it permits to think about values that are in between both true and false, while classical logic only works with values, which are either true or false or 0 or 1. Table 1 shows the main distinctions between these two types of platforms. The philosopher Aristotle came up with the idea of bivalence, or bivalence which serves as the basis of classical logic. This principle says that any statement can be true or false. This strict foundation is useful in fields such as math's and computation, in which accuracy has become very important. But it has trouble with situations where the data has become incomplete or unclear, particularly whenever trying to figure out what medical conditions possess symptoms that are similar to each other. The use of fuzzy logic, on the other hand, is intended to permit different levels of truth exist at once. It does not place inputs into an exact yes/no category; instead, it gives each one a membership value between 0 and 1. This number shows how tightly the input fits into a certain group (Baker et al., 1974). It is perfect for applications, which require to operate like human beings, like smart automation, risk evaluation, and decision-making that is driven by AI. Fuzzy-based systems tend to be more adaptable in fields like healthcare, climate control, and robotics since they allow for gradual changes between categories instead of sudden ones. This is an essential tool in the field of current artificial intelligence since it enables to arrive at more accurate predictions and operate with challenging information with lesser difficulty.

3 Risk Assessment in Healthcare Using Fuzzy Logic

3.1 Traditional Risk Assessment

Traditional risk assessment methods within the healthcare industry primarily employ mathematical frameworks, set standards, and the opinions of medical professionals to figure out what might be dangerous. Although a lot of people use these approaches, they ought to have a lot of problems that make them less effective while confronting multifaceted and unclear medical data. Perhaps one of the biggest concerns they endure is that they require accurate and complete information. It can be challenging to classify individuals into high-risk or low-risk groups due to the variability in the severity, frequency, and progression of symptoms associated with numerous medical

Table 1 Classical versus fuzzy logic systems

Feature	Classical logic	Fuzzy logic
Nature	Rigid, binary-based reasoning	Flexible, multi-valued reasoning
truth values	Only two values: 0 (false) and 1 (true)	Infinite values between 0 and 1
Handling of uncertainty	Cannot manage ambiguity or partial truths	Designed to handle imprecise and uncertain data
Decision making	Based on strict conditions (yes/no)	Uses gradual transitions and approximate reasoning
Mathematical model	Based on set theory and crisp logic	Based on fuzzy set theory with membership functions
Suitability for real-world problems	Limited, as most real-life situations are not strictly binary	Highly applicable to complex and vague scenarios
Processing of inputs	Requires precise numerical inputs	Works with linguistic variables and vague inputs
Application areas	Circuit design, digital computing, formal verification	Control systems, AI, robotics, medical diagnosis, decision support systems

conditions. This can make it hard to put patients into one of the above categories. Conventional models have had a hard time dealing with these kinds of modifications, which can lead to wrong diagnosis or an interruption in their use. Another important limitation to keep in mind is the reality that standard assessment frameworks tend to be very flexible (Brenneman et al., 1988). The vast majority traditional methods employ binary or deterministic choice making, which means that conditions are categorized into groups based on set thresholds. For instance, an individual with a blood sugar level slightly lower than the diabetic range may be deemed healthy, despite the presence of additional risk factors. Because of this lack of adaptability, the gradual transition between health statuses doesn't appear to recorded, which makes it more likely that people will be wrongly classified. These strategies typically are unsuccessful, since they fail to incorporate a number of other factors that have a direct impact on the things (ISO, 2022). The healthcare professionals conduct risk assessments; they ought to look at a number of things, such as predisposition to disease, ways of life, and environmental factors. Conventional approaches have a hard time looking at and comparing all of these different factors, resulting in the risk assessment too simple. The programmes are unable to effectively handle inadequate or ambiguous data, a common issue in real medical records. Neglecting bad information or making wrong assumptions regarding other information could render risk estimates less accurate. The limitations of traditional methods have been highlighted by the escalating complexity of diseases and the diversity of patient populations. Traditional frameworks cannot deliver ongoing monitoring and flexible risk frameworks that are essential for the management of chronic conditions like cancer and cardiovascular diseases. These problems show that humans need more advanced techniques like fuzzy logic and machine learning that can better deal with uncertainty and give us risk assessments that are more accurate and tailored to our needs (Zadeh, 1965).

3.2 Fuzzy Logic in Medical Risk Analysis

Accurate and flexible methods must be developed for medical risk analysis to deal with the difficulties of predicting diseases and evaluating patients. Common methods often use fixed threshold values and deterministic models which can miss important changes in health conditions. A lot of diseases have symptoms that cannot be classified into clear categories. This makes it hard to figure out the level of the risk. To get around these issues, it requires sophisticated computer methods which can handle uncertainty and inaccuracy. In clinical practice, information about patients can frequently be incomplete, subjective, or inconsistent. The genetic predisposition, lifestyle choices, and external variables all play a role in health risks; however, it is hard to figure out the specific ways they work. Traditional approaches have a hard time dealing with this kind of variation that may contribute to either oversimplification or misclassification of risks. To make diagnoses more precise, it requires an approach that is more adaptable that takes into account health indicators which overlap and risk levels that fluctuate gradually. The risk assessment becomes more like actual medical situations as soon as it is adding a reasoning system that permits for truths that are incomplete. This method examines at the amount of vulnerability a patient demonstrates as opposed to simply stating whether or not they have an illness or condition. In particular, a level of cholesterol found to be slightly higher than normal might not promptly indicate heart disease. But if paired with additional risk factors, the risk increases. This method makes sure that the evaluation will be more thorough, that lowers the risk of incorrect diagnosis or delayed treatment. The addition of smart models to clinical decision support systems makes them better at predicting things (Saravanakumar et al., 2024). These models help physicians in evaluating disease risks using multiple variables, even in the absence of certain data points or while uncertainty exists. This method is useful for early disease detection, personalized treatment planning, and long-term health monitoring as it enables the change the evaluations on the spot. This will ultimately contribute to better treatment for patients along with health outcomes.

3.3 Based Risk Models for Disease Prediction

The latest intelligent risk assessment models that use soft computing techniques have been a more advanced way to predict diseases as they deal with unclear and wrong medical data. These systems employ a degree of the truth instead of strict numerical limitations, thereby making it easier to assess health risks in a more adaptable and flexible way. This flexibility becomes particularly useful in healthcare, in which symptoms often intersect and patient data may not be complete or clear. These models work in three primary phases: turning numbers into other numbers, employing rule-based reasoning, and developing clear risk assessments. Initially, information about patients such as age, cholesterol levels, and lifestyle choices are organized into a structured format that can handle various degrees of seriousness. As an example, instead of simply indicating that a blood pressure reading has become "high" or "normal", it provides a value that shows the proximity it falls within either of those categories. This method reduces serious labelling mistakes and makes sure that health problems can be identified correctly. The second level involves making inferences based on rules established by experts that indicate "if this occurs, subsequently that happens". These conditions look at a lot of health markers at once to figure out how likely someone has become to get sick. A rule might say, "If cholesterol levels have been high and blood pressure has become moderately high, then the risk of heart disease has become high". This way of thinking has similarities to the way people make a selection, which makes it easier to do more complex assessments of a risk. The last step turns the identified risk level into an arrangement that is easy to comprehend which helps the healthcare professionals to arrive at smart decisions. These models have been successfully employed in predicting chronic conditions such as diabetes, cardiovascular diseases, and hypertension. They improve early diagnosis, make preventative care more accessible, and improve overall patient outcomes by combining many indicators of wellness and dealing with uncertainty well. Their ability to improve risk assessments makes them an essential part of modern healthcare analytics (Lee, 1990).

4 Fuzzy Logic in Early Disease Prediction

4.1 Fuzzy Systems in Handling Uncertain and Incomplete Data

The fuzzy systems provide a strong way to deal with the uncertainty and a missing data in medical risk assessment. These systems work well with ambiguous, insufficient, or missing information. In contrast to the rigid models that need exact inputs. They permit the move between different levels of a risk gradually, thereby rendering them more useful in real life while symptoms and test outcomes rarely fall into strict categories. The fuzzy-based models provide a thorough analysis by taking into account a wide range of the elements, such as qualitative and a subjective input such as lifestyle factors or a pain reported by patients. This improves accuracy in forecasting, reduces down on incorrect classification, and enables medical professionals make more accurate decisions, which leads to better patient outcomes and more customized healthcare solutions. The fuzzy-based systems use to offer a

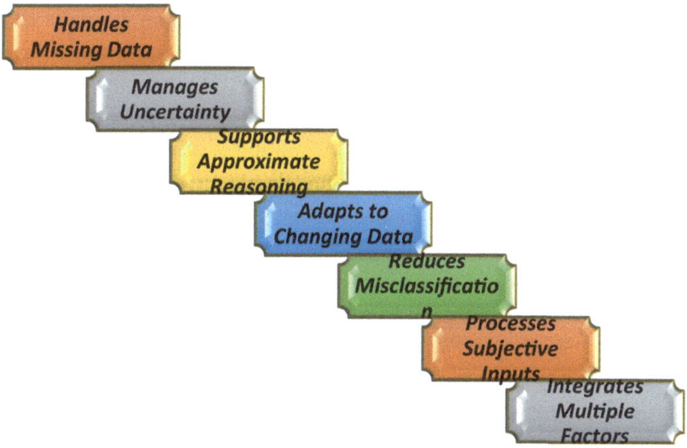

Fig. 1 Benefits of fuzzy systems for uncertain and incomplete data

more adaptable and dependable approach to medical risk analysis by tackling the unpredictability, insufficient information, and a complicated relationships among risk factors, which leads to an enhanced early disease detection and a superior patient care. Figure 1 shows how fuzzy systems may be beneficial when the information is uncertain or incomplete.

- *Handles Missing Data*: Medical records are often incomplete due to missing test results, unrecorded symptoms, or patient-reported gaps. Traditional models either discard incomplete data or make rigid assumptions that may lead to inaccurate conclusions. Fuzzy-based systems, however, can process missing values by assigning degrees of relevance to available information, ensuring a more reliable risk assessment even with partial data sets. This capability is especially useful in emergency care, where quick decisions must be made despite incomplete patient histories.
- *Manages Uncertainty*: Many diseases, such as diabetes and hypertension, do not have strict symptom boundaries. Patients may exhibit varying degrees of risk factors that do not fit into predefined categories. Classical models struggle with such cases, often misclassifying borderline conditions. Fuzzy-based approaches allow for partial memberships in multiple risk categories, capturing subtle variations and improving diagnostic precision. This is particularly beneficial in diseases where early symptoms are vague or progress over time.
- *Supports Approximate Reasoning*: Medical professionals often use qualitative terms like "moderate risk" or "slightly elevated" rather than precise numerical values. Traditional models require exact thresholds, making decision-making rigid and less reflective of real-world scenarios. Fuzzy-based models incorporate linguistic terms and allow for gradual transitions between risk levels, enhancing the interpretability of results. This flexibility helps doctors make better-informed decisions, especially when dealing with ambiguous or borderline cases.

- *Adapts to Changing Data*: Health conditions are dynamic, with risk factors evolving due to lifestyle changes, medication effects, or disease progression. Conventional risk models are often static, unable to adjust to new data in real time. Fuzzy-based systems, on the other hand, continuously update input parameters, ensuring that risk predictions remain relevant and accurate as patient conditions change. This adaptability is crucial in chronic disease monitoring and personalized treatment planning (Sharma & Obaid, 2020).
- *Reduces Misclassification*: Fixed-threshold models classify patients into strict categories, which may lead to misclassification, particularly in cases where health indicators fall near cutoff points. For example, a patient with a cholesterol level just below the "high-risk" threshold may be labelled as "normal" despite showing other warning signs. Fuzzy-based assessments consider a wider range of contributing factors, assigning appropriate risk levels and reducing the chances of misdiagnosis or delayed treatment.
- *Processes Subjective Inputs*: Some health parameters, such as pain levels, stress, or fatigue, are inherently subjective and difficult to measure numerically. Traditional models struggle to incorporate such qualitative data into risk assessments. Fuzzy-based techniques, however, can translate subjective inputs into meaningful risk evaluations, making them highly effective in areas like mental health assessment, pain management, and lifestyle-based disease prediction.
- *Integrates Multiple Factors*: Diseases often result from a combination of factors, including genetic predisposition, lifestyle habits, environmental conditions, and medical history. Traditional risk models typically analysed each variable separately, which can lead to an oversimplified evaluation. Fuzzy-based systems integrate multiple risk factors simultaneously, capturing interactions between variables and providing a more comprehensive assessment of a patient's health status. This holistic approach improves accuracy and ensures that all relevant information is considered (Fig. 1).

5 Implementation and Computational Aspects

5.1 Designing a Fuzzy Expert System for Healthcare

To create an expert system for a healthcare, it is necessary to take a structured approach that combines the medical knowledge with a computer intelligence. These systems help the healthcare professionals to determine out which illnesses a patient possesses, how harmful they are to their health, and which treatments to suggest, all while navigating uncertainty and insufficient medical data. To design a system, it needs to figure out what the problem involves, determine the right input parameters, establish rules, and then set up a deduction system to draw useful inferences. The initial phase is figuring out which specific healthcare issue the system is attempting to overcome. This could be anything from predicting diseases to helping healthcare professionals determine out what is wrong with a patient to finding the best way to treat them. You should set clear goals, like making diagnoses more accurate, reducing false positives and negatives, and making sure that the tests can be used on different types of patients. To make a system, which fulfils clinical requirements, it is essential to comprehend the context of medicine. Identifying the right input variables has significance for getting a precise evaluation. These variables can be made up of physiological parameters including blood pressure, glucose levels, cholesterol, and body temperature, alongside qualitative data such as reported by patient's symptoms, lifestyle habits, and family history. This method works especially well for combining numbers and phrases, which makes this perfect for dealing with subjective medical information. Following figuring out the input variables, the next step has become to make rules and membership functions. These rules are based on expert medical expertise and clarify the way symptoms and possible diagnoses have been related. The functions of membership give different categories different levels of belonging that allows the system sort patient conditions in an easier manner than traditional binary decision-making. An inference mechanism must be utilized by the system to take inputs and make medical decisions. The inference engine relies on the rules that have already been set up to evaluate patient data and give results which demonstrate risk levels, possible diagnoses, or treatment suggestions. A well-designed expert system helps healthcare professionals make decisions by giving them a reliable way to deal with ambiguity and improve patient outcomes (Gallab et al., 2019).

5.2 Data Collection and Fuzzy Rule Development

High-quality information as well as clear rules have been what makes an expert system in healthcare work (Bowles & Peláez, 1995). Gathering information means getting patient records, outcomes of clinical trials, detector results, and opinions from experts. To be accurate and helpful in many scenarios, these data sets need to be diverse and encompass various demographics, patterns of illness, and environmental factors. The Electronic health records (EHRs), outcomes from wearable devices, and actual patient inputs from questionnaires or consultations are all possible sources of data (Gargama & Chaturvedi, 2011). This has great significance to make sure that the data is correct. This means doing things including normalizing, dealing with values that are missing, and getting rid of discrepancies. After collecting information, the next step has become to create rules which transform medical knowledge through logical ways to make decisions. These rules clarify the way symptoms, risk factors, and possible health problems have been related to each other. Expert input has become very important for making these standards. It usually comes from clinical guidelines, past instances, and the experiences of medical professionals. The set of rules must be able to evolve as fresh medical information comes to light or patient trends change. Development of membership functions has become an important part of building rules since it decides how input values are grouped. For instance, a blood pressure reading might be divided into the "low," "normal," and "high" groups based on the ranges instead of a strict limit. This flexibility makes it easier to accurately (Sreedhar et al., 2025) describe health conditions that cuts down on misclassification. Making certain that the rules are correct has been an important aspect of making sure the system is accurate (Pandey & Pandey, 2025). To improve the clinical decision-making framework, the developed model has been evaluated towards historical medical cases and real-time patient data. It is also possible to add continuous learning mechanisms that change the rules based on new information about healthcare, which makes the system more flexible over time.

6 Comparative Analysis with Other Predictive Models

This is necessary to compare expert systems in healthcare to other predictive models, such as statistical methods, machine learning algorithms, and rule-based expert systems, in order to determine how well they work. Every approach has advantages and disadvantages, thereby rendering it better or worse for different healthcare applications. The logistic regression model and Bayes networks tend to be two examples of traditional statistical models that depend on set mathematical relationships between the variables (Pandey et al., 2024). These models function well for problems that have been clearly defined, but they have trouble with data that does not seem clear or certain. Expert systems, on the other hand, tend to be more flexible as they can handle partial truths and approximate reasoning. This makes them more appropriate for complicated medical situations. Artificial neural networks, decision trees, and support vector machines have been all examples of machine learning models that have become widely utilized because they can learn patterns from large amounts of medical data. These mathematical representations are often very accurate, but require a lot of labelled data and computational resources. They work as "black boxes", which makes it hard for healthcare professionals to understand their methods to make decisions. On the other hand, expert systems tend to be more transparent and simpler to understand, so this makes them better for medical decision-making. Similar to expert-driven models, rule-based expert systems rely on rules that have already been set up. But they cannot be modified easily because rule sets need to be updated by hand while new medical knowledge emerges out. Adaptive models, on the other hand, are able of handling the changing information sets through incorporating in real-time inputs and changing the decision parameters when necessary (Gargama & Chaturvedi, 2011). By looking at the pros and cons of the different types of the predictive techniques. An expert-driven models stand out as a useful tool for the healthcare professionals, especially when an uncertainty, qualitative inputs, and explainability have been important. They are a good choice for the risk assessment, disease prediction, and a personalized treatment planning since they may combine expert knowledge with computer-based reasoning.

7 Conclusion

The implementation of expert-driven systems in healthcare has shown significant potential in improving risk assessment for disease forecasting, and clinical decision-making. These approaches provide a versatile and the comprehensible means of addressing uncertainty and ambiguous medical data, that transcending the limitations of traditional statistical and a machine learning methodology. In contrast to the traditional methods that rely on rigid thresholds or require huge data sets, these systems offer a flexibility and that openness that makes them an ideal for use in the medicine. The consequences of these advancements include not only improved disease forecasting but also comprehensive improvements within healthcare. The data-driven expert models are capable of looking at the complicated patient data to find the early warning signs. This allows medical professionals take immediate action that lowers the number of a hospital stays and improves the patient outcomes. Combining them in telemedicine, wearable devices, and personalized treatment could enhance to preventive care by finding an individual who are at risk of getting a serious illness before they happen. These systems can help medical professionals make informed decisions by giving them access to current patient data and expert opinions. This will lead to a more effective and a compassionate healthcare system. Although the current implementations show potential, an additional study is required to refine these models as well as expand their scope of an application. Future research ought to concentrate on an enhancing adaptability by incorporating the immediate learning systems that modify decision-making criteria in accordance with evolving medical knowledge. The cooperation between medical professionals, data scientists, and AI researchers from the different fields will assist to make rules and make sure that these systems meet a real-time medical requirement. For widespread adoption, it will be important to deal with a problem related to the ethics, data protection, and complying with the rules. By continuing to improve an expert-driven approach, healthcare systems can progress towards more intelligent, more efficient, and increasingly personalized ways to care for patients.

References

Baker, S. P., O'neill, B., Haddon, W. J., & Long, W. B. (1974). The injury severity score: A method for describing patients with multiple injuries and evaluating emergency care. *Journal of Trauma and Acute Care Surgery, 14*, 187.

Bowles, J. B., & Peláez, C. (1995). Fuzzy logic prioritization of failures in a system failure mode, effects and criticality analysis. *Reliability Engineering and System Safety, 50*, 203–213.

Brenneman, F. D., Boulanger, B. R., McLellan, B. A., & Redelmeier, D. A. (1988). Measuring injury severity: Time for a change. *Journal of Trauma and Acute Care Surgery, 44*, 580.

Chen, L., Li, Y., Huang, C., Li, B., Xing, Y., Tian, D., Li, L., Hu, Z., Na, X., Li, Z., et al. (2022). Milestones in autonomous driving and intelligent vehicles: Survey of surveys. *IEEE Transactions on Intelligent Vehicles, 8*, 1046–1056.

Gallab, M., Bouloiz, H., Alaoui, Y. L., & Tkiouat, M. (2019). Risk assessment of maintenance activities using fuzzy logic. *Procedia Computer Science, 148*, 226–235.

Gargama, H., & Chaturvedi, S. K. (2011). Criticality assessment models for failure mode effects and criticality analysis using fuzzy logic. *IEEE Transactions on Reliability, 60*, 102–110.

Gennarelli, T. A., & Wodzin, E. A. I. S. (2005). A contemporary injury scale. *Injury, 2006*(37), 1083–1091.

ISO/SAE 21434 (2021). Road Vehicles—Cybersecurity engineering. international organization of standardization, society of automotive engineers. Geneva, Switzerland; Warrendale, PA, USA, 2021.

ISO 21448. (2022). Road vehicles—Safety of the intended functionality. International Organization of Standardization: Geneva, Switzerland.

Lee, C. C. (1990). Fuzzy logic in control systems: Fuzzy logic controller. I. *IEEE Transactions on Systems, Man, and Cybernetics, 20*, 404–418.

Macher, G., Sporer, H., Berlach, R., Armengaud, E., & Kreiner, C. (2015). SAHARA: A security-aware hazard and risk analysis method. In *Proceedings of the 2015 Design, Automation & Test in Europe Conference & Exhibition, Grenoble, France, 9–13 March 2015* (pp. 621–624).

Pandey, B. K., Pandey, D., & Lelisho, M. E. (2024). Face mask identification with enhanced cuckoo optimization and deep learning-based faster regional neural network. *Scientific Reports, 14*(1), 29719.

Pandey, B. K., & Pandey, D. (2025). Securing healthcare medical image information using advance morphological component analysis, information hiding systems, and hybrid convolutional neural networks on IoMT. *Computers in Biology and Medicine, 185*, 109499.

Saravanakumar, R., TamilSelvi, T., Pandey, D., Pandey, B. K., Mahajan, D. A., & Lelisho, M. E. (2024). Big data processing using hybrid Gaussian mixture model with salp swarm algorithm. *Journal of Big Data, 11*(1), 167.

Sharma, S., & Obaid, A. J. (2020). Mathematical modelling, analysis and design of fuzzy logic controller for the control of ventilation systems using MATLAB fuzzy logic toolbox. *Journal of Interdisciplinary Mathematics, 23*, 843–849.

Sreedhar, C., Kallam, S., Ghantasala, G. P., Anthoniraj, S., Kumarganesh, S., Sagayam, K. M., Pandey, B. K., & Pandey, D. (2025). Enhancing healthcare data security using RFE and CRHSM for big data. *Computers in Biology and Medicine, 190*, 110063.

Sun, F. R., & Zhang, P. (2021). A survey on cyber-security of connected and autonomous vehicles (CAVs). *IEEE Transactions on Intelligent Transportation Systems, 23*, 6240–6259.

Zadeh, L. A. (1965). Fuzzy sets. *Information and Control, 8*, 338–353.

AI-Based Clinical Decision Support Systems for Smart Healthcare

Manish Rai, Shishir B. Nuti, V. Purushothama Raju, Pallavin Shetty, Kamasaisvm, Joshuva Arockia Dhanraj, and Hassan Khalid Abozibid

Abstract The use of intelligent decision support systems in healthcare has marked an improved clinical decision-making. Resulting a greater diagnostic precision, tailored treatment approaches, and an effective patient management. These systems utilize an extensive dataset, predictive analytics, and a real-time monitoring to enhance the medical processes and to assist healthcare professionals in providing prompt and evidence-based care. Their influence transcends a singular clinical environment that providing solutions for early disease identification, remote patient surveillance, and the resource optimization, especially used in the underprivileged areas. Although they possess transformative potential, issues such as data privacy, algorithmic bias, and regulatory compliance must be resolved to guarantee ethical deployment. The standardization and interoperability are considered as an essential item for efficient data interchange among healthcare systems, that facilitating a more

M. Rai (✉)
Department of Computer Science and Engineering (AI&ML), Manipal University Jaipur, Jaipur, India
e-mail: manishrai2587@gmail.com; manish.rai@jaipur.manipal.edu

S. B. Nuti
BGS Global Institute of Medical Sciences, Bengaluru, India

V. P. Raju
CSE, Shri Vishnu Engineering College for Women, Bhimavaram, Andhra Pradesh, India
e-mail: praju@svecw.edu.in

P. Shetty
NMAM Institute of Technology, Nitte (Deemed to Be University), Karkalla Taluk, Udupi District, Karnataka, India
e-mail: pallavirjsh@nitte.edu.in

Kamasaisvm
KL College of Law, Koneru Lakshmaiah Education Foundation Vaddeswaram, Guntur District, Andhra Pradesh, India

J. A. Dhanraj
Research and Development Cell, Lovely Professional University, Jalandhar-Delhi, Phagwara, Punjab, India

H. K. Abozibid
Al-Zahrawi University College, Karbala, Iraq

D. Pandey et al. (eds.), *Smart Healthcare*,
https://doi.org/10.1007/978-981-95-8828-2_13

integrated and cooperative approach to patient care. The establishment of transparent and accountable frameworks is crucial for fostering the trust in these technologies and alleviating a danger linked to the automated decision-making. The fundamental functions, technological innovations, and practical applications of an intelligent clinical decision support systems that emphasizing their influence on the future of global healthcare. By harmonizing innovation with ethical considerations and regulatory supervision, these systems can substantially enhance medical efficiency, minimize errors, and improve overall patient outcomes.

Keywords Clinical decision support · Predictive analytics · Medical data integration · Healthcare interoperability · AI

1 Introduction

The making of clinical decisions as traditionally depended on the expertise and experience of healthcare providers, in conjunction with medical guidelines, diagnostic tests, and histories of patients. Healthcare providers and other experts use their expertise to examine at symptoms, investigate at lab data, and decide on treatment based on prevailing medical standards. This strategy has performed well, but it is limited by the extent to which people are able to think, how influenced they might have been, and the way different practitioners make decisions. The conventional approaches might require a long time and are incapable of taking into account the vast and the constantly growing body of the medical information. The process of digitizing healthcare systems has made electronic health records (EHRs) possible, which makes it easier to document and find patient information. The growing complexity of illnesses along with the large amount of medical literature. The requirement for precision medicine have shown that individuals need the better decision support tools. This need has culminated in the use of artificial intelligence (AI) in making decisions about healthcare. The AI-powered Clinical Decision Support Systems (CDSS) employ machine learning, natural language processing (NLP), and big data analytics in order to assist healthcare professionals diagnose illnesses, recommend treatments, and predict how patients will do with more accuracy. AI-driven Clinical Decision Support Systems are capable of looking at large datasets all at once, find patterns that human medical professionals might miss, and give data driven insights that help doctors make decisions based on evidence. This is different from traditional methods and these algorithms are always learning and changing as they look at more patient data. The AI-driven decision-making signifies a revolutionary advancement in the contemporary healthcare by diminishing human errors, decreasing misdiagnoses, and optimizing clinical workflows, thereby facilitating more intelligent, efficient, and personalized medical care.

1.1 AI in Modern Healthcare Systems

The use of cutting-edge computer technology has changed a lot about the medical services that are available today. These systems use big datasets and complicated algorithms to make diagnoses accurate enough to speed up dealing with administrative duties, and improve the care that patients are given. The medical community has the ability to make smart decisions since they can quickly understand complicated information. This cuts down on mistakes and presents a more treatment options. Prevention of diseases earlier in life is probably the most important thing these smart solutions are used over at the moment. The pattern recognition algorithms examine imaging data, test results, and patient histories to find illnesses that include cancer, heart problems, and neurological diseases via more accuracy. This ability facilitates the step in shortly which could mean that more patients survive treatment and that drugs work better. These technologies make personalized healthcare possible by letting doctors change treatment plans based on each patient's genetics, lifestyle, and medical history. The assessment of large-scale clinical data (Tian et al., 2019) aids physicians in recommending optimal treatments for individual patients, thereby minimizing side effects and expediting recovery. This method can be very helpful in medical treatment for cancer, where picking the right mix of drugs can have a big impact on the way patients respond to treatment. An essential component of running a hospital and making sure that patients and staff get along is making sure that computers work. The virtual assistants and interactive platforms might be able to help with more than simply making appointments, urging people to take their prescribed medications, and looking for early signs of illness. Healthcare facilities may utilize better use of their resources by using predictive models to figure out the number of individuals will be admitted. This helps make sure that medical facilities are used correctly and lowers the chances of them getting too crowded. The study of pharmaceuticals and the discovery of new drugs is a further significant consideration. The research community are able to employ computer simulations to look at molecular structures, anticipate the manner in which drugs will work together, and speed up the search for new drugs. This has been shown to be very useful during global health emergencies, while quick action and the development of effective treatments are very important. There have been a number big steps ahead, but there are still problems that need to be fixed, such as data privacy, moral dilemmas, and following the rules. It is important to deal with any possible biases while ensuring sure that automated processes for making decisions have been clear. So that people are capable of trusting those systems. These advances in technology, on the other hand, have been developed, to make medical services substantially better by making them more accurate, faster, and easier to get to. Numerous individuals anticipate that this revolution will keep going because it will continue to get better (Nasr et al., 2021).

2 Fundamentals of AI-Powered CDSS

2.1 Core Functionalities of CDSS

A Clinical Decision Support System (CDSS) is a complex digital tool that helps healthcare professionals make quick and accurate clinical decisions. The CDSS enhances diagnostic precision, therapeutic methodologies, and a comprehensive patient care by the leveraging extensive medical data, clinical guidelines, and a real patient scenario. Figure 1 shows the main functions of a CDSS. These modern innovations help healthcare providers make fewer mistakes, operate more efficiently, and follow proven medical procedures. The Clinical Decision Support System (CDSS) might function on its own or be added to Electronic Health Record (EHR) systems. It helps doctors make decisions in real time at the point of care. The people usually divide them into two groups that knowledge-based systems, that incorporate established medical protocols, and non-knowledge-based systems, and this use machine learning and predictive analytics to give adaptive insights.

1. *Data Processing and Integration*: The CDSS collects and a processes data from a number of sources, such as electronic health records (EHRs), lab results, imaging reports, genomic data, and medical literature. The system integrates these the datasets to create a full and current patient profile that ensuring that the healthcare providers have all the information they must have to make good decisions. The

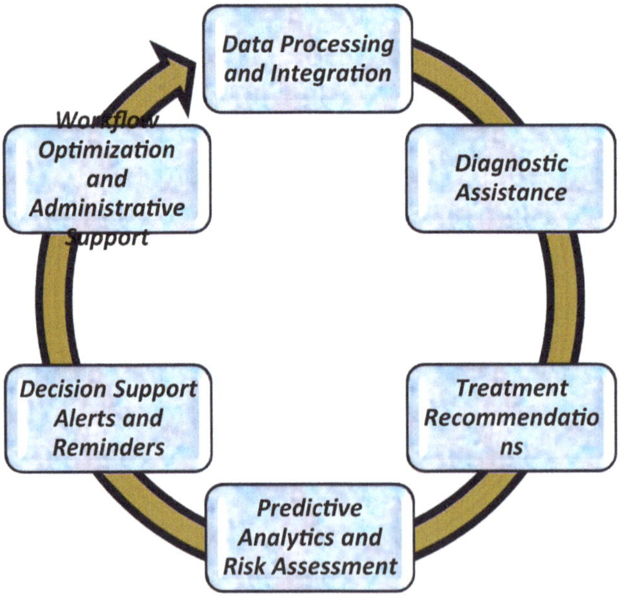

Fig. 1 Key functions of CDSS

ability to combine large amounts of data that is both structured and unstructured reduces error rates, cuts down on duplication, and makes clinical assessments more reliable. The data in real-time synchronization ensures that changes happen all the time, so medical professionals always have the most recent data available.

2. *Diagnostic Assistance*: The Clinical Decision Support System that uses an advanced pattern recognition algorithms to examine at a patient's symptoms, test results, and past medical records to make diagnoses that are more precise. The system makes a differential diagnosis through ranking possible conditions based on the clinical guidelines and a statistical probability. This feature has been particularly helpful for finding rare diseases, figuring out complicated illnesses, and lowering the number of wrong diagnoses. AI-powered image analysis also helps radiologists and pathologists find problems in medical scans including X-rays, MRIs, and CT scans. This cuts down on mistakes made by people and helps find diseases earlier (Chaudhary et al., 2022).
3. *Treatment Recommendations*: The CDSS makes personalized suggested therapies by looking at a variable like a patient age, medical history, genetic profile, and laboratory findings. It indicates the right medicines to determine the right doses and then informs medical professionals about the possible drug interactions, contraindications, and the allergic reactions. When there are additionally, other treatment options available that comprising lifestyle changes or non-drug therapies. The system gives guidance based on evidence. This makes sure that each patient gets the best and safest treatment plan that is right for them.
4. *Predictive Analytics and Risk Assessment*: The CDSS uses a predictive modelling to assess the disease progression, in order to anticipate complications, and also to identify patients at high risk of developing serious conditions. By analysing an historical patient data and the population health trends. The system helps clinicians to implement the preventive strategies to reduce hospital readmissions and manage the appearing chronic diseases in a more effective manner. For example, it can able to predict the likelihood of a patient with diabetes developing complications such as kidney disease, cardiovascular disorders and prompting the early intervention. Additionally, real-time monitoring capabilities enable early detection of critical conditions such as sepsis, stroke, or cardiac arrest, allowing timely medical responses.
5. *Decision Support Alerts and Reminders*: To enhance patient safety and ensure adherence to medical best practices. A CDSS generates an automated alerts and reminders for the healthcare professionals. These notifications include a warning for the abnormal lab results, missed screenings, medication dosage errors, and the required follow-up appointments. The physicians may able to receive reminders for an overdue preventive screening to ensure that patients undergo in the necessary tests for an early disease detection. Similarly, a CDSS can flag potential surgical risks, ensuring that preoperative checklists are followed to minimize complications. By providing real-time decision support, these alerts improve patient outcomes and reduce the risk of medical errors.

6. *Workflow Optimization and Administrative Support*: In addition to the supporting clinical decision-making, a CDSS enhances healthcare facility operations by streamlining administrative tasks. The automated documentation features are used to generate structured clinical notes, discharge summaries, and prescription reports that help for reducing the time of the clinicians and also spend on a manual data entry. The system also optimizes resource management by predicting the patient admissions, ensuring efficient allocation of hospital beds, medical staff, and equipment. The CDSS facilitates the telemedicine services by providing a real-time decision support to a remote healthcare providers for improving accessibility and efficiency in a virtual consultations.

2.2 Traditional and AI-Driven CDSS

The machine learning methods and clinical guidelines are often used in traditional decision support systems. To help the healthcare providers. These systems examine patient data and provide suggestions based on decision trees and IF THEN rules that people have put together by hand. The organization work well in circumstances that are straightforward, but they have trouble with more complicated cases that need adaptive learning and real-time data processing. Implementing conventional models has become hard work for medical professionals since they have to do it by hand. Given that they are so rigid, they are unable to adapt to new medical procedures, methods, and discoveries. Artificial intelligence powered devices learn from huge amounts of patient information, real-time health data, and medical literature employing advanced machine learning and deep learning models. These new methods find patterns and connections that human specialists could have overlooked, which makes them more accurate than systems that only use regulations. The capacity for adaptability keeps guidance up to date with medical knowledge and lets them deal with more difficult issues. Machine learning frameworks can take in new research and suggestions for changes, which gives doctors the most up-to-date information. Another difference is how data is processed and combined. Structured data, like patient demographics, lab results, and medication history, is what traditional models look at. They have a hard time figuring out the use clinical notes, wearable device signals, gene sequencing, and also the unstructured medical images. AI-based methods get around this problem by using big data analytics and natural language processing to look at data from many different places (Solanas et al., 2017). Advanced algorithms can find signs of illness in genetic data or get important information from radiological scans. This makes treatment completer and more personalized. Combining different types of data makes it easier to predict diseases, diagnose them early, and tailor treatment to each person. Conventional systems make suggestions based on set medical standards without taking into account how different patients are. This often leads to a one-size-fits-all approach that could prove unsuccessful for the entire population. Artificial intelligent models make personalized medicine possible by changing treatment to fit the unique requirements of every patient. The organization look at genetic profiles, the extent to which previous treatments worked, lifestyle factors, and environmental factors to make treatments more effective. The latest technologies use data from individual patients to make therapy more effective and reduce side effects, which leads to better health outcomes. Traditional alert systems operate on rules and send out a lot of notifications, which tend to make healthcare workers tired of getting them. Numerous signals, including false positives, cannot be very important in a clinical setting, so healthcare providers may not pay attention to them or ignore them. The artificial intelligence-based systems can use predictive analytics to put high-risk patients first and get rid of unnecessary notification messages. The latest algorithms can predict medical events consisting of strokes and sepsis instead of just finding abnormal test results. This permits healthcare providers act before a disease gets progressively worse. Machine learning-based frameworks maintain patients safer and help workers get more done by cutting down on interruptions and focusing on important alarms. An additional significant distinction has been that decision support seems automated. The conventional techniques require clinicians to assess suggestions and relevance manually (Chui et al., 2017). This could lead to different decisions being made in stressful places like emergency rooms. The artificial intelligence helps doctors make decisions faster by giving them ranked proposals, confidence rankings, and visual statistics. Certain advanced solutions use NLP to summaries patient histories, analyse physician notes, and create automated clinical reports. The result takes some of the mental work off of healthcare workers. Conventional real-time monitoring methods employ retrospective analysis to determine treatments. This strategy is useful, but it doesn't give you quick feedback in important situations. The AI-integrated systems keep an eye on the vitals of individuals, lab values, and other health indicators in real time to find early signs of deterioration. AI can analyse continuous electrocardiogram (ECG) recordings to forecast the cardiac arrest hours in advance and facilitating the medical intervention. Preventive care improves patient outcomes and the use of resources, which means fewer hospital readmissions and unnecessary surgeries (Olawade et al., 2023).

2.3 AI in Clinical Reasoning and Decision-Making

Advanced computational tools have evolved the manner in which doctors think by making medical decisions more accurate and faster. Conventional diagnostic approaches depend on physician proficiency, established medical instructions and accessible patient information. However, as diseases get more complicated and there is more medical information accessible to people, it gets harder to process and understand data correctly. Artificially intelligent systems help solve this problem by looking at massive amounts of data, finding trends, and giving scientific proposals. This helps healthcare providers make decisions that are more accurate and promptly. A number of the best things about these technologies is the fact that they can combine and analyses data from different sources about people with illnesses. The conventional approaches mostly deal with structured data like lab results and patient history.

These contemporary decision support devices on the reverse hand can also use unstructured data like imaging scans, gene sequences, physician notes, and contemporaneous physiological data from wearable devices. By putting together so much details, these systems help find early signs of illness, see patterns that might be neglected, and guess whatever might go wrong. This wider view makes it possible to take a more thorough approach to diagnosis and treatment (Xie et al., 2021). In differential diagnosis, computational models assist clinicians by comparing patient symptoms, diagnostic results, and imaging findings with comprehensive medical databases. For instance, radiology tools with pattern recognition capabilities can find strange things in X-rays, MRIs, and CT scans with amazing accuracy. This helps the radiologists to find diseases like cancer, fractures, or neurological conditions. In the identical way, a predictive model that use genetic and an epidemiological data can help to figure out the spread of certain diseases. This allows the doctors to intervene early and create the personalized preventive strategies. Artificially intelligent systems help with personalized treatment planning by looking at the various variables like medical history, genetic predispositions, and possible drug interactions, in addition to the diagnosis. These solutions are more than standard treatment procedures; instead, they make personalized recommendations based on each individual's unique traits. For example, in oncology, computational models examine tumour genetics and the extent to which treatments work to suggest the best therapies. This improves patient outcomes while reducing unnecessary procedures and side effects. The use of predictive analytics is also very important for figuring out health risks and stopping problems from happening (Paul et al., 2021). These systems can find early warning signs of serious conditions like sepsis, stroke, or cardiac arrest by looking at real-time physiological data. This prompts timely actions. The hospitals can use this information to better use their funds to cut down on emergency patient admissions and make patients safer overall. The technology also helps people to make better decisions by making their work more efficient. The automation of routine administrative tasks like getting medical literature, summarizing patient records, and managing electronic health data makes life easier for healthcare workers. The conversational agents and virtual assistants make the process even easier by giving the instant access to clinical guidelines and recommending the right tests. Due to this efficiency, healthcare providers can spend more time taking care of patients directly instead of doing paperwork. The principles related oversight is still extremely significant. The computational models make things more accurate and efficient, but they do not belong to perfect. The medical community need to carefully consider automated recommendations to make sure they fit with their own clinical judgement and the needs of each patient. To keep trust and reliability in a healthcare setting, these systems need to be open to follow the ethical guidelines, and be checked on a regular basis.

3 AI Technologies in CDSS

An advancement in the intelligent systems has transformed medical decision-making by improving the diagnostic precision, treatment planning, and patient monitoring. Various technologies are as shown in Fig. 2, which contribute to this progress by analysing complex data, recognizing patterns, and providing real-time recommendations.

- *Predictive Models*: Predictive analytics employs machine learning (ML) and deep learning to determine out the state of wellness, the manner in which their disease will progress, along with what the best treatments are for that individual. The machine learning, or ML algorithms, on the other hand, keep improving their forecasting abilities each time they get new data. These models examine at both structured data, like lab test results, medical history, and genetic markers, and unstructured data, like radiology imaging findings and clinical notes. The use of deep learning, especially convolutional neural networks (CNNs), has improved image-based diagnostics a lot better by finding problems in medical images with a lot of exactness. Recurrent neural networks (RNNs) and transformers analyse data in time series, like ECG readings, to identify heart arrhythmias or forecast stroke risks. The ensemble learning techniques also combine several models to provide medical predictions more reliable and robust (Panesar et al., 2019).
- *Language Processing*: Natural language processing (NLP) has become very important for getting useful information from huge amounts of unstructured medical text. Electronic health records (EHRs), physician notes, and published research contain significant data. Although their unstructured format renders the manual analysis more challenging. The NLP algorithms turn this information into a structured information, which makes it is easy to find and to comprehend. The primary application of NLP in healthcare includes a computerised documentation that makes it easier for medical professionals to do their assigned duties. Speech recognition models write down what healthcare professionals and patients say to each other, summarise the most important points, and automatically update

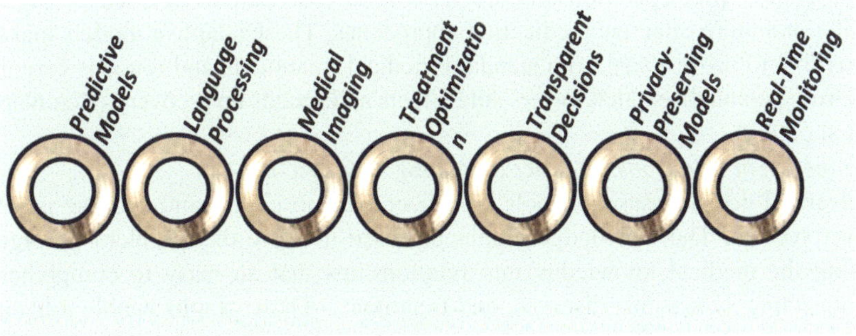

Fig. 2 AI technologies in CDSS

patient records. Clinical chatbots and virtual assistants also use NLP to support healthcare workers by suggesting tests, finding relevant research, and pointing out possible drug interactions. Sentiment analysis within patient-reported outcomes serves in evaluating mental health conditions and the efficacy of treatments. NLP models may identify signs of depression, anxiety, or medication side effects in patient feedback by looking at the language patterns.

- *Medical Imaging*: The computer vision has changed medical imaging by automating the process of finding and classifying diseases in radiological scans. In the past, the medical professionals had to look over X-rays, MRIs, and CT scans by using their hands, which made it more likely that mistakes would be made. The modern vision based models now help doctors find lung nodules, fractures, brain tumours, and the retinal diseases with a great accuracy. In oncology, An AI-powered imaging tools look at histopathological slides to tell the difference between benign and the malignant tumours. These models help radiologists make faster and more accurate diagnoses by comparing new scans to huge databases of labelled medical images. In dermatology, image recognition systems look at skin lesions to see if they are at risk for melanoma. This lets doctors find the disease early and treat it quickly. 3D reconstruction techniques that use computer vision go beyond diagnostics by giving detailed anatomical models that help with planning before surgery, making surgery more accurate, and lowering the risk of complications.
- *Treatment Optimization*: Personalised treatment planning is an essential for enhancing the patient outcomes. The Reinforcement Learning (RL) is being increasingly utilised to refine therapeutic strategies. RL systems learn through trying things out and changing their treatment advise based on the manner in which the patient reacts, rather than traditional models which utilise static datasets. The most common use of RL is in cancer treatment, in which chemotherapy treatments can be changed based on the extent to which a person can handle them in addition to how quickly the tumour has become expanding. RL models improve ventilator settings in Intensive Care Units (ICUs) to make sure that oxygen is delivered quickly and with minimal harm to the lungs as possible. Personalised drug dosing models additionally consider into account things such as metabolism and genetic predisposition that are specific to each patient in order to suggest safer and more effective medication approaches. These adaptive models make it possible to move away from standard medical treatments and towards care that is truly personalised, that lowers side effects and speeds up recovery (Renukappa et al., 2022).
- *Transparent Decisions*: In order to making sure that, the
- advanced decision support tools have been easy to understand and use is for a big problem. The knowledge graphs are used to solve this problem by organising the medical knowledge into relationships that are easy to comprehend, connecting symptoms, diseases, and treatments. These graphs enable a healthcare professional to see the way computerised suggestions have been created, that makes them more trustworthy and an easier to comprehend. The Explainable AI (XAI) makes things even clearer by showing the manner in which models

make decisions. Shapley Additive Explanations (SHAP) a Local Interpretable Model-agnostic Explanations (LIME) are two methods that show which patient-specific factors had the biggest impact on a diagnosis or treatment suggestion. This makes sure that doctors and nurses can carefully look at AI-driven suggestions before using them in real-life situations. These solutions deal with worries about "black-box" AI models by making them easier to understand. They also make sure that decision support tools follow medical guidelines and ethical standards (Kamruzzaman, 2020).

- *Privacy-Preserving Models*: The use of patient data for the training of a predictive models presents a significant privacy and the security challenges. The Federated Learning (FL) provides a solution by allowing institutions to collaboratively train models without sharing the raw patient data. Instead of centralizing a data, this decentralized approach enables an algorithm to learn from multiple sources while maintaining the confidentiality. For example, a hospital across different regions can able to contribute to the training of the diagnostic models without exposing to a sensitive patient information. This not only enhances the data security but also improves the generalizability of a models by incorporating the diverse patient populations. In addition to federated learning, an homomorphic encryption and differential privacy techniques are further use to protect the patient confidentiality. By ensuring that, the data remains anonymized during processing. These advancements make it possible to leverage large-scale healthcare data without compromising an ethical and legal requirements.
- *Real-Time Monitoring*: The wearable devices and Internet of Things (IoT) sensors collect the health data from patients at the time. This enables healthcare professionals take action before any serious problems take place. The use of edge computing helps to speed up this process. By processing data on the device itself, as opposed to in the cloud. This minimises latency time and also speeds up the response times. The smart watches equipped with the ECG sensors can able to identify the early signs of atrial fibrillation. The users and healthcare providers be informed, so that they can act promptly. Continuous glucose monitors (CGMs) monitor blood sugar levels in real time, which helps people with diabetes more effectively control their condition. In hospitals, continuous monitoring systems continually keep an eye on the vital signs of ICU patients in an attempt to anticipate problems like sepsis or respiratory failure. These predictive alerts enable medical staff intervene in before things get worse, which lowers the number of deaths and hospital readmissions. The medical community can move from reactive care to a more preventive and personalised approach by combining real-time analytics with clinical workflows (Jiang et al., 2017).

4 Advanced Implementations of AI-Powered CDSS

Intelligent systems in clinical environments have contributed to the precision and efficacy of decisions in medicine. In addition to supporting with medical evaluation, other uses include personalized planning of therapy, early diagnosis of illness, robotic-assisted therapies, and precision healthcare. The aforementioned new ideas make things better for individuals, reduce the price of healthcare, and make things less difficult for medical staff. The combination of genetics, lifestyle, and pre-existing health issues are capable of rendering traditional therapy techniques less effective for some people. Intelligent systems decision support technologies provide tailored therapeutic solutions by analysing particular to the patient data. These systems employ health information, genetic markers, and responses to therapy to make sure that the procedures have been effective and as little invasive as possible. In oncology, predictive models examine the characteristics of tumours along with the way patients respond to chemotherapy drugs to suggest the best treatment. The cardiologists use risk assessments to figure out which treatment would be best for a patient: medication, lifestyle changes, or surgery. These methods help doctors choose the best treatments to lower the risk of side effects and improve the participant's outlook. Advancement in decision support technology is also helping a lot with early disease detection. In standard diagnostic tests, symptoms may not show up until later in the disease's progression. Through looking at large datasets, sophisticated models can find early signs of cancer, neurological disorders, and metabolic conditions. This makes it possible to do medical procedures ahead of time, which increases survival rates and lowers down on healthcare costs. The robotics of surgeries have benefited from an intelligent decision support system. Robotic devices that guide the surgeons to get better at their occupations and make fewer mistakes (Lytras et al., 2019). These technologies help make repairs and to protect tissue by analysing the anatomy in real time. Robotic-assisted rehabilitation programmes change therapeutic activities based on patient data (Tayefi et al., 2021), which speeds up recovery for people with musculoskeletal and neurological problems. Advanced implementations are also changing how doctors make decisions in precision medicine. By combining genomic data with real-time patient data, smart algorithms can suggest treatments that are tailored to each person's genetics. Genetic differences can change how drugs are broken down in pharmacology. Personalized drug prescriptions make therapy safer and more effective by lowering side effects and increasing effectiveness. Real-time monitoring (Ali et al., 2020) helps people make better decisions about critical care and managing chronic illnesses. Wearable and implanted sensors maintain an eye on physiological data thus letting doctors know about possible problems before they get worse. Early detection and management can save lives for people with diabetes, heart disease, and lung disease. Medical professionals can give better, more personalized care by adding these new technologies to healthcare systems. The use of predictive modelling, robotic-assisted therapies, precision medicine, and real-time monitoring are all changing modern healthcare for the better, making patients better and clinical procedures better.

5 Data Integration and Interoperability

The effective implementation of an intelligent decision support systems in healthcare that relies significantly on seamless data integration and interoperability. The healthcare organizations able to gather a lot of patient data from electronic health records (EHRs), diagnostic imaging, wearable devices, and the lab results (Saravanakumar et al., 2024). To make accurate and timely clinical decisions. They need to be able to combine and also process all of this information. But problems like the data fragmentation, inconsistent formats, and security worries often make it is hard for different healthcare systems to share data quickly and easily (Sreedhar et al., 2025). A substantial component of integration is putting together different data sources into one platform. It is hard for doctors to get a full medical history because patient records, imaging scans, and lab results are often stored in different databases. Advanced data management methods make sure that structured and unstructured data, such as healthcare notes, genetic information, and real-time sensor readings, are all in sync so that you can get a full picture. Standardized protocols that include Health Level Seven (HL7) and Fast Healthcare Interoperability Resources (FHIR) make it easy for different platforms and institutions to share medical information without any problems. The ability to communicate is very important for making sure that different healthcare systems and software can talk to each other. As long as there is no standardization, hospitals and clinics that use different EHR systems may have trouble collaborating effectively, which makes it harder to share patient information promptly (Kumarganesh et al., 2025). Healthcare providers may enhance coordination between specialists, primary care doctors, and emergency responders by using universal data standards and cloud-based infrastructures. This will allow them to share an important information in a real time. As soon as combining medical information from different places, a data security (Pandey et al., 2024) and privacy are considered as a very important pillar. As more people use cloud storage and networked medical devices, it's more important than ever to keep private patient information safe from breaches and unauthorized access. The information stays safe, due to advanced encryption methods, blockchain technology, and the federated learning approaches. These additionally enable different healthcare organizations to work together to analyse the data. The Health Insurance Portability and Accountability Act (HIPAA) and the General Data Protection Regulation (GDPR) are the two examples of regulatory frameworks that used to set rules for keeping data private while applying it in a moral way. The combination of real-time data obtained from wearable devices and the remote monitoring systems makes the decisions even better by giving a constant health information. An automated alerts that enable healthcare providers know about the problems assists patients with chronic conditions like diabetes or high blood pressure get the care required quickly. Healthcare professionals can better track how a disease is getting worse and change treatment plans as needed by combining real-time sensor data with past medical records. Thorough data integration and interoperability (Pandey et al., 2021) not only make work easier. However, they also improve the quality of care for patients by making sure that medical decisions can be made on the most complete and up-to-date information possible. As healthcare systems keep evolving, it will be important to use strong data-sharing tools to improve predictive analytics, precision medicine, and overall clinical efficiency.

6 Conclusion

The advancement of an intelligent decision support systems has transformed, a clinical practice by enhancing the diagnostic accuracy, enhancing the methods of treatment, and improving the overall patient care. This conversation has demonstrated that, by using a modern technology in medical decision-making makes the workflows better and the provision of healthcare more personalized and effective. These systems use large databases, predictive models, and the real-time monitoring to give proactive treatments that lower mistakes and improve the patient outcomes. These smart systems have the power to change the manner, in which healthcare is done around the world. By solving important problems such as limited resources, predicting illnesses, and managing patients from a far. These technologies help bridge the gap in care by providing an evidence-based guidance and facilitating the telemedicine possible in areas where access to specialist medical knowledge is completely restricted. The ability to analyse large amounts of medical data in a real time, makes it easier to find diseases early and keep an eye on epidemics, which in turn makes public health programmes more effective. It is still very important to make sure that intelligent decision-making systems are developed and controlled in an ethical way. As these technologies become more self-sufficient, it is required to pay more attention to problems like a data privacy, algorithmic bias, and who is responsible for the making decisions. By putting in place strong rules and ethical standards. It also requires to ensure that these tools work in a fair, safe, and open way. To make sure they are accurate and avoid unintended results, like unfair healthcare recommendations based on incomplete or biased datasets, these systems need to be watched and updated all the time.

References

Ali, F., El-Sappagh, S., Islam, S. R., Kwak, D., Ali, A., Imran, M., & Kwak, K. S. (2020). A smart healthcare monitoring system for heart disease prediction based on ensemble deep learning and feature fusion. *Information Fusion, 63*, 208–222.

Chaudhary, S., Kakkar, R., Jadav, N. K., Nair, A., Gupta, R., Tanwar, S., Agrawal, S., Alshehri, M. D., Sharma, R., Sharma, G., et al. (2022). A taxonomy on smart healthcare technologies: Security framework, case study, and future directions. *Journal of Sensors, 2022*, 1863838.

Chui, K. T., Alhalabi, W., Pang, S. S. H., Pablos, P. O. D., Liu, R. W., & Zhao, M. (2017). Disease diagnosis in smart healthcare: Innovation, technologies and applications. *Sustainability, 9*, 2309.

Jiang, F., Jiang, Y., Zhi, H., Dong, Y., Li, H., Ma, S., Wang, Y., Dong, Q., Shen, H., & Wang, Y. (2017). Artificial intelligence in healthcare: Past, present and future. *Stroke and Vascular Neurology, 2*.

Kamruzzaman, M. (2020, July 6–10). Architecture of smart health care system using artificial intelligence. In *Proceedings of the 2020 IEEE international conference on multimedia & expo workshops (ICMEW)* (pp. 1–6). London, UK.

Kumarganesh, S., Murugesan, M., Ganesh, C., Santhiyakumari, N., Thangavel, M., Jayaram, K., Martin Sagayam, K., Pandey, B. K., & Pandey, D. (2025). Hybrid plasmonic biosensors with deep learning for colorectal cancer detection. *Plasmonics, 20*(7), 4895–4909.

Lytras, M. D., Chui, K. T., & Visvizi, A. (2019). Data analytics in smart healthcare: The recent developments and beyond. *Applied Sciences, 9*, 2812.

Nasr, M., Islam, M. M., Shehata, S., Karray, F., & Quintana, Y. (2021). Smart healthcare in the age of AI: Recent advances, challenges, and future prospects. *IEEE Access, 9*, 145248–145270.

Olawade, D. B., Wada, O. J., & Ling, J. (2023). Using artificial intelligence to improve public health: A narrative review. *Frontiers in Public Health, 11*, 1196397.

Pandey, B. K., Pandey, D., Wariya, S., & Agarwal, G. (2021). A deep neural network-based approach for extracting textual images from deteriorate images. *EAI Endorsed Transactions on Industrial Networks and Intelligent Systems, 8*(28), e3.

Pandey, B. K., Pandey, D., & Lelisho, M. E. (2024). Face mask identification with enhanced cuckoo optimization and deep learning-based faster regional neural network. *Scientific Reports, 14*(1), 29719.

Panesar, S., Cagle, Y., Chander, D., Morey, J., Fernandez-Miranda, J., & Kliot, M. (2019). Artificial intelligence and the future of surgical robotics. *Annals of Surgery, 270*, 223–226.

Paul, D., Sanap, G., Shenoy, S., Kalyane, D., Kalia, K., & Tekade, R. K. (2021). Artificial intelligence in drug discovery and development. *Drug Discovery Today, 26*, 80.

Renukappa, S., Mudiyi, P., Suresh, S., Abdalla, W., & Subbarao, C. (2022). Evaluation of challenges for adoption of smart healthcare strategies. *Smart Health, 26*, Article 100330.

Saravanakumar, R., TamilSelvi, T., Pandey, D., Pandey, B. K., Mahajan, D. A., & Lelisho, M. E. (2024). Big data processing using hybrid Gaussian mixture model with salp swarm algorithm. *Journal of Big Data, 11*(1), 167.

Solanas, A., Casino, F., Batista, E., & Rallo, R. (2017, September 11–13). Trends and challenges in smart healthcare research: A journey from data to wisdom. In *Proceedings of the 2017 IEEE 3rd international forum on research and technologies for society and industry (RTSI)* (pp. 1–6). Modena, Italy.

Sreedhar, C., Kallam, S., Pradeep Ghantasala, G. S., Anthoniraj, S., Kumarganesh, S., Martin Sagayam, K., Pandey, B. K., & Pandey, D. (2025). Enhancing healthcare data security using RFE and CRHSM for big data. *Computers in Biology and Medicine, 190*, 110063.

Tayefi, M., Ngo, P., Chomutare, T., Dalianis, H., Salvi, E., Budrionis, A., & Godtliebsen, F. (2021). Challenges and opportunities beyond structured data in analysis of electronic health records. *Wiley Interdisciplinary Reviews: Computational Statistics, 13*, Article e1549.

Tian, S., Yang, W., Le Grange, J. M., Wang, P., Huang, W., & Ye, Z. (2019). Smart healthcare: Making medical care more intelligent. *Global Health Journal, 3*, 62–65.

Xie, S., Yu, Z., & Lv, Z. (2021). Multi-disease prediction based on deep learning: A survey. *CMES-Computer Modeling in Engineering and Science, 128*, 489–522.

Machine Learning in Medical Imaging: Enhancing Diagnosis and Treatment

Aparna Pandey, P. Tamilselvi, Kawerinder Singh Sidhu, Chinnem Rama Mohan, Kavita Khatana, M. K. Sharma, and Ali Ihsan Alanssari

Abstract Machine learning has been employed in medical visualization, and this is changing the method in which medical professionals diagnose and treat patients in the modern health care system. By employing advanced algorithms and predictive models, medical professionals are able to generate diagnoses with greater precision, drastically cut down the time it takes to interpret outcomes and identify patterns that traditional methods have overlooked. The advancement of medical imaging technologies along with vital machine learning methodologies, consisting of supervised, unsupervised, deep, reinforcement, and transfer learning. The importance of these approaches in changing the manner in which diagnostic workflows. Real-life situations have shown that tools powered by AI can help healthcare providers find diseases earlier and improve patient outcomes in many different fields of medicine. Although it has many advantages, there are still problems that make it hard to use in a lot of

A. Pandey (✉)
Computer Science and Engineering, Bhilai Institute of Technology, Raipur,, Chhattisgarh Swami Vivekanand Technical University, Bhilai, Chhattisgarh, India
e-mail: aparna95pandey@gmail.com

P. Tamilselvi
Department of Computer Science and Engineering, Sathyabama Institute of Science and Technology, Chennai, Tamil Nadu, India

K. S. Sidhu
Uttaranchal Institute of Management, Uttaranchal University, Dehradun, Uttarakhand, India

C. R. Mohan
Department of Computer Science and Engineering, Narayana Engineering College, Nellore, Andhra Pradesh, India

K. Khatana
Department of Applied Sciences and Humanities (Chemistry), G.L. Bajaj Institute of Technology and Management, Greater Noida, India

M. K. Sharma
Mathematics, Chaudhary Charan Singh University, Meerut, Uttar Pradesh, India

A. I. Alanssari
Al-Nisour University College, Nisour Seq. Karkh, Baghdad, Iraq
e-mail: ali.ih.eng@nuc.edu.iq

D. Pandey et al. (eds.), *Smart Healthcare*,
https://doi.org/10.1007/978-981-95-8828-2_14

clinical settings. These problems include lacking adequate information, models that are not easy to understand, bias, and problems with laws and regulations. To get the most out of machine learning in imaging, it is necessary to do something about these problems. These technologies will greatly change the future of healthcare by making precision medicine easier and giving patients better care that is more focused on them.

Keywords Machine learning · Medical imaging · Deep learning · Healthcare AI · Reinforcement learning · Precision medicine · Diagnosis

1 Introduction

Over the last one hundred years, medical imaging has developed a lot and has grown into an important part of clinical practice. At first, medical professionals used physical examinations and basic lab tests in order to figure out what might have been wrong with a patient. Wilhelm Roentgen discovered X-rays in 1895, and they made it possible to see inside things without breaking them wide open. This new idea made it possible for more advanced imaging methods. The field of radiation therapy progressed rapidly alongside technological advancements. In the 1970s, Computed Tomography (CT) changed diagnostic medicine by giving medical professionals cross-sectional body images with detail and contrast that had never been seen previously. Magnetic resonance imaging (MRI) subsequently employed magnetic fields and radio waves to get precise images of soft tissue for evaluation. These methods might help medical professionals find diseases earlier and more accurately, and that would be better for patients. In real time, the ultrasound became popular because it is trustworthy, lightweight, and affordable. It was very important in obstetrics, cardiology, and emergency medicine. PET made it possible to see the manner in which the human body's metabolic and biochemical processes work, which is important in neurology and oncology. The use of digital technology has made imaging better. The transition from film to digital made it easier to store, share, and analyse images. The PACS made it easier for healthcare workers to manage and interpret scans, which made imaging more readily available and beneficial. The combination of computer science and medical imaging has generated new ways to process and analyse images. AI and machine learning have made it easier to reconstruct images, find problems, and make clinical decisions. PET/CT and PET/MRI are other options. They combine information about the body's structure and function in one scan. These improvements have made it possible to customize therapy by using accurate imaging data to change the manner in which treatments are given. In most medical fields, medical imaging is very important for diagnosis, treatment planning, and monitoring. Imaging has become a key part of modern healthcare because it has gotten better at resolution, speed, and accuracy. This has changed the way physicians find and treat illnesses.

1.1 The Rise of AI in Medical Imaging

Artificial intelligence has undergone shifts the method by which healthcare professionals think about diagnosing and planning treatment in the field of medical imaging. The radiologist and other medical professionals have always been in charge of interpreting complex images from X-rays, CT scans, and MRIs. Subsequently, the huge increase in imaging data and the growing demand from clinics have created it even more important to have intelligent technologies that work with human expertise. The latest advancements in machine learning and deep neural networks have unlocked new possibilities in the field. Highly sophisticated algorithms, especially those based on convolutional techniques, are now capable of identifying same patterns and problems in the medical images that might not be noticed during busy clinical workflows (Bajwa et al., 2021). These systems are not meant to take the place of radiologists; instead, they are meant to help them do their jobs better and faster. The latest diagnostic tools are making things easier in emergency rooms and other acute care settings by putting the most important cases first. For example, the suspected strokes or internal bleeding can be flagged in seconds, which enables healthcare professionals act more quickly and helps patients get better. These kinds of technologies have caused a big change in the way things work, in which machines help sort through and analyses huge amounts of data in real time. Artificially intelligent systems have become more important for more than just diagnostics. They are also helping to improve image quality and reduce interference. They are also helping to plan treatments through the use of the predictive analytics. By considering data and imaging results that are specific to each patient. The medical professionals can make more personalized and effective care plans. These tools are also considered as a very important for closing the gap in a healthcare. In rural or under-resourced areas in which it is hard to get specialist interpretation, cloud-based platforms and automated solutions serve to close the gap by providing timely and accurate preliminary reports. There are clear benefits to intelligent imaging devices, but they also bring up new issues about data privacy, following the rules, and using them in an ethical way. To make sure that these new technologies are used responsibly, it is still important to have transparency, explainability, and trust between technology and practitioners (Kuwaiti et al., 2023).

1.2 Machine Learning in Medicine

The data-driven algorithms have changed the manner in which healthcare diagnoses, treats, and manages patients. The move from approaches based on rules to adaptive systems that learn from massive data sets has contributed to medicine more accurate and efficient. These intelligence technologies that were only used in research facilities. These sophisticated algorithms attempt to identify hidden patterns and connections in a genetic data, medical imaging, lab tests, and patient records. These approaches are based on data and get better with additional information, thereby rendering them useful in the unpredictable world of medical treatment. The use of predictive analytics proved to be one of the first things that worked. The automated risk assessment systems help hospitals and clinics detect people that may be at risk for long-term diseases like cancer, diabetes, and heart disease (Mohammed et al., 2022). These predictive abilities enable doctors start taking steps to prevent problems early, which is good for long-term health. AI has made a big difference in diagnostic imaging. The latest technology helps radiologists and pathologists find cancers, fractures, and diseases that only affect certain organs by pointing out and categorizing unusual things. The programs have decreased the number of mistakes in diagnosis and made workflows run more smoothly, especially in places where facilities are limited. The algorithmic insights have also made personalized medicine better. Artificial intelligence systems propose treatments based on an individual's medical history and clinical information, which makes treatment more personalized. In the pharmaceutical field, these models help to speed up the process of finding the new drugs, identifying molecules, and improving the design of clinical trials. The healthcare workers employ automation to make the best use of hospital resources, patient flows, and administrative tasks. These technologies make healthcare better and easier to get by predicting whenever patients will need to come back and facilitating telemedicine platforms. Even with the changes made, there are still problems. The medical community needs to deal with issues like data privacy, algorithmic transparency, and biases in training datasets. For these technologies to be useful and ethical, they need to be integrated in a way that lasts. The use of learning-based systems makes medicine a lot better. Their effects are already making a healthcare better around the world by speeding it up, making it more accurate, and tailoring treatment to each person (Wang et al., 2021).

1.3 Synergy Between AI and Diagnostic Imaging

The combination of an advanced computer systems and the medical imaging have provided up a whole novel field related to clinical diagnostics. This synergy has enhanced the manner in which a medical professional able to see, comprehend, and utilize the complex anatomical and pathological data. The requirement for intelligent support systems has increased a lot as imaging technologies including CT, MRI, ultrasound, and PET continue to generate huge amounts of data with high resolution. The tools for diagnosis currently cannot operate alone any more. Healthcare professionals are able to obtain deeper insights faster and more accurately compared to ever before by putting learning algorithms onto imaging platforms. A computerized system image analysis finds tiny imperfections, sorts connective tissue, and points out important areas that could have been missed, particularly if there are quite a lot of them to examine. In consequence of these factors, medical professionals are capable of making decisions swiftly and with additional details and the chances of missing a diagnosis have been lower. These smart systems have made image reconstruction and enhancement quicker and more effective in addition to recognizing patterns. Techniques such as noise reduction, artefact correction, and resolution enhancement that used to need a lot of manual input are now accomplished automatically. This has made images clearer, examinations faster, and less radiation exposure for patients in CT and other imaging techniques. A further big step forward is in functional medical imaging, in which complex models are employed to combine structural and physiological data. By combining results from different types of imaging techniques like PET/CT or PET/MRI, healthcare providers are able to look at both anatomical features and metabolic activity at the same time. This makes it easier to make an accurate diagnosis for the complicated conditions like cancer staging or the neurological disorders. The collaboration between medical professionals and a smart imaging platforms is also changing the manner in which diagnostic results are communicated. The systems now give preliminary reports, suggest different diagnoses, and suggest follow-up actions. This helps healthcare professionals prioritize urgent cases and make busy medical settings run more smoothly. This collaboration has made it easier for people in underserved areas to get expert-level diagnostic support. The artificial intelligence-based imaging solutions and remote platforms have made this possible for establishments in rural or low-resource areas to get computerized evaluations and real-time consultations. This has helped to close the healthcare gap (Sharma et al., 2021).

2 Key Medical Imaging Techniques

Medical imaging has been an important part of modern diagnosis. Figure 1 shows that there are many different ways to do the procedure, each one designed for a specific clinical need. X-rays are now a quick and easy way to take pictures of broken bones and problems with the chest. CT scans give cross-sectional images that are very important for finding injuries and cancers inside the body. MRI is particularly effective at imaging soft tissue, which makes it easier to check the nervous system and muscles and bones. An ultrasound constitutes a type of imaging which does not use radiation and is used a lot in obstetrics and cardiology. PET scans demonstrate the manner in which the body is using energy, which is important for diagnosing cancer and doing research on the brain. Mammography has been utilized to find breast cancer early, whereas fluoroscopy and SPECT provide dynamic and functional imaging that is important for therapies and confirming whether or not organs work. *X-ray Imaging*: X-ray imaging is the most established and widely accessible diagnostic tool in medical practice. It works by passing ionizing radiation through the body to create two-dimensional images that differentiate tissues based on density. Dense materials like bones appear white, while softer tissues show up in varying shades of grey. X-rays are most commonly used to identify fractures, infections (such as pneumonia), dental problems, and joint abnormalities. Their quick turnaround and affordability make them essential in emergency medicine, orthopaedics, and dentistry. Portable

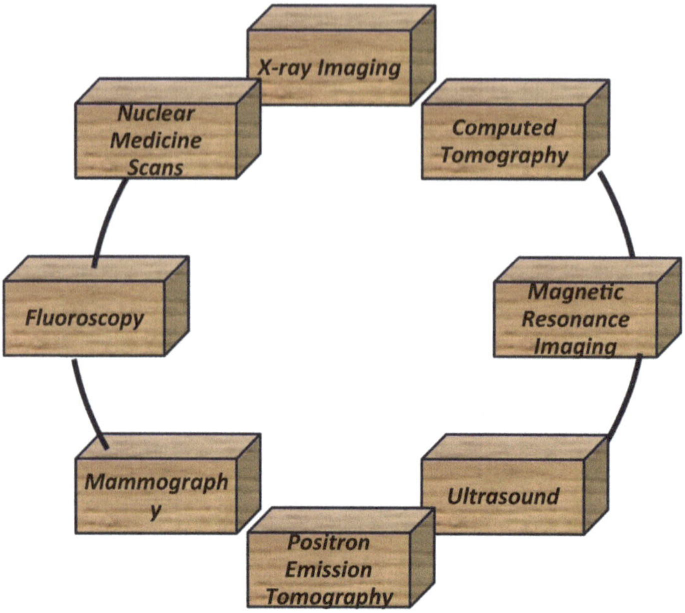

Fig. 1 Techniques in medical imaging

X-ray units further extend their utility to bedside imaging in hospitals and rural healthcare settings, allowing for rapid diagnosis even in critical care environments.

1. *Computed Tomography* (CT): CT scans are constructed on the same ideas as regular scanned images. However, they take numerous images from different angles to make cross-sectional slices of the body. This type of imaging gives much more detail than regular radiation, which makes it very useful for trauma, cancer detection, and heart health checks. CT can be utilised to see bleeding inside the human body, find tumours, and inspect for injuries to bones and tissues that are soft. The latest CT systems can make 3D models of organs and blood vessels, which at first can help with planning surgery. The inclusion of contrast media allows it to become even better at highlighting blood vessels, tumours, and tissues that are damaged, thereby making it more accurate for diagnosing conditions in fields comprising oncology and cardiology.
2. *Magnetic Resonance Imaging* (MRI): MRI has become a type of imaging which will not inconvenience someone and uses powerful magnets and radiofrequency waves in order to make clear pictures of soft tissues and internal organs. It does not utilise ionizing radiation like CT or X-rays employ, which makes it safer to use over and over again. MRI is great at showing the structure of the mind, the spinal cord, muscles, ligaments, and organs like the heart and liver. It proves to be very important tool for finding neurological problems like tumours in the brain or multiple sclerosis and musculoskeletal injuries which include torn ligaments. The functional magnetic resonance imaging technique has become very important in

neuroscience and pre-surgical brain mapping because it facilitates scientists and medical professionals map brain activity by determining changes in blood flow (Sreedhar et al., 2025).

3. *Ultrasound* (Sonography): Ultrasound imaging incorporates sound waves with high frequencies to make visualizations of organs and tissues in real time. It is commonly employed in obstetrics for foetal development tracking and its uses also include cardiology (e.g. echocardiography), abdominal imaging, and musculoskeletal evaluations. Perhaps the best things about ultrasound is that it is safe because it does not employ radiation, thus rendering it great for people who are pregnant or young in age. It is also very useful in emergencies and in developing areas because it is easy to carry and cheap. Doppler ultrasound, a type of technique that is used to check blood flow and find problems with the blood vessels, such as deep vein thrombosis.
4. *Positron Emission Tomography* (PET): PET has become a type of nuclear medicine imaging that shows the manner in which tissues are metabolizing. PET scans can identify areas of increased or decreased metabolic function by using radioactive tracers such as fluorodeoxyglucose. It works especially well in oncology, as it helps find tumours, keeping an eye on the way cancer progresses, and see the way treatment has become working. PET can be utilised in cardiology to check the health of the heart muscle and in neurology to learn more about diseases like Alzheimer's and epilepsy. This hybrid imaging provides both anatomical and functional information in conjunction with CT or MRI (for example, PET/CT). This makes it easier to diagnose complicated cases.
5. *Mammography*: Mammography represents a type of low-dose X-ray imaging that is only used on breast tissue. It is very important for finding breast cancer beforehand because it can often find tumours or microcalcifications before they are readily detected. Digital mammography and 3D tomosynthesis constitute two modern methods that make images clearer, which cuts down on false positives and the need for unnecessary biopsies. For regular checkups, medical practitioners endorse screening mammograms. For specific circumstances, like lumps or nipple discharge, medical practitioners use diagnostic mammograms. Mammography has played a big role in lowering the number of deaths from breast cancer by finding it early.
6. *Fluoroscopy*: Fluoroscopy allows it to see moving structures inside the body by taking images taken with X-rays in real time. It is often used in treatments that involve putting in catheters, taking pictures of blood vessels, and studying the digestive system, such as barium swallow tests. This type of imaging is very useful in both diagnostic and therapeutic settings because it permits to see how the body works in the present moment, particularly during a swallow or blood flows. This method is often used by radiologists and surgeons to help with minimally invasive procedures, indicating that fewer open surgeries are needed. However, because it involves constant exposure to radiation, safety measures have been required to protect both patients and healthcare workers.

7. *Nuclear Medicine Scans* (e.g. SPECT): The radioactive substances are used in Single Photon Emission Computed Tomography (SPECT) and other nuclear medicine normally scans to take a peek at the way the organs are working and the body works. People often use the SPECT to check the flows of the blood to the heart, find bone infections, and find any neurological disorders like Parkinson's illness. SPECT is an important tool for functional imaging since it illustrates the way organs are working, which is different from structural imaging techniques. Healthcare professionals can find functional problems with anatomical accuracy by using SPECT and CT together. These scans are very helpful for customizing medications, keeping an eye for when the disease is getting worse, and arriving at clinical decisions, especially in complicated cases of cardiology and oncology.

3 ML Techniques Powering Medical Imaging

3.1 Supervised Learning Models

To make diagnosing of a patients in medical facilities more accurate. An artificial intelligence models which employ the labelled datasets have become extremely essential. These computers are able to identify and classify the diseases with astounding precision by inspecting labelled medical images, in which doctors have able to found cancers, fractures, or additional health issues. Numerous individuals employ a computational model, especially convolutional neural networks (CNNs) to perform things like detect the tumours, classify diseases, and identify an organ. They help medical professionals by automatically checking mammograms to tell the difference between malignant and benign tumours. They frequently accomplish this with more sensitivity and specificity than traditional methods. Their capacity to quickly look at large numbers of images has become very important, particularly in fields like oncology, cardiology, and neurology that are in high demand. These algorithms have become commonplace in CT and MRI to find small patterns that may be linked to cancer, strokes, or heart problems. Automated techniques that identify ischemia zones in minutes have dramatically enhanced stroke diagnosis. This makes it more likely that patients will get immediate medical care and better outcomes. In busy medical environments, these AI-powered tools can assist radiologists make decisions by pointing out strange areas or deviations in images. This assists them put urgent patients beginning at the top of their list. This improvement to the workflow reduces cognitive load, minimizes the chance of human error, and speeds up the time required to report. Their growing use in emergency rooms and telemedicine systems demonstrates the way they can be used to contribute to healthcare more scalable (Zou et al., 2022).

3.2 Unsupervised Learning

Unsupervised learning plays a unique and useful role in medical imaging since it detects hidden patterns and structures in datasets that have no clear labels. These algorithms operate on their own, identifying relationships and categories that medical professionals may not have been able to observe. This is different from algorithms that are trained on data that has been labelled. This method works particularly well whenever there are a lot of unclassified images simply because it facilitates someone to find new features and connections without making any conclusions beforehand. To look into the fundamental structure of complex imaging collections of data, these individuals frequently employ techniques such as clustering, dimensionality reduction, and anomaly detection. One of the best things about unsupervised methods is the fact that their bodies can sort medical images into different categories based on their pixel intensities, texture, or shape. In one instance, clustering algorithms can differentiate brain MRI scans into normal tissue, grey matter, white matter, and possible abnormalities, although there are no specific diagnostic labels. These kinds of insights often serve as the first step in more research or the basis for later supervised models (Fu et al., 2019). Healthcare professionals are able to comprehend the manner in which diseases progress, identify rare diseases, and even find new types of diseases by combining similar images or structures. The Principal Component Analysis (PCA) and t-Distributed Stochastic Neighbour Embedding (t-SNE) constitute two common reductions of dimension methods that make highly dimensional imaging data easier to work with by turning the information into simpler forms that are easier to observe and recognize. These techniques may identify out small differences among groups of patients or within sets of data, thereby making it easier to find pattern outliers, or unusual patterns. The unsupervised approach can assist with personalized treatment planning in cancer research by examining imaging indicators to find tumour heterogeneity. A further significant application involves discovering unusual patterns. These algorithms are capable of discovering unusual characteristics in new scans that might mean early-stage illnesses or rare pathologies by learning exactly what healthy anatomical structures typically appear. In radiology, these kinds of systems have grown more and more useful for screening large datasets given that it might not be possible for a person to take a glance at every image. This type of learning is employed for a multitude of clinical purposes. It is also used to improve data preprocessing, for example removing noise from images, making segmentation more accurate, or making synthetic data to add to existing datasets. Although these models do not directly give specific diagnoses, they contribute to diagnostic workflows by showing hidden patterns in medical imaging data that give us more information. These methods will become very important for making information-based findings and supporting precision medicine initiatives as the number and complexity of imaging studies keep going up (Li et al., 2014).

3.3 Deep Learning and the Role of CNNs

Deep learning is influencing the manner in which medical images are generated and the convolutional architectures have been considered at the centre of this evolution. These networks have been developed to process visual information. Thereby making them perfect for understanding a complicated medical images including CT scans, MRIs, X-rays, and the ultrasounds. They develop hierarchical patterns from raw pixel data on themselves, starting with simple edges and shapes and moving on to more complex features such as tumours or tissue structures which are not normal. This ability to automatically extract useful features has become much better than older methods that needed people to manually engineer image characteristics. Those working in the medical field use these systems a lot to classify images, find objects, and divide them into categories. For example, they are able to identify the difference among healthy and diseased tissues, identify important findings including lung nodules, or draw tumour boundaries with pixel-level accuracy. The application of them spans a variety of disciplines, from oncology, where tumour segmentation can be useful for planning treatment, to neurology, where finding brain lesions assists with stroke diagnosis and monitoring. A further advantage about these deep learning frameworks is the manner in which their bodies can work with large datasets, which makes them very flexible for different types of patients and imaging techniques. In clinical workflows, their bodies are often built into computerized diagnosis platforms, which give radiologists the ability to automatically assess and priorities difficult cases. This extra layer of support assists in making medical assessments more accurate by lowering the number of different diagnoses. These models do more than simply to identify things, they ought to also help quantitative imaging by getting biomarkers or other useful metrics. For instance, within cardiology an automated analysis of echocardiograms assists healthcare professionals to figure out how well the heart is working and find problems like left ventricular dysfunction or valve disorders. Their effectiveness is strongly related to the availability of high-quality training data. They could be susceptible to image distortions or variations from different scanners. Healthcare professionals frequently desire enhanced interpretability to fully trust model outputs, which drives continuous research into explainable deep learning solutions (Matey et al., 2022).

3.4 Reinforcement Learning

Adaptive decision making systems have begun to change in the manner, in which imaging operations can be carried out and have transformed better. These intelligent agents acquire the knowledge by interacting with their environment and gradually enhancing their actions to reach particular objectives, like improving image quality or simplifying workflows. This technique has been increasingly employed in medical imaging to enhance parameters during the process of an immediate image acquisition. In MRI imaging procedures, machines that operate independently may modify the pulse sequences, field gradients, or resolution settings to make images clearer and evaluations faster. This makes sure that the patient has become comfortable and the diagnosis has become correct. In radiation-based imaging, like as CT scans, this aspect method personalizes radiation levels for individual patients through dynamically altering technical parameters such as tube current or voltage. The result provides superior images with less radiation exposure, and this is important for reducing risk over time in those most susceptible, such as children and patients requiring multiple scans. They may eliminate artefacts, improve features, or reduce noise on their own, resulting in images that are easier to understand and diagnose. These models add significant information that standard algorithms could overlook whenever data is hard to see because of blurred motion or poor contrast. In clinical settings with substantial workloads, intelligent solutions assist in organizing workflow by putting urgent cases ahead of others. By analysing patient data and health history, their bodies help get important images to specialists faster, which cuts down on interruptions in diagnoses that need to happen rapidly, like strokes or trauma-related injuries. To make sure that reward systems are accurate as well as that systems are reliable within unpredictable healthcare settings, meticulous design and testing will be required. Before being used in real-life situations, these models frequently undergo through a lot of training in simulated settings. This makes sure that patients get the best care possible while making it easier to make decisions. This new technology has produced imaging platforms that automate processes and always adapt to new clinical needs. As these systems become better, they ought to reduce down on inefficiency, lower operational costs, and help radiologists by taking care of repetitive or technical work. This will free up healthcare professionals to focus on more complex case analyses.

3.5 Leveraging Pre-trained Models

Transfer learning has proven to be an extraordinarily effective methodology in a medical imaging. By enabling the utilization of a knowledge that derived from models. Initially trained on extensive datasets for novel, domain-specific tasks and instead of building algorithms from scratch, which often requires a lot of resources. The healthcare professionals and investigators are capable of employing smaller, customized datasets to change existing networks to solve the medical problems. This method substantially decreases the time and computational resources required to complete model construction, which makes it particularly beneficial in healthcare, in which annotated medical images tend to be limited. By fine-tuning models which were initially developed on large image datasets like ImageNet. The experts may generate diagnostic tools that can find problems in X-rays, MRIs, CT scans, and various other types of imaging. They may alter an algorithm that was trained on millions of natural images to find things like animals or cars so that this can find lung nodules, brain tumours, or retinal problems. This method operates by reusing features like edges, textures, and shapes that can be common in both natural and medical images. It also improves the representation of the model's deeper layers to focus on patterns that are specific to clinical settings. Obtaining a tagged medical image usually requires the help of medical professionals and takes a lot of time, so transfer learning helps improve existing datasets. This has been particularly important in fields like medical pathology, in which deep models can be modified changed to find cancerous cells in histological slides, and ophthalmology, where pre-trained networks have been used to find diabetic retinopathy in retinal scans (Moorthy & Gandhi, 2022). This method can be employed for diagnosing diseases, as well as for image segmentation, classification, and predicting the manner in which diseases will progress. Fine-tuned models are frequently implemented in systems for clinical decision-support to help medical professionals find minor issues and make the whole process more efficient. Transfer learning possesses a lot of benefits, although it can also be challenging. It means that models trained on datasets that are not medical or related to healthcare could not be able to be generalized well to specialized healthcare settings. As a result, these solutions need to be carefully validated and calibrated before they can be used in healthcare settings.

4 ML Transforming Medical Imaging

- *Enhanced Diagnoses*: AI-driven models are changing the manner in which radiologists examine medical images by finding small patterns that people might miss. These technologies enable it to be easier to tell the difference between benign and malignant tumours with more accuracy, which results in fewer false positives and false negatives. In addition to classifying conditions, these models help find early signs of diseases like cancer, heart disease, and neurodegenerative disorders, thus making it easier to get treatment quickly. Predictive techniques analyse images of patients and clinical data to seek out exactly what might happen in the future including whether the disease might get worsening. This helps healthcare professionals make better decisions about treating their patients.
- *Accelerated Workflows*: Machine learning makes healthcare operations better by automating tasks that are done repeatedly over and over that includes the image segmentation, annotation, and early reporting. The radiologists may employ algorithms to find anatomical parts or outline tumours that cuts down on the time needed to do these things by a lot. This automation makes people more productive and less fatigued, which lessens the chances of making mistakes while accomplishing the same thing over and over. These smart solutions help healthcare workers by taking care of fundamental responsibilities, which at first frees up more time for them to work on complicated cases and correspond to patients. This makes care delivery better overall.
- *Expedited Analysis*: Advanced algorithms have made it possible to process and understand images much faster. It used to take an hour of manual work to do operations. But now they can be done in minutes even with large datasets such

as comprehensive CT scans or multiple MRI. Fast processing has become very important in emergency rooms and intensive care units, where quick test results are needed. Artificial intelligence-based analysis makes it easier to do large screening programs, like breast and lung cancer screenings, by quickly going through a lot of scans and picking out the ones that need immediate care.

- *Customized Therapies*: Machine learning enhances personalised medicine by extracting quantitative biomarkers from imaging data, providing clinicians with an individualized insights regarding the patients. These genetic markers help the medical professionals decide the manner in which to treat a patient, such as which chemotherapy regimen will work best and the best way to plan radiotherapy based on the malignancy's exact location and size. Imaging driven models offer flexible treatment plans that change as new scans are taken, making sure that treatments stay in line with the fact that the individual's condition has been changing. This level of personalization allows a clinician to deliver a precise care tailored to the specific patient attributes (Hussain et al., 2021).
- *Reduced Errors*: Artificial intelligence-based methods reduce the differences between radiologists by information evaluations. These models help doctors to make a decision by finding problems that could not have been found otherwise. Giving them a very important second opinion. This reduces the risk of losing something especially in complicated or unclear situations. The objective nature of computerised result fosters consistent reporting and improves collaboration among interdisciplinary teams, consequently leading to safer and more reliable diagnostics.

This technology makes it possible to quickly and accurately understand complicated imaging data that leads to earlier disease detection as well as improved diagnosis. As soon as medical professionals can use algorithms that are capable of discovering small patterns in scans like X-rays, MRIs, and CT images. They can arrive at better decisions while making fewer mistakes whenever diagnosing patients. Figure 2 shows the manner in which machine learning contributes to modern medical imaging through automating and improving the procedure by which medical professionals make diagnoses. Machine learning further makes workflows more efficient through reducing the number of manual tasks and speeding up image processing. These new ideas not solely help patients get better, but they also make the most of the resources available in the healthcare system. This leads to the door for more specific and data-driven approaches in clinical practice.

5 Real-World AI in Diagnostics

Artificial intelligence is benefiting healthcare within tangible manners through improving diagnostic accuracy, efficiency, and patient outcomes improved. A number of instances demonstrate the manner in which these technologies have influenced

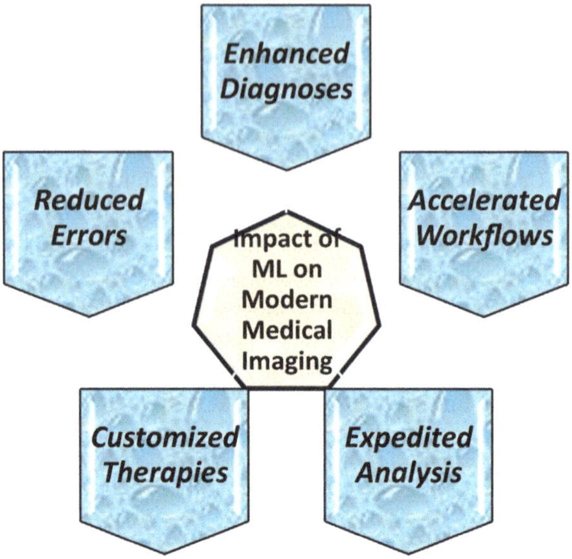

Fig. 2 Impact of machine learning on modern medical imaging

medical imaging within a variety of specialties and clinical settings. In oncology, AI-powered tools have been implemented added to mammography screening programs to help find breast cancer before it becomes serious. A notable instance has been the use of algorithms based on deep learning to accurately flag unusual lesions in mammograms, comparable to the method experienced radiologists accomplish it. In a large study, employing AI assistance helped find tumours in the dense breast tissue sooner and cut down on the number of missed diagnosis. The result not simply helped more people survive, but it additionally decreased down on unneeded biopsies, that helped patients feel less anxious and made better use of healthcare assets. In cardiology, machine learning models have been employed to read echocardiograms and CT angiograms. This is an additional significant illustration. AI tools are currently used at some of the best healthcare facilities to find warning signs of heart disease, like left ventricular dysfunction or blockages in the coronary arteries, regardless of whether these issues are very small in scale. These tools enable cardiologists' figure out which individuals have a higher risk by examining imaging data along with their demographics and histories of illness. This helps them make decisions concerning when and when to treat patients (Ker et al., 2018). AI has shown remarkable accomplishments in the field of neuroscience by quickly diagnosing acute ischemic strokes with brain CT and MRI scans (Aljuaid & Anwar, 2022). The algorithms can able to identify large vessel blockages and measure the cerebral perfusion deficits that cuts down on the time required to get treatment. This has contributed to faster decisions about thrombolysis or mechanical thrombectomy in an emergency situation, in which every minute counts, which has helped the patients to recuperate and remain alive longer. AI-driven diagnostics (Rädsch et al., 2022) are additionally employed in eye care to find diabetic retinopathy by looking at images of the retina. The automated systems have already been used successfully in community clinics and remote healthcare settings to identify patients for this visually impaired condition, especially in areas where there is a shortage of health care professionals. These tools enable healthcare providers who are not specialists flag patients requiring immediate vision restoration, thereby making it easier for people to get early treatment.

6 Barriers to ML in Imaging

There are many big problems that need to be solved prior to machine learning can be used more frequently in the field of a medical imaging. A significant challenge is getting an accurate data and ensuring that it is publicly accessible. High-performing models require a large number of labelled medical imagery, but these datasets are often limited by issues with confidentiality, scattered data sources, and the requirement for expert annotations. The differences in technology for imaging, techniques, and patient attributes could result in data that is inconsistent, preventing the development of models that translate effectively across various healthcare settings. A significant issue is that it is hard to explain matters. Many artificial intelligence systems (Pandey et al., 2024), particularly deep learning models, operate like "black boxes," giving predictions without explicitly clarifying the reason behind them. This lack of transparency makes professionals who additionally are used to knowing why diagnostic conclusions become nervous. Without clear results, medical professionals might not want to have complete confidence or use these tools in important parts of treatment, particularly if patients' lives have been put at stake. Legal and regulatory problems are making it harder for AI to become more commonly utilized (Pandey & Pandey, 2025). Getting certified by regulatory agencies such as the FDA or EMA has become hard because machine learning models must undergo through a lot of evaluations to prove that their algorithms are safe and effective. Given that these algorithms are capable of learning and changing following the time they are put into application, they make it harder for traditional approval procedures that are meant for healthcare equipment that are resistant to change. Another cause for concern is that, an AI application (Saravanakumar et al., 2024) might be prejudiced and inequitable. The models that have been trained on datasets that are not representative of the whole population that, might unintentionally accomplish worse on a category that are not accurately represented, such as certain age or racial categories. This could cause differences in the accuracy of diagnoses and health results, possibly making the current health inequality worsening. To deal with this problem, it is necessary to make different, encompassing datasets and cautiously check over fairness while developing models. To add machine learning technologies to current hospital systems such as PACS (Picture Archiving and Communication Systems) or electronic health records, an enormous amount of technical and infrastructure changes need to be implemented. Training for clinicians and change management tend to be essential, as a healthcare personnel member accustomed to traditional diagnostic methods that can impede the adoption of new technologies.

7 Conclusion

Machine learning is altering the manner, in which medical imaging works and starts a new era that fosters creativity in health care. Machine learning has demonstrated immense potential for improving accuracy, speeding up processes, and helping with clinical decision making throughout the practical diagnostics. Deep learning that includes the supervised, unsupervised learning, and reinforcement learning have been all ways to analyse the images accurately, which leads to earlier disease detection and improved treatment for patients. AI-powered solutions have improved diagnostic results and changing the manner in which patients are cared for in many medical fields, including oncology and neurology. The use of machine learning is expected to play a much bigger role in healthcare in the near future. This will still be able to help with predicted diagnosis and customized treatment plans because it can examine large amounts of imaging and clinical data. This progress will undoubtedly render medical services faster and better in general. As explainable AI and model transparency improve, medical professionals are going to develop confidence on these systems. These advantages in ethical AI frameworks will help to make sure that people from different backgrounds are able to employ these technologies without discrimination. Intelligent algorithms that enhance human expertise and make it easier to make decisions based on data will continue to have an increasing impact on the future of medical imaging. There are numerous problems like data limits, complicated rules, and problems with integration that need to be solved by working together by healthcare providers, researchers, and technology developers. The growing cooperation between machine intelligence and clinical experience might alter our ability to diagnose and treat patients all over the world, thereby making care safer, faster, and more customized.

References

Aljuaid, A., & Anwar, M. (2022). Survey of supervised learning for medical image processing. *SN Computer Science, 3*, 292.

Bajwa, J., Munir, U., Nori, A., & Williams, B. (2021). Artificial intelligence in healthcare: Transforming the practice of medicine. *Future Healthcare Journal, 8*, e188–e194.

Fu, Y., Lei, Y., Wang, T., Curran, W. J., Liu, T., & Yang, X. (2019). Deep learning in medical image registration: A review. *Physics in Medicine and Biology, 65*, 20TR01.

Hussain, A., Malik, H., & Chaudhry, M. U. (2021). Supervised learning based classification of cardiovascular diseases. *Proceedings of Engineering and Technology Innovation, 20*, 24–34.

Ker, J., Wang, L., Rao, J. P., & Lim, T. C. C. (2018). Deep learning applications in medical image analysis. *IEEE Access, 6*, 9375–9389.

Kuwaiti, A. A., Nazer, K. H. A., Al-Reedy, A., Al-Shehri, S. Z., Al-Muhanna, A. F., Subbarayalu, A. V., Muhanna, D. A., & Al-Muhanna, F. A. (2023). A review of the role of artificial intelligence in healthcare. *The Journal of Personalized Medicine, 13*, 951.

Li, Q., Cai, W. T., Wang, X., Zhou, Y., Feng, D. D., & Chen, M. (2014, December 10–12). Medical image classification with convolutional neural network. In *Proceedings of the 2014 13th international conference on control automation robotics and vision (ICARCV)* (pp. 844–848). Singapore.

Matey, V., Chauhan, N., Mahale, A., Bhistannavar, V., & Shitole, A. (2022, December 15–17). Real estate price prediction using supervised learning. In *Proceedings of the 2022 IEEE Pune section international conference (PuneCon)* (pp. 1–5). Pune, India.

Mohammed, M. A., Mohammed, M. A., & Mohammed, V. A. (2022). Impact of artificial intelligence on the automation of digital health system. *International Journal of Software Engineering and Applications, 13*.

Moorthy, J., & Gandhi, U. D. (2022). A survey on medical image segmentation based on deep learning techniques. *Big Data and Cognitive Computing, 6*, 117.

Pandey, B. K., & Pandey, D. (2025). Securing healthcare medical image information using advance morphological component analysis, information hiding systems, and hybrid convolutional neural networks on IoMT. *Computers in Biology and Medicine, 185*, 109499.

Pandey, B. K., Pandey, D., & Lelisho, M. E. (2024). Face mask identification with enhanced cuckoo optimization and deep learning-based faster regional neural network. *Scientific Reports, 14*(1), 29719.

Rädsch, T., Reinke, A., Weru, V., Tizabi, M. D., Schreck, N., Kavur, A. E., Pekdemir, B., Ross, T., Kopp-Schneider, A., & Maier-Hein, L. (2022). Labelling instructions matter in biomedical image analysis. *Nature Machine Intelligence, 5*, 273–283.

Saravanakumar, R., TamilSelvi, T., Pandey, D., Pandey, B. K., Mahajan, D. A., & Lelisho, M. E. (2024). Big data processing using hybrid Gaussian mixture model with salp swarm algorithm. *Journal of Big Data, 11*(1), 167.

Sharma, A. K., Nandal, A., Dhaka, A., & Dixit, R. (2021). Medical image classification techniques and analysis using deep learning networks: A review. In *Health informatics: A computational perspective in healthcare*. Springer.

Sreedhar, C., Kallam, S., Ghantasala, G. P., Anthoniraj, S., Kumarganesh, S., Sagayam, K. M., Pandey, B. K., & Pandey, D. (2025). Enhancing healthcare data security using RFE and CRHSM for big data. *Computers in Biology and Medicine, 190*, 110063.

Wang, S., Cao, G., Wang, Y. L., Liao, S., Wang, Q., Shi, J., Li, C., & Shen, D. (2021). Review and prospect: Artificial intelligence in advanced medical imaging. *Frontiers in Radiology, 1*, Article 781868.

Zou, J., Gao, B., Song, Y., & Qin, J. (2022). A review of deep learning-based deformable medical image registration. *Frontiers in Oncology, 12*, 1047215.

Securing Healthcare Data Using AI-Driven Approaches to Privacy and Compliance

Snehal Dipak Chaudhary, K. Jose Reena, Kawerinder Singh Sidhu, Pamarthi Satyanarayana, E. Sweety Bakyarani, Joshuva Arockia Dhanraj, and Hassan Khalid Abozibid

Abstract As a healthcare becomes increasingly computerized, the amount and sensitivity of patient data have also increased. This makes. it is harder to protect privacy while also adhering to the rules. This work looks at an artificial intelligence technique to make a healthcare data more secure, while also making sure that HIPAA and GDPR rules are observed. Machine learning, natural language processing, and federated learning have been among the numerous examples of the AI technologies that are changing the manner in which healthcare companies keep an eye upon to protect and handle sensitive data. These systems automate reporting and auditing, identify problems in real time, enforce security rules, and keep patient data safe without getting in the way of medical procedures. The primary issue is how systems powered by AI will achieve a balance between privacy, innovation, and rules. The

S. D. Chaudhary (✉)
Department of Information Technology, Bharati Vidyapeeth (Deemed to Be University) College of Engineering, Pune, Maharashtra, India
e-mail: sdchaudhary@bvucoep.edu.in

K. J. Reena
Department of Computer Applications, B.S. Abdur Rahman Crescent Institute of Science and Technology, Chennai, Tamil Nadu, India

K. S. Sidhu
Uttaranchal Institute of Management, Uttaranchal University, Dehradun, Uttarakhand, India

P. Satyanarayana
School of Law, VelTech Rangarajan Dr. Sagunthala R&D Institute of Science and Technology, VelTech University, Avadi, Tamil Nadu, India

E. S. Bakyarani
Department of Computer Science, Faculty of Science and Humanities, SRM Institute of Science and Technology, Kattankulathur, Chengalpattu, India
e-mail: sweetye@srmist.edu.in

J. A. Dhanraj
Research and Development Cell, Lovely Professional University, Jalandhar-Delhi, Phagwara, Punjab, India

H. K. Abozibid
Al-Zahrawi University College, Karbala, Iraq

D. Pandey et al. (eds.), *Smart Healthcare*,
https://doi.org/10.1007/978-981-95-8828-2_15

federated learning enables people work together to build AI models while not sharing patient data, which lowers the risk of data breaches. The businesses can respond to changing risks and rules with AI-based adaptive access controls and predictive compliance solutions. It is hard to find a balance between making data easy to get to, keeping it safe, and adhering to the rules in rapidly changing healthcare and technologically driven settings. Using AI and human oversight together to build data management systems that are clear, strong, and abide by the rules. The automation of important compliance processes and giving healthcare providers early insights into regulatory trends gives them an edge over their competitors while getting rid of human error and administrative roadblocks. AI that is strategically integrated may help privacy-first healthcare organizations, allowing businesses to provide safe, ethical, and effective patient care in a digital world.

Keywords AI · Healthcare · Data privacy · Compliance · Cybersecurity · Anomaly detection · Federated learning · Patient data · ML

1 Introduction

As healthcare organizations perform a growing portion of their work to the internet, it is growing harder to keep the sensitive patient information safe and secure. The traditional security methods sometimes fail to the protect well against a new cyber threat and the complicated regulations that come with them. Innovative technologies are now at the forefront of addressing these problems by improving privacy protections and making compliance easier. Machine learning models have been very important for finding strange things in a large amount of the healthcare data. These systems assist in preventing data breaches and unauthorized access prior to they happen by spotting strange patterns or suspicious actions. A further significant application is automating data elimination, which employs algorithms to swiftly eliminate or hide personally identifiable information from clinical notes, patient records, and research datasets. This keeps information confidential while allowing secure sharing. Automation tools are changing the manner in which healthcare providers follow rules like HIPAA and GDPR especially when it comes to regulatory compliance. These systems maintain an eye on legal changes all the time, do audits in real time, and generate reports that help businesses maintain their paperwork up to date and avoid monetary penalties. Smart access control systems are being used that change user permissions based on things like behavior, location, and role. This risk-based approach limits access to sensitive data so that it can only be accessed when it is safe to do so. Many individuals continue to be concerned about the ethical use of these kinds of technologies. For instance, there can be a risk of bias in automated selections, a lack of transparency, as well as a need for better data governance. As soon as incorporated to existing systems in an intelligent manner, these tools can help safeguard privacy, increase healthcare institutions more resilient to threats, and make sure that they stay compliant in a digital world that keeps growing more complicated.

1.1 Data Security in Healthcare

Data security in healthcare is very important because patient information is very private. This includes medical histories, diagnoses, treatment plans, and personal identification information. In the event this data is stolen or accessed without permission from the person, this could lead to serious problems like identity theft, insurance fraud, losing money, and losing confidence in patients. Cyberattacks frequently target healthcare organizations because medical data is worth more on the black market than many other types of personal information. Healthcare professionals face both cyber threats and internal hazards such as data leaks and employees using data in ways that are not allowed. Maintaining strong security measures in place protects the confidentiality of patients while also making sure that medical services are always available and confidential. Ransomware attacks, for instance, may disrupt important healthcare operations that can delay treatment and even put lives at risk. HIPAA in the USA and GDPR in Europe constitute two laws that require healthcare data to be kept safe. If you fail to comply with the rules, it could face big fines, harm to the brand, and loss of recognition. As the healthcare industry becomes more digital through electronic health records (EHRs), telemedicine, and health information exchanges, the need for strong data security systems has become even more important. To keep patient trust, make sure that medical professionals act ethically, and protect public health infrastructure, this is important to keep confidential data secure (Murdoch, 2021).

1.2 AI in Healthcare Data Management

In recent years, the utilization of an artificial intelligence in managing healthcare data has grown quickly. This is because medical information is becoming more complex and readily available. The healthcare organizations, clinics, and research facilities produce an enormous quantity of the data in every single day that encompassing electronic health records (EHRs), imaging data, genomic information, and administrative records. It has become challenging to manage and protect this data effectively, and traditional systems often fail to perform a good job of keeping it safe. Healthcare systems are implementing AI technologies like machine learning and the natural language processing to automate and improve many parts of the data management. These applications help the healthcare providers to organize, process, and get a data back faster and with fewer mistakes. For instance, smart algorithms can able to organize medical documents, pull useful information out of unstructured clinical notes, and point out inconsistencies in the patient records. AI has implications for keeping sensitive information safe as well as making the operations to run more efficiently. Advanced models can find strange patterns concerning the way data is accessed or employed, which helps businesses find and deal with security threats right away. Automation powered by AI additionally assists healthcare providers follow the rules by helping them keep track of data flows, ensure that every piece of documentation is in order, and follow the rules of privacy regulations like HIPAA and GDPR. The utilization of AI in managing healthcare data is additionally helping patients get better results. AI helps with clinical choice making to make personalized treatment plans easier and also speeds up the administrative tasks, giving medical professionals more time to care for patients. As AI keeps developing, its role in managing data is expected to grow as well. This will give healthcare organizations novel approaches to balance efficiency, security, and complying with the rules in a world, which is becoming more digital (Reddy et al., 2019).

2 The Landscape of Healthcare Data Privacy

2.1 Sensitive Healthcare Data

Healthcare organizations deal with a wide range of private information that is necessary for the treatment of patients. This information encompasses more than merely basic medical records. It also includes the personal, financial, and a clinical information that could lead to identity theft, insurance fraud, or putting patient safety at risk if it were obtained. Figure 1 shows the different types of sensitive health data. As the healthcare sector increasingly digitizes records and adopts the networked systems such as electronic health records, telemedicine platforms, and health information exchanges, the amount and variety of sensitive data are growing. To protect these records is important task for keeping patient confidence, following the law, and keeping the public health infrastructure safe from cyberattacks.

1. *Electronic Health Records (EHRs)*: EHR systems are central to modern healthcare delivery, enabling real-time access to patient information across departments and even between different healthcare institutions. They improve clinical outcomes by reducing medical errors, supporting evidence-based care, and streamlining workflows. However, the interconnected nature of EHR systems also increases the attack surface, making them a prime target for cybercriminals and requiring advanced cybersecurity measures (Morley et al., 2019).
2. *Personally Identifiable Information (PII)*: PII serves as the foundation for linking patient identities to their medical and financial records. Because it is used in both administrative and clinical systems, its compromise can have wide-reaching consequences, including fraudulent insurance claims, phishing attacks, and privacy violations. The value of PII on the black market is high, which is why healthcare organizations implement strict access controls and encryption to protect this data.
3. *Protected Health Information (PHI)*: PHI is critical for processing insurance claims, coordinating care, and medical research. It is often stored and transmitted through multiple systems such as EHRs, billing platforms, and health information exchanges. Due to its sensitive nature, regulations mandate safeguards like data

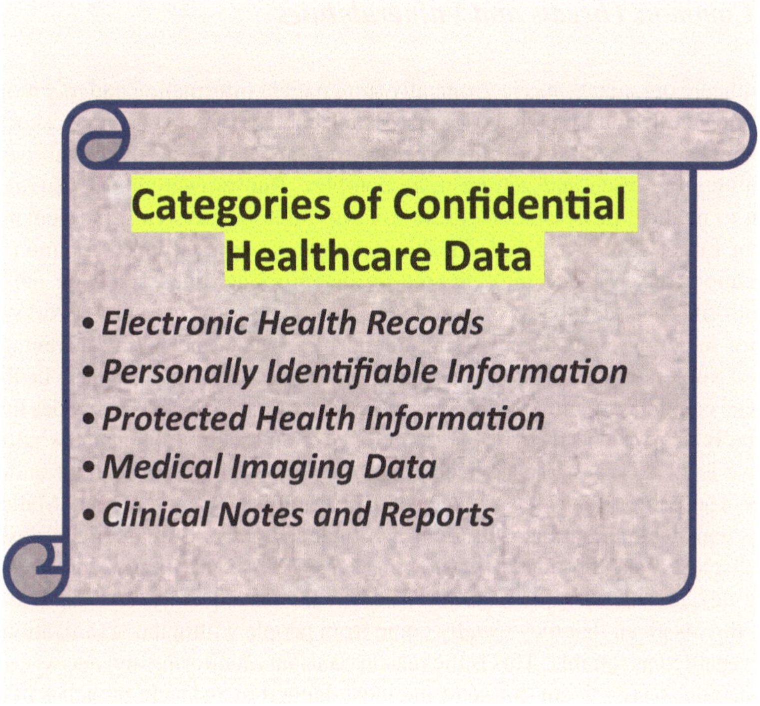

Fig. 1 Types of sensitive healthcare data

encryption, secure access protocols, and regular auditing to prevent unauthorized disclosures and breaches.

4. *Medical Imaging Data*: Imaging files are large, often shared across networks for remote consultations and AI-based diagnostic tools. The integration of imaging systems with AI solutions for faster and more accurate diagnoses has improved patient care, but also presents cybersecurity risks. Hackers may exploit vulnerabilities in Picture Archiving and Communication Systems (PACS) or DICOM protocols, potentially gaining access to both image data and patient metadata.
5. *Clinical Notes and Reports*: These records provide crucial insights into patient conditions, physician decision-making, and treatment plans. Since clinical notes are often free-text and subjective, they may contain sensitive information not found elsewhere in structured fields. Natural Language Processing (NLP) tools are increasingly used to extract meaningful data from these notes, but improper handling or storage can expose confidential patient narratives to unauthorized access.

2.2 Common Threats and Vulnerabilities

As healthcare organizations electronically store patient information and rely more on interconnected systems that they face increasing amounts of dangers and weaknesses. Cyberattacks have been one of the biggest problems at present given that they are happening more often and getting more complex. Ransomware attacks frequently happen to medical professionals, preventing up important systems and demanding payment to get access restored. Phishing campaigns have become common. The organization trick workers into clicking on inappropriate links or giving out their login information, and that can then be used to break into internal networks. The m aware infections, attacks involving denial of service, and taking advantage of outdated vulnerabilities in software can all cause problems for medical facilities, and these can delay treatments and put the safety of patients at risk. Insider threats are equally scary since they involve employees, contractors, or business partners that have legal access to private health information but might use it in a fraudulent manner. These threats may have been deemed intentional or unintentional. Malicious insiders can steal patient data for their own financial gain, while negligent insiders could disclose data through not following safe cybersecurity procedures such as leaving devices unlocked or handling private files inadequately. It is hard to spot insider threats given that they usually come from people within the organization that can be regarded as reliable. This is the reason constant monitoring and access control have become so significant. Some of the most dangerous risks are breaches of data, and this can happen because of attacks from outside sources or mistakes made by staff members (Prakash et al., 1914). A data breach takes place when someone gets access to shares or steals electronic health records (EHRs), financial information, or different kinds of protected health information (PHI) with no permission. The healthcare sector is an ideal target since medical data possesses a high resale value on the black market, which might be used for identity theft, medical fraud, and other illegal activities. Aside from the financial effects, breaches can make patients lose trust and lead to lawsuits and fines under data protection laws like HIPAA, GDPR, or local privacy laws. The attack surface has gotten bigger because more people are using telehealth services, cloud storage, mobile health apps, and connected medical devices. Cybercriminals can easily get into these technologies because they don't always have standard security protocols. The healthcare industry poses even more risk given that it still uses old systems that have not been renovated or replaced. An organization have to employ a layered security strategy that involves employee training, encryption, multi-factor authentication, regular security audits, and AI-driven threat detection tools that identify and resolve risks in real time (Wang et al., 1878).

2.3 Balancing Data Accessibility and Privacy

Healthcare companies continually have to contend with the problem of making sure that patient data is quickly available while also keeping it safe from people who ought not to possess it. Healthcare professionals need quick and safe access to patient data, such as electronic health records (EHRs), lab reports, and imaging information, in order to reach important decisions that can save lives. Creating access faster and easier will occasionally weaken safeguards for confidentiality, leading to sensitive information more likely to be accessed. One of the main problems involves creating systems which are both easy for healthcare workers to understand and strong enough to keep them protected. Access restrictions that have been excessive can slow into clinical workflows, and this can lead to longer wait times for treatment and diagnosis. On the contrary, allowing data too easy to get without proper permission protocols increases the likelihood of insider threats and data breaches. The growing use of platforms based on the cloud, telemedicine, and health applications for mobile devices have rendered the balance even more unstable. These technologies enable easier for medical professionals to interact with each other and share data from a far, however they also add more access areas, leading to it being harder to keep apprised of that is able to view or modify patient data at any given time (Khalid et al., 2023). If there cannot be strict security rules and role-based access restrictions, people who ought not to be able to use these systems might be able to gain access. Afterward the rules add another level of challenging. The legal requirements like HIPAA and GDPR stipulate that healthcare providers must protect patient data, while also making it is straightforward for authorized the workforce to get to it when they required. It can turn out hard to meet both criteria at the same time, especially when handling a lot of data or combining other services. Emergencies and unexpected medical situations often require a rapid and adaptable access to the information about patients, which could give rise to the bypassing of a conventional security measure. In these situations, businesses need to carefully evaluate the safety of patients toward any privacy risks. To find an appropriate balance, this needs to a combine technological advances, policy, and ongoing training to feed a staff. To make sure that healthcare professionals are able to access crucial information while protecting patient privacy, innovations such as authentication using multiple factors, AI-driven obtain monitoring, and adaptive safeguards have been implemented (Zarifis et al., 2020).

3 AI-Powered Security Solutions in Healthcare

3.1 Cybersecurity and Compliance Automation

In the modern healthcare industry, in which cybersecurity and regulatory procedures have become more sophisticated, technological advancements have grown more and more significant. These systems are capable of quickly processing enormous quantities of information, leading to this easier for them to spot unusual activities like unauthorized access or leakage of information. A few of the numerous advantages of using machine learning techniques is the fact that they can find minute patterns and strange things that would typically pass unnoticed in person surveillance. Machine learning has additionally made this much easier to adhere to the regulations. Nowadays, regular audits, risk evaluations, and enforcement of regulations are capable of being done with very little help from staff members. Thus, this less probable that people will make mistakes, as well as also helps businesses remain in compliance with regulations like HIPAA and GDPR. In cybersecurity, sophisticated instruments are capable of rapidly deal with attacks by isolating harmed accounts or systems. This minimizes damage prior to it gets much worse. These systems can also keep a watch on networks and devices for weaknesses all the time, so they can correct problems or report them right away. Natural language processing makes it easier to work with unstructured data including medical notes and reports. This ensures that private information has become properly labeled and handled according to privacy rules. Furthermore, predictive models have advantages for security teams given that they can warn them about threats which are getting worse. This allows healthcare providers improve the defenses in a preventive manner. These improvements help healthcare organizations strike a balance between being efficient, protecting data well, and adhering to the regulations (Richardson et al., 2021).

3.2 Machine Learning (ML) for Anomaly Detection

The search for anomalies has become an important part of keeping the healthcare systems secure. Modern algorithms can be taught from past data to set a baseline over that constitutes typical behavior on networks, devices, and applications. A change to this standard, such as logging in to an odd times, transferring of the data without a permission, or accessing files without having proper permission, may trigger off the warnings and contribute to an additional investigation. This approach is considerably more adaptable than traditional security standards since it changes along with the way healthcare operations develop. The system is capable of quickly identifying the difference among harmless anomalies and a serious danger, and this greatly cuts down on false alarms and speeds up the incident response. The identification of anomalies is a very useful in places with a lot of networks like healthcare centers or hospitals that use a lot of different systems and the medical devices. This technology maintains an eye on complex ecosystems in a real time, identifying threats that human teams or simpler security solutions could have overlooked. People frequently employ an unsupervised learning method such as clustering or dimensionality reduction to find the exploitable weaknesses and unknown threats. Healthcare organizations can stop risks from turning into full-blown data breaches by ensuring they can find small, obscure actions. Overall, this innovative approach helps keep sensitive patient data secure, makes sure the system functions properly, and helps with ongoing efforts for satisfying regulatory requirements (Pereira et al., 2021).

3.3 Natural Language Processing (NLP) for Data De-Identification

Natural Language Processing is changing the manner in which healthcare organizations handle private patient information. Names, addresses, birth dates, and contact information are frequently concealed in unorganized material within clinical records, physician notes, and medical transcriptions. B y employing NLP techniques, these identifiers are detected automatically and eliminated or replaced with undetectable tokens that are anonymous. By streamlining this procedure, businesses may significantly decrease the chance of sharing data sets for studies, analytics, or collaborative initiatives that contain confidential medical data. This enables organizations comply with privacy laws like HIPAA while still making useful clinical data available for various other purposes. Even when identifiers have been concealed in sentences with a lot of context or phrasing, which is not clear, advanced models are capable of comprehending huge quantities of complicated data. The system can also work with different terms in medicine and document formats, allowing it to sure that all datasets have been fully protected. This method not simply protects patient privacy, but additionally also makes operations more efficient by reducing the need for manual information removal, which takes a lot of time and is easy to make mistakes (Rahman et al., 2022). Healthcare continues to produce a lot of unstructured data, but automated removal of identities through NLP makes absolutely certain that sensitive data continues to remain safe without getting in the way of work.

3.4 AI in Adaptive Access Control Systems

Adaptive access control systems employ smart algorithms to control the manner in which users have access to sensitive healthcare data. These systems move beyond conventional permissions assigned by roles that are static by constantly checking variables like user conduct, device type, location, and time of access. In case any unusual events take place, including a healthcare worker trying to get to patient data from a device or location they do not recognize, the system may quickly initiate extra authentication procedures or block access completely. By employing this dynamic method makes certain that access to electronic health records (EHRs) and other important information will remain safe without interfering with normal business. Adaptive controls, for example, may provide authorized medical workers greater authority throughout emergencies while maintaining an eye on their conduct to make sure they are not misusing their access. These systems may enhance their responses over time through learning from past patterns. This allows healthcare providers find an acceptable compromise between the need for privacy and the need for data to be available. While they see strange conduct, like trying to access something outside of work hours or failing to sign in multiple times, they ought to put in place stricter controls, creating insider threats even less likely. They also reduce internal risks through setting stricter controls within place. These solutions are adaptable which means that businesses may adhere to privacy rules while still being able to change how they do things quickly. They can also work well with additional safety precautions, like encryption and tools for finding hazards to give it better protection against unwanted unauthorized access to information (Elhoseny et al., 2021).

4 AI and Regulatory Compliance Automation

The automation of AI and regulatory compliance is changing the manner in which healthcare companies handle a complicated legal obligation. Figure 2 shows artificial intelligence tools for compliance in the healthcare. An automated systems able to enhance items more efficient through creating the tasks like monitoring, auditing, and providing the information in a simpler form that means less time is spent on manual tasks that are prone to a mistake. These advanced technologies contribute to keeping up with requirements like HIPAA and GDPR by quickly identifying problems while making sure that policies are carried out in a consistent way on all platforms. The process of an automation improves operations more efficiently by frees up employees from administrative duties, and helps to make sure that data protection measures are always correct and up to date. As healthcare rules evolve, artificial intelligence based applications allow the companies to quickly react, making both security and accountability better without stopping any important medical services.

- *Automated Auditing*: AI simplifies the generation of audit logs by automatically collecting and correlating data from multiple sources such as clinical systems, billing platforms, and user activity records. It ensures that reports are formatted according to regulatory standards, ready for both internal review and external regulatory inspections. It also highlights anomalies and suggests remediation steps.
- *Risk Assessment*: By evaluating threat intelligence feeds, historical incident data, and current system vulnerabilities, AI provides continuous risk scoring. It predicts the likelihood and potential impact of data breaches or non-compliance events.

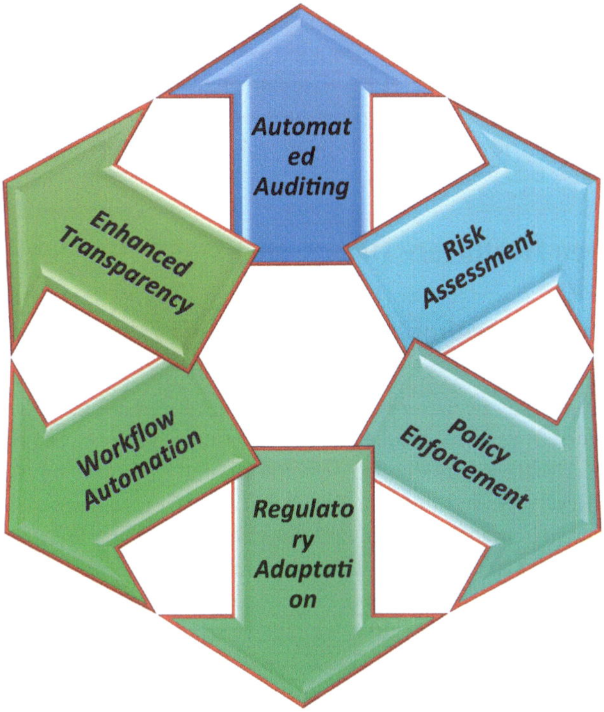

Fig. 2 AI-powered compliance tools in healthcare

Healthcare providers can prioritize mitigation actions based on these insights, focusing on high-risk areas such as legacy systems or third-party vendors.

- *Policy Enforcement*: AI enforces both external regulations (like HIPAA, GDPR) and internal security policies by automating rule application across users and devices. For example, it can automatically block unauthorized file transfers, enforce multi-factor authentication, or encrypt data in transit and at rest. It also audits employee behavior against internal codes of conduct and usage policies.
- *Regulatory Adaptation*: Healthcare regulations frequently change based on technological advances, emerging threats, or legal reforms. AI helps organizations stay updated by integrating regulatory updates directly into compliance workflows. It automatically adjusts system configurations and security controls, ensuring that the healthcare organization always aligns with the latest legal requirements (Alabdulatif et al., 2022).
- *Workflow Automation*: From onboarding new employees to reviewing user permissions, AI automates repetitive and critical compliance-related processes. For example, it can automate monthly access control reviews, data lifecycle management (such as archiving or deleting outdated records), and trigger incident response procedures when a breach is suspected.

- *Enhanced Transparency*: AI-driven tools provide a centralized, easily accessible view of compliance operations. Detailed visual reports, interactive dashboards, and audit trails make it easier for both technical teams and management to understand compliance status at any given moment. This level of visibility is crucial during legal inquiries, external audits, or stakeholder reporting.

5 AI-Driven Healthcare Data Security

5.1 Federated Learning in Protecting Data Privacy

Federated learning has been very important for keeping data private in the healthcare field because it permits people train models together without distributing raw data (Xu et al., 2020). AI models possess traditionally needed centralized datasets for learning effectively, and this is a significant privacy risk, particularly whenever handling private patient information. Federated learning solves this problem through permitting a training to take place in many places concurrently. With this method, the information stays in a local servers or devices, like hospital databases or medical devices. Simply model updates, like weights or gradients, are needed to transmit to a central server (Keshta, 2022). This method significantly reduces the chance of the data breaches, since patient records never leave their original location. Although someone listens in on the conversation channels, but the information that is sent does not give away any private information. Federated learning also helps people follow the privacy laws like HIPAA and GDPR, which require strict rules about the manner data can be shared and processed (Sreedhar et al., 2025). Federated learning enables healthcare organizations to work together around the world to build strong AI models (Kumarganesh et al., 2025) while not putting the safety of patients at a risk. For instance, hospitals in various fields may collaborate together to make diagnostic models for rare diseases whereas still keeping control of their individual information. This is especially helpful for making models with diverse, representative datasets because it makes them more accurate and less skewed. Federated learning is often used with other privacy-protecting methods, like differential privacy and secure multiparty computation, to make data protection even better. These additional components ensure that even the updates to the aggregated model refrain from giving away an information about the specific data points. Federated learning enhances AI-driven medical services more ethical and safer by keeping information private and promoting safe collaboration. It permits healthcare organizations leverage the power of large-scale AI without giving up the privacy of patient information (Saravanakumar et al., 2024).

5.2 *AI Forecasting for Regulatory Changes*

Artificial intelligence-driven predictive tools help the healthcare organizations to predict that which novel regulations and developments are likely to take place in the near future. As opposed to responding to new laws or modifications shortly after they occur, these processes examine an abundance of regulating data, legal documentation, policy revisions, and global healthcare trends in order to determine a term that could occur in the future. This preparedness strategy assists the healthcare providers to prepare themselves ahead of time and avoid the costly problems that come due to failing to comply with the rules. AI (Pandey et al., 2024) forecasting methods can find the patterns in past updates to the regulations and look at changes in healthcare governance around the world to give early warnings about the compliance problems that are starting to happen. Changes to data privacy, telemedicine, AI ethics, or cross-border data sharing can be predicted ahead of the time. This helps businesses make sure that their internal rules and the technical systems are in synchronized form before new laws go into the effect. AI models used for forecasting combine machine learning algorithms and the natural language processing to look at unstructured legal documents, government publications, and an industry data. These solutions give compliance teams and an executive to predictive insights that help them make smart choices about changes to the policies, investments in technology, and training for the employees. In the fast changing world of healthcare, where data security and privacy are always under scrutiny, it is important to stay up to date on the changes to the law. Companies can avoid operational problems caused by sudden changes in compliance by using proactive forecasting. By showing a proactive approach to governance and risk management.

6 Conclusion

The use of artificial intelligence approaches in a healthcare data security and a compliance has become an important way to deal with the growing difficulty of keeping a sensitive patient information secure. The research presented here shows the modern technologies that enhance data protection by additionally automating compliance procedures within an environment that is heavily regulated. Artificial intelligence facilitates to keep an eye on things all the time to the find unusual patterns that help to protect the confidentiality of an individuals. AI makes things much safer and faster, but healthcare companies need to carefully balance new technology, patient privacy, and following the rules. An excess of automation without enough control could lead to new security holes or moral problems, while not enough automation could slow down operations and make patient care worse. AI usefulness in this area depends on making systems that are safe, clear, and able to adapt to changing rules. Additionally, the healthcare organizations should use an integrated strategy to get the most out of an artificially intelligent privacy and compliance solutions. This includes putting money into the federated learning and the privacy preserving technology. Healthcare providers can build a strong system that protect private information, follow rules, and build trust with patients and other stakeholders by combining the AI capabilities with an human experience.

References

Alabdulatif, A., Khalil, I., & Rahman, M. S. (2022). Security of blockchain and AI-empowered smart healthcare: Application-based analysis. *Applied Sciences, 12*, 11039.

Elhoseny, M., Haseeb, K., Shah, A. A., Ahmad, I., Jan, Z., & Alghamdi, M. I. (2021). IoT solution for AI-enabled privacy-preserving with big data transferring: An application for healthcare using blockchain. *Energies, 14*, 5364.

Keshta, I. (2022). AI-driven IoT for smart health care: Security and privacy issues. *Informatics in Medicine Unlocked, 30*, Article 100903.

Khalid, N., Qayyum, A., Qayyum, A., Al-Fuqaha, A., & Qadir, J. (2023). Privacy-preserving artificial intelligence in healthcare: Techniques and applications. *Computers in Biology and Medicine, 158*, Article 106848.

Kumarganesh, S., Murugesan, M., Ganesh, C., Santhiyakumari, N., Thangavel, M., Jayaram, K., Martin Sagayam, K., Pandey, B. K., & Pandey, D. (2025). Hybrid plasmonic biosensors with deep learning for colorectal cancer detection. *Plasmonics, 20*(7), 4895–4909.

Morley, J., Machado, C. C. V., Burr, C., Cowls, J., Taddeo, M., & Floridi, L. (2019). The debate on the ethics of AI in health care: A reconstruction and critical review. *Social Science Research Network*.

Murdoch, B. (2021). Privacy and artificial intelligence: Challenges for protecting health information in a new era. *BMC Medical Ethics, 22*, 122.

Pandey, B. K., Pandey, D., & Lelisho, M. E. (2024). Face mask identification with enhanced cuckoo optimization and deep learning-based faster regional neural network. *Scientific Reports, 14*(1), 29719.

Pereira, T., Morgado, J., Silva, F., Pelter, M. M., Dias, V., De Cássia Nogueira Barros, R., De Freitas, C., Negrão, E., De Lima, B. F., Da Silva, M. C., et al. (2021). Sharing biomedical data: Strengthening AI development in healthcare. *Healthcare, 9*, 827.

Prakash, S., Balaji, J. N., Joshi, A., & Surapaneni, K. M. (1914). Ethical conundrums in the application of artificial intelligence (AI) in healthcare—A scoping review of reviews. *Journal of Personalized Medicine, 2022*, 12.

Rahman, A., Hossain, M. S., Muhammad, G., Kundu, D., Debnath, T., Rahman, M. S., Khan, M. S. I., Tiwari, P., & Band, S. S. (2022). Federated learning-based AI approaches in smart healthcare: Concepts, taxonomies challenges and open issues. *Cluster Computing, 26*, 2271–2311.

Reddy, S., Allan, S., Coghlan, S., & Cooper, P. (2019). A governance model for the application of AI in health care. *Journal of the American Medical Informatics Association, 27*, 491–497.

Richardson, J. W., Smith, C., Curtis, S., Watson, S. E., Zhu, X., Barry, B. A., & Sharp, R. R. (2021). Patient apprehensions about the use of artificial intelligence in healthcare. *NPJ Digital Medicine, 4*, 140.

Saravanakumar, R., TamilSelvi, T., Pandey, D., Pandey, B. K., Mahajan, D. A., & Lelisho, M. E. (2024). Big data processing using hybrid Gaussian mixture model with salp swarm algorithm. *Journal of Big Data, 11*(1), 167.

Sreedhar, C., Kallam, S., Ghantasala, G. P., Anthoniraj, S., Kumarganesh, S., Sagayam, K. M., Pandey, B. K., & Pandey, D. (2025). Enhancing healthcare data security using RFE and CRHSM for big data. *Computers in Biology and Medicine, 190*, 110063.

Wang, C., Zhang, J., Lassi, N., & Zhang, X. (1878). Privacy protection in using artificial intelligence for healthcare: Chinese regulation in comparative perspective. *Healthcare, 2022*, 10.

Xu, J., Glicksberg, B. S., Su, C., Walker, P. B., Bian, J., & Wang, F. (2020). Federated learning for healthcare informatics. *Journal of Healthcare Informatics Research, 5*, 1–19.

Zarifis, A., Kawalek, P., & Azadegan, A. (2020). Evaluating if trust and personal information privacy concerns are barriers to using health insurance that explicitly utilizes AI. *Journal of Internet Commerce, 20*, 66–83.

Predictive Financial Modelling for Personalized Healthcare Plans Using AI

Mercedes Huerta-Soto, Edwin Hernan Ramirez, Edwin Asnate Salazar, Diego Villegas-Ramirez, and Carmen Cardenas Lara

Abstract The utilization of predictive financial modelling in improving tailored healthcare programmes. The project seeks to enhance healthcare cost forecasting, resource allocation, and patient care management through the integration of sophisticated machine learning methodologies and extensive data sources. A substantial emphasis is focused on the convergence of healthcare, finance, and artificial intelligence, highlighting how data-driven methodologies can enhance decision-making processes for providers, insurers, and politicians. The cost-effectiveness analysis to identify ideal healthcare interventions for various demographic groups, maintaining affordability and increasing health outcomes. The suggested intelligent financial planning framework utilizes predictive models to evaluate risks, project future healthcare costs, and create customized plans, so ensuring optimal resource allocation. The capacity of machine learning and prediction algorithms to develop more egalitarian, cost-efficient, and sustainable healthcare systems. It emphasizes the necessity of

M. Huerta-Soto
Universidad Nacional Santiago Antúnez de Mayolo, Huaraz, Perú
e-mail: mhuertas@unasam.edu.pe

E. H. Ramirez (✉)
Universidad Tecnologica del Perú, Lima, Perú
e-mail: C30120@utp.edu.pe

E. A. Salazar
Department of Computer Science and Engineering, Universidad Nacional Santiago Antunez de Mayolo, Huaraz, Peru
e-mail: edwin_johny@unasam.edu.pe

D. Villegas-Ramirez
Universidad Nacional Mayor de San Marcos, Lima, Peru
e-mail: 11150017@unmsm.edu.pe

C. C. Lara
Universidad Católica de Trujillo Benedicto XVI, La Libertad, Peru
e-mail: c.cardenas@uct.edu.pe

D. Pandey et al. (eds.), *Smart Healthcare*,
https://doi.org/10.1007/978-981-95-8828-2_16

amalgamating clinical, financial, and behavioural data to produce precise predictions and enhance overall healthcare provision. The study seeks to diminish healthcare expenses and improve patient welfare by providing significant insights for individualized treatment. Implementing predictive technology can revolutionize healthcare finance, enhancing accessibility, affordability, and customization for various populations, hence facilitating future developments in the field.

Keywords AI · Predictive modelling · Personalized healthcare · Financial forecasting · ML · Resource allocation · Patient care

1 Introduction

The combination of an advanced data analytics and healthcare finance is changing the manner people get and pay for a health services. As medical needs become more complicated and treatment costs expand, there is a greater need for smarter and more personalized financial solutions. Traditional health plans often rely on broad data that limits their flexibility and does not do a good job of taking into account the specific requirements of every patient. On the other hand, a modern computer models are capable of looking at a wide range of a factors that include from clinical records to lifestyle choices to come up with flexible and personalized financial solutions. These smart algorithms use large datasets to find patterns, determine what might have will happen next in healthcare, and determine to the amount it will expense. This ability to make predictions helps healthcare providers and insurers forecast plans that are both inexpensive and specific to each individuals risk profile and treatment needs. For patients, it means their bodies will have a better understanding of their future medical costs and be better prepared to handle subsequent healthcare financial obligations. These models use machine learning techniques to make their predictions better over time by using new data, thereby making them more accurate. Someone who additionally has had a chronic illness, is incapable of moving around much, or has certain genetic markers may need more frequent monitoring and care. Predictive modelling can take these things into account and change the structure of plans as required. This adaptability leads to better resource allocation with quicker action and possibly big savings for both patients and providers. Using smart forecasting in the financial planning makes the healthcare system more fair and open. By getting rid of the uncertainty and a generalization that come with traditional insurance models. The stakeholders can get useful information about future costs and coverage needs. It also opens up new possibilities for dynamic pricing which are adjusted for risks premiums, and continual policy customization. Integrating these technologies into existing healthcare and insurance systems is consider as a very difficult task. Data privacy, model transparency, and ethical decision making are all very important issues that need to be carefully thought about it. The shift to automated personalization in healthcare funding shows that people are moving towards care planning models that are more sustainable, inclusive, and efficient.

1.1 The Intersection of AI, Finance, and Healthcare

The integration of modern data science with financial and healthcare systems is creating new opportunities in the funding and management of medical services. In the past, the financial parts of the healthcare system, including structuring insurance, predicting costs, and billing, have worked on independently. By using actuarial data and past trends to arrive at decisions. At the same time, healthcare delivery has improved to use more personalized methods that put prevention, early intervention, and personalized therapy top of mind. It is now possible to combine different fields and create systems that work more effectively together and respond with greater speed, due to advanced computer tools. Modern analytical models are capable of discovering patterns in large amounts of health and financial data that human planners had difficulty recognizing before. This makes more straightforward to predict treatment costs more accurately, assess risks better, and come up with coverage agreements that are very specific to each person. Insurers are able to employ more than simply age and income to make premium plans that are fairer and more realistic. They can also use health behaviour, pre-existing diseases, and lifestyle data. This personalized plan is good for both people that get better and cheaper options, and providers and insurers, who can better manage their resources and cut down on waste. At the same time, the healthcare industry is under more pressure to cut costs and improve results. It is very important to be accurate when making financial plans, especially in public health systems and accountable care settings. Intelligent technologies facilitate the alignment of clinical objectives with financial sustainability through real-time decision-making, automated budgeting, and the early identification of expense conditions. The combination of technology, money, and medicine is not only making operations more effective, but it is also changing the way we think about care. Adding cost modelling to patient journeys makes the system more proactive, based on data, and ultimately more caring about health and money (Wachter & Brynjolfsson, 2024).

1.2 Growing Demand for Personalized Healthcare Solutions

The demand for personalized healthcare has risen substantially in recent years, due to advancements in health care technology, improved patient awareness and an increasing number of chronic diseases. Modern patients expect care that is both effective and tailored to their unique biological, moral, as well as socioeconomic traits. The traditional one-size-fits-all approach is becoming a less effective that often leading to worse outcomes and the higher healthcare costs. The healthcare systems have begun to shift towards models that put the patient foremost and also focus on the individualized therapeutic strategies and specific methods to avoid illness. This movement is closely related to the way easy it is to get detailed health data, such as genomic information from electronic medical records and real-time data from wearable devices (Zhang & Boulos, 2023). This information gives a lot of understanding of the likelihood of getting sick, their capacity to respond to treatment, and their overall way of life. Whenever used correctly, it helps healthcare providers provide more accurate diagnoses, offer targeted treatments, and better predict future wellness requirements. Personalization also includes the money side of healthcare. Patients differ not only in their medical needs but also in their financial capabilities, risk tolerance, and expectations concerning health insurance coverage. As a result, more and more people are trying to come up with financial plans that reflect these traits. The goal is to make healthcare easier to get to, more open, and easier to manage by using variable insurance premiums, tiered coverage, and budgeting tools that can predict costs. Trends in demographics, including an ageing population, better healthcare knowledge, and more people using digital health platforms, are also pushing the shift to personalized healthcare. The public are taking more control of their health and seeking solutions that fit their own goals and values. As this demand grows, the healthcare industry needs to change by using tools and structures that enable it possible to give truly personalized care, both medically and financially (Zaballa et al., 2023).

1.3 The Role of Predictive Financial Modelling

The predictive financial modelling has become an important component of the change that has taken place in the manner in which our team plan and manage healthcare costs. By employing these mathematical models, healthcare providers, insurers, and patients are capable of figuring out the amount their future medical bills are going to cost through looking at a lot of data about both individuals and groups of people. This makes it possible to make personalized health plans that could give one the most coverage for the least amount of money. The use of predictive modelling also helps find people who are at a high risk, which makes it possible to intervene early and avoid costly treatments in the future. It makes it easier to make decisions in real time by giving financial information right away during patient care. This leads to better financial planning and more sustainable healthcare delivery. Figure 1 shows the different ways that predictive financial modelling can be employed.

- *Cost Forecasting*: Predictive financial modelling employs health data from individuals and groups to predict the amount medical care will cost in the future. These models can predict both expected and unexpected medical expenses by analysing historical trends, socioeconomic information, and factors related to lifestyle. For instance, an individual with diabetes or another chronic condition may have more expensive medical expenses over their lifetime. Predictive modelling can help you figure out the amount these costs will amount to ahead of time. This information helps the two patients and insurers create more effective choices, lowering the chance of unanticipated expenses. Insurance companies can set premiums more

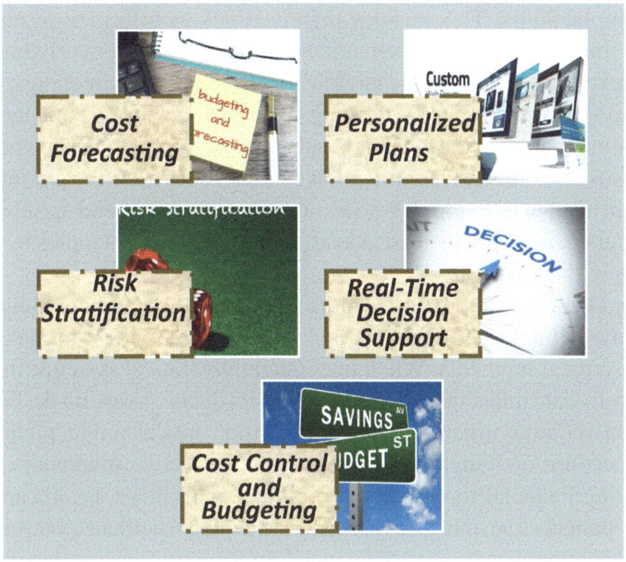

Fig. 1 Financial predictions and their function

accurately, and patients can become ready for treatments and medical events that are most likely to take place in future years. Furthermore, it helps healthcare providers prepare for their individual monetary requirements ensuring that resources are being utilized in the best way possible. Being effortlessly capable to predict costs permits healthcare managers be more prepared, and this in the end helps both individuals and healthcare organizations economically (Tan et al., 2023).

- *Personalized Plans*: Predictive financial modelling allows for the creation of highly personalized healthcare plans by analysing a variety of individual data points, including medical history, family health risks, and lifestyle choices. Traditional insurance models often group patients into broad categories based on age or gender, which can lead to over- or under-insurance. However, predictive modelling takes a more refined approach by factoring in specific risk indicators, such as the likelihood of developing certain conditions. This ensures that coverage matches an individual's actual needs rather than a generalized template. For example, a smoker may require higher coverage for respiratory diseases, while someone with a family history of heart disease might need additional cardiovascular coverage. By tailoring the plan to the patient's unique profile, the system can optimize costs, offer only necessary coverage and avoid unnecessary services, which improves both affordability and satisfaction (Ooi et al., 2023).
- *Risk Stratification*: Risk stratification helps insurers and healthcare providers identify individuals who are at a higher risk for expensive medical treatments. Predictive models assess a wide range of factors such as pre-existing conditions, age, lifestyle habits, and genetic predispositions to estimate the likelihood of future

health complications. This enables organizations to prioritize resources effectively. For instance, high-risk individuals can be targeted for early interventions, such as preventive care, lifestyle modifications, or regular screenings, which may reduce the overall cost of care in the long term. By focusing on patients most likely to need significant care, these models help healthcare systems become more efficient and sustainable. Risk stratification enables more accurate pricing for health plans, ensuring that individuals who are at lower risk do not end up subsidizing the costs of higher-risk patients. It also leads to better health outcomes by addressing issues before they escalate.

- *Real-Time Decision Support*: Real-time decision support powered by predictive financial modelling allows patients and healthcare providers to make informed choices at critical moments. When integrated into clinical systems, these models provide up-to-date financial insights as treatment decisions are made. For example, if a patient requires urgent surgery, a real-time model might predict the cost of the procedure and suggest alternative, cost-effective treatment options. By incorporating financial forecasting into clinical workflows, healthcare providers can offer patients the most economical care plans without compromising on quality. This immediate access to financial information ensures that decisions are aligned with both medical needs and budget constraints. For patients, it provides transparency about the cost implications of different treatment options, helping them make better-informed choices. For insurers and healthcare providers, it enhances resource allocation by prioritizing interventions that are both clinically and financially optimal (Nova, 2023).
- *Cost Control and Budgeting*: Cost control and budgeting through predictive financial modelling help both individuals and healthcare organizations manage healthcare expenses over time. By forecasting both short-term and long-term medical costs, patients can set aside the necessary funds for anticipated treatments, reducing the likelihood of unexpected financial strain. For example, if a model predicts the need for multiple doctor visits or a prolonged hospital stay, patients can prepare in advance by adjusting their savings or exploring flexible insurance coverage options. Healthcare providers also benefit from these predictive tools by ensuring that funds are allocated to the most cost-effective care pathways. For insurers, predictive models can help refine pricing strategies, ensuring premiums are accurately adjusted based on the patient's future healthcare needs. These models can also identify opportunities for cost-saving measures, such as preventive care programmes, which help mitigate the need for expensive interventions later. This comprehensive approach leads to better financial outcomes for all parties involved.

2 Existing Knowledge and Technological Advancements

2.1 Financial Modelling in the Healthcare Sector

Healthcare financial modelling has changed because healthcare delivery is more complicated and better financial management is needed. Early healthcare financial models used past data and general financial assumptions to plan budgets and divide costs. The main uses of these early models were for hospital budgets, reimbursement rates, and insurance compliance. They did not possess the skills to deal with the fact that healthcare services are always changing and that companies are under more pressure to offer affordable care. As healthcare systems grew and evolved, financial modelling got better. Integrating patient demographics, treatment histories, and resource use made it possible to do a more comprehensive financial analysis. This led to more advanced models that were capable of figuring out the amount that it would cost to treat a patient and provide healthcare. ICD-10 (International Classification of Diseases) and other diagnostic and procedural coding systems helped figure out what patients needed and the amount that they ought to cost, which made financial estimates better. The next big step forward was managed care systems in the 1990. The healthcare industry used adjusted for risk capitation models to reduce costs. These models used demographic data and risk variables to figure out the amount that healthcare would cost for the whole population. This change was made to cut down on unnecessary treatments and make things run more smoothly. The financial models of this time included ideas from the management of population health, which helped healthcare providers figure out the amount that it would cost to prevent and treat chronic diseases. In the early 2000, better data analytics and computing power made financial modelling better. As health data and EHRs became more widely available, it became possible to track and predict finances in real time (Miao et al., 2023). Healthcare companies are able to examine at huge amounts of data to better guess what will happen to patients, which patterns will happen, and what resources they will require. In this day and age, clinical decision support systems and financial modelling included cost estimates in the treatment strategies. The most recent step is to add AI and ML to healthcare financial modelling. These technologies let predictive models work with huge amounts of complicated data, find hidden patterns, and accurately estimate the amount healthcare is going to expense. AI models can look at risk factors, predict the manner in which diseases will progress, and make the best use of resources all at the same time. As value based care models become more common and it need more advanced financial models that use both clinical and financial data to better control costs and improve patient outcomes (Ullah et al., 2022).

2.2 Personalized Healthcare and Precision Medicine

The personalized healthcare and precision medicine focus on customizing medical care based on elements such as genetics, environment, and lifestyle. The goal is to cease using the old one-size-fits-all approach and instead offer treatments that work better while causing fewer side effects. Personalized healthcare utilizes detailed patient information, like genetic profiles to make individualized treatment plans. This helps to ensure sure that each patient gets care that is right for their unique biological makeup. Genetic profiling is an important part of precision medicine since it helps find genetic predispositions and mutations that could affect the manner in which a person responds to certain treatments. This genetic information helps medical professionals find out the likelihood that someone will get certain diseases and develop methods to stop them or treat them early. Also, targeted therapies are used in precision medicine to treat certain genetic mutations or molecular markers. This makes treatments work better and hurt healthy cells less. Biomarkers and diagnostic tools are also very important for precision medicine. Biomarkers are measurable signs, including proteins or genetic variants that help find diseases early and keep track of the way treatments are working. These diagnostic tools help healthcare professionals find diseases accurately and make smart choices about the best treatments. The treatment strategies include beyond genetic factors, but also lifestyle and environmental factors. This gives an extensive understanding of the condition of the individual health. The personalized healthcare is all about using data to make decisions. The utilization of big data that include the electronic health records (EHRs) and real time health monitoring helps people arrive at better decisions and get treatment that is right for them at the moment. As precision medicine develops, the focus is on more than simply treating diseases; it is also on proactive and preventive healthcare. Healthcare systems can take steps to stop diseases from starting by learning about genetic risks and environmental factors. For precision medicine to work, individuals with different fields need to work together. Healthcare professionals, geneticists, bioinformaticians, and pharmacologists must collaborate to ensure that treatments are scientifically valid, tailored, and efficacious (Malik et al., 2022).

2.3 Artificial Intelligence in Financial Forecasting

The use of advanced computer techniques in financial forecasting has changed how healthcare organizations plan and manage their money. These systems use algorithms that can observe large databases to produce more accurate and flexible financial predictions. These systems use past financial data, patient records, treatment costs, and other information to make projections that change in real time, which helps people develop better decisions. Machine learning algorithms that are a type of these systems are very good at predicting long-term healthcare costs as well as expenses for individual patients. These models are designed to find hidden patterns and connections in large datasets, and thus make it easier to predict future costs or find groups of people who are at greatest risk. Predictive models are able to look at the medical records of an individual and determine out the type of care they need as well as how much it will run them in the future. This makes it easier to make more personalized financial plans. These computer models help save money by finding patterns and problems. By looking into the way patients move through the system, the manner in which resources are being utilized, and the amount that treatment costs, they ought to can suggest methods to cut down on waste while also making better use of resources. This helps healthcare companies improve their budgeting processes while ensuring they can still provide high quality care without spending too much money. Using modern computing algorithms enables someone to perform analyses on data in real time. The healthcare providers are able to maintain an eye on the patient data. As it is being collected, consequently making it easier to quickly change treatment plans or financial plans. These changes made in real time to ensure that the costs always match the needs of the patients, which makes the business more financially stable. Implementing computer models to predict healthcare costs opens up new ways to be creative. These systems not only predict costs by combining a lot of patient and financial data, but they also suggest ways to improve patient care and operational efficiency, thereby aiding the healthcare industry keep moving forward (Saravanakumar et al., 2024).

3 Investigation and Model Construction

3.1 Data Acquisition and Preparation

To develop a reliable and an accurate financial model in the personalized healthcare. It is necessary to be able to get and prepare data well. During this stage, the datasets that are used for generating predictions and decisions have been gathered, cleaned, organized, and safeguarded. As soon as it comes to predicting healthcare finances, numerous amounts of different types of data need to be gathered and combined to get a full picture of every single individual medical and financial situation. The main types of data used in personalized healthcare financial modelling are clinical, financial, and behavioural data. The clinical information is made up of physician notes, electronic health records (EHRs), results of diagnostic tests, and treatment histories. This information gives you an idea of the medical history of a patient, diagnoses, current conditions, and suggested therapies. Insurance claims, billing histories, treatment costs, and coverage details are all examples of financial data. These datasets are useful for assessing the economic burden of treatments and predicting healthcare expenditures at both individual and population levels. It is also important to look at behavioural data, like the number of times people exercise, the food they eat, the amount that they smoke or drink, and the social factors that affect their health. This kind of data can have a big effect on health outcomes and is often used to make cost and risk predictions more accurate. Combining these data sources gives us an improved understanding of patient profiles, which permits us make better and more accurate predictions. When dealing with sensitive health and financial information, individual must follow the strict rules about privacy, security, and ethics. In the USA, HIPAA and in Europe, GDPR are able to protect the personal health information by requiring data protection practices and limiting access to it without permission. To keep patient information protected. It is important to use an encryption, anonymization, and the secure storage protocols. The ethical issues must be taken into account to make sure that the data is collected alongside informed consent and used in an appropriate manner. Advanced analytics must also be free of bias and fair, particularly if they are used to make predictions that affect financial decisions or care recommendations. To keep trust in these systems, it is essential to be open regarding the way data is used and to enable people choose whether or not to have their data collected (Bugaj et al., 2023).

3.2 AI Models and Predictive Algorithms

The application of advanced computer models to predict healthcare costs gives very accurate, data-driven insights. Normally, the health care professionals and insurers can use predictive algorithms to figure out the amount that treatment is going to cost, how susceptible to infection a patient appears, and the best way to make a personalized financial strategy. Different machine learning and deep learning methods have been employed and each one has its own benefits depending on the kind and structure of the data. The public often use linear and logistic regression models to find out the amount that healthcare will cost and the manner in which that certain medical events will happen in the future. They help us figure out the effect of different factors that includes the age, diagnosis, and treatment costs, are related to each other. The Support Vector Machines (SVM) are used for classification of the tasks, like finding high-risk patients by looking at their past health and the financial data. These models use labelled datasets to train the system. So, they perform best when the results (like cost or treatment success) are already known. The neural networks and other deep learning models are considered as appropriate for working with the complicated, highly dimensional information like medical imaging or electronic health records. They can learn features from a raw data on their own that makes them great for personalized healthcare apps. The Recurrent Neural Networks (RNNs) and Long Short-Term Memory (LSTM) networks are used to work with series of data like patient histories or records of an ongoing treatment. These models are great at finding patterns over time, which is important for figuring out how much continuous therapy will cost and the manner in which a disease will progress (Ghebrehiwet et al., 2024).

3.3 System Architecture and Workflow

The AI-driven financial forecasting in healthcare, the system architecture and workflow are designed to ensure that data can be easily integrated, analysed, and output is generated accurately. The first step is to identify and collect an important input variable, such as clinical records such as medical history and treatment data, financial information which include billing and insurance claims. The technique of feature engineering is applied to refine this raw data into meaningful inputs for modelling. This involves processes like normalization along with encoding and creating composite variables that take into account the patient age and the health. These engineered features improve the model better and also offering the accurate and useful predictions. The core system then uses predictive algorithms to process this structured data and also provide outputs such as estimated healthcare costs, risk categories for the patients, and prospective budget forecasts. The Hospitals, insurance companies, and the public health organizations need these outputs to make better and smart financial plans. The organization help to predict the treatments patients are likely to require, determine the best use of resources, and create individualized payment or treatment strategies. Dashboards or decision support systems provide an output in the real time to healthcare professionals and administrators. Robust model evaluation methods have been utilized to ensure the accuracy of these predictions. The Mean Absolute Error (MAE), Root Mean Squared Error (RMSE), and Mean Absolute Percentage Error (MAPE) constitute significant measures which appear at model accuracy from various perspectives. To ensure the model performs effectively across various datasets and to mitigate the risk of over fitting. The cross validation and other methods have been utilized. This continuing examination, combined with regular recalibration also ensure that the forecasting system stays up to current with changes in treatment methods, costs, and patient demographics. This integrated process lets healthcare providers make informed financial decisions and gives patients better treatment at the same time.

4 Cognitive Model for Strategic Financial Planning

A Cognitive Model for Strategic Financial Planning helps the healthcare industry make the most of its financial planning. The framework shown in Fig. 2, uses advanced machine learning algorithms and methods for making choices that are similar to the way people make decisions. This model makes decisions better by imitating in which individuals think and taking into account a number of factors, such as the patients' risk, the effectiveness of the treatment, and the budget. It is capable of looking at situations that are both complicated and changing and it allows for better guesses regarding whatever will happen next. This plan not only helps support proactive financial initiatives. But it also makes better use of resources, predicts costs more accurately, and gives each patient better care. By learning from past data and

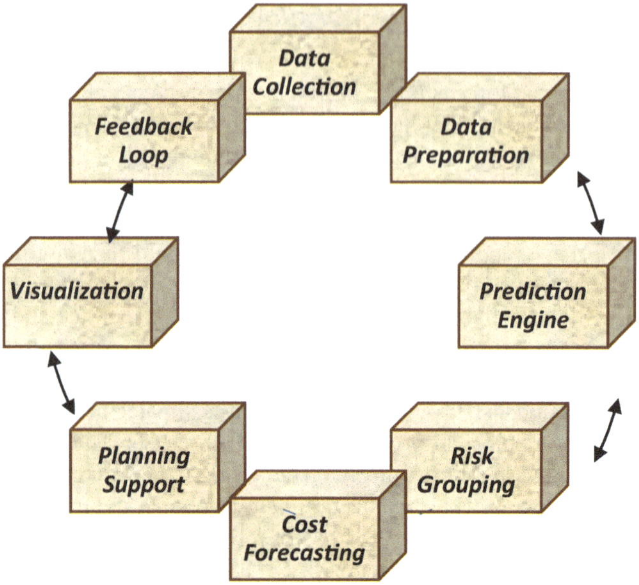

Fig. 2 Smart framework for financial planning

getting feedback from users, the model can keep getting better at making proposals for strategic healthcare financial management.

1. *Data Collection*: The data collection is considered as the starting point of an intelligent financial planning in healthcare. It involves the gathering of a structured and unstructured data from multiple sources such as electronic health records (EHRs), insurance claims, wearable devices, lab reports, and the behavioural data. The clinical data may include the diagnosis codes, lab results, treatment records, and the prescriptions. The behavioural data that includes activity levels, sleep patterns, diet, and the utilization of the substance helps in building a more holistic view of the patient. These inputs offer a 360-degree view necessary for personalized financial predictions. The data is usually pulled out from the databases, APIs, IoT-enabled health devices, and even the patient surveys. High-quality data at this stage, ensures the predictive models receive accurate and relevant information. Without a strong foundation of reliable data, later steps in the framework such as modelling and risk prediction may yield flawed results. Hence, this phase also involves data validation to confirm the accuracy and completeness of each data stream (Preiksaitis & Rose, 2023).
2. *Data Preparation*: The information has to be processed, organised, and put into a format that the predictive models will be comprehend, after this has been gathered. This step basically involves the fixing data entry mistakes, addressing of inadequate or incorrect values, changing of units, and encoding variables with a category. The development of features is an important part of this stage. It means making new variables features that give you more information or better show the

problem. For instance, by putting together age, BMI, and cholesterol levels could help to show how likely someone is to have heart problems. Time continuum characteristics, which include the frequency of medical appointments in the past year, may additionally be significant. The normalization process ensures that different types of data are on an identical magnitude, thereby helping the model work more effectively. This step might additionally employ dimensionality reduction methods to get rid of extra or insignificant variables that might mislead the model. The public often use SQL, Python (Pandas), and automated data pipelines in the cloud (like Azure and AWS). Thoroughly collected and clean data assures sure that the machine learning models work with adequate data inputs, which has a direct effect on the precision and dependability of the predictions possess.

3. *Prediction Engine*: The predictive engine is the fundamental component of the intelligent planning framework. It uses advanced algorithms to determine the things will happen in the future. This engine uses machine learning methods like regression modelling, support vector machines (SVM), decision trees and neural networks. These models develop the ability to identify trends in historical data that will allow them to predict the amount that healthcare will be administered, precisely how much it will cost, as well as the expected outcomes. For instance, it can predict the amount that a diabetic person might spend in the next year or the probability that likely they are going to be hospitalised in the next 30 days. LSTM (Long Short-Term Memory) and other time series models have been great at finding patterns over time. To avoid excessive overfitting, the model must be trained, validated, and tested alongside cross validation. It should also be updated periodically to include the most recent information and advancements in healthcare. The engine is the location where data turns into knowledge. It helps healthcare providers, insurers, and policymakers estimate future needs and use resources wisely. By finding people who are at high risk and high cost early on, interventions are frequently quick and cheap.
4. *Risk Grouping*: In the aftermath of arriving at predictions, the system organizes patients or users into groups based on the probability they are to be at risk. Risk stratification is the term that is designated as an important part of a proactive healthcare management. Patients are frequently put into low, moderate, or elevated risk categories based on the quantity of money they ought to must contribute, the complexity of their medical condition, or the way likely they are to have an acute occurrence. For example, a patient whose work is likely to need a lot of hospitalization and expensive treatment might be put in a group with a high risk. This grouping facilitates it possible to create targeted interventions, like personalized treatment strategies or disease management programmes. It also helps healthcare systems decide the manner in which to best use their financial assets. This information could help insurance companies change the manner in which they charge premiums or make health plans that are more specific to certain groups of people. Furthermore, predictive risk scoring could assist with population health management by finding groups or communities that are particularly at risk of getting chronic diseases or epidemics. It improves patient outcomes

and lowers healthcare costs by allowing for early intervention and better use of medical resources.

5. *Cost Forecasting*: The cost forecasting procedure takes place when someone make financial predictions using the models outputs. This figures out the amount that healthcare expenses will be for individuals and companies in the short and long terms. These forecasts may include the costs of drugs, hospital stays, outpatient visits, surgeries, as well as rehab. It additionally takes into account possible emergencies along with ways to manage chronic diseases. These predictions enable insurance companies create unique payment structures and coverage choices. The hospitals are able to utilize the data to make expenditures, employ the right number of staff, and estimate the amount of inventory their bodies will have to purchase. Policymakers may employ this on a larger scale to decide the manner in which to spend the national health budget. Estimating also helps people determine out the amount they might have to pay out of their own pockets, thus making simpler to prepare ahead or sign up for the right health plans. Medical professionals may prevent financial surprises, reduce the risk of getting into debt, and continue to keep their operations going by using accurate cost predictions. It gives everyone involved the details needed to formulate smart and strategic monetary decisions.
6. *Planning Support*: This is the phase in which the ideas that come from models are transformed into plans which must be put into action. The healthcare administrators, insurance analysts, along with patients can obtain help from the system in real time. The dashboards and decision support tools provide stakeholders suggestions for care pathways, techniques to save money on medical care, approaches to stop issues prior to develop, or modifications to the budget. A healthcare professional could, for instance, get informed that a patient is probably going to fail to make payments and provide a plan which is more flexible. Medical facilities are able to alter the number of staff they have based on the number of patients they anticipate treating, and health insurance companies might change the manner in which benefits are administered. The system additionally allows it to run "what-if" experiments to determine the way various financial or clinical strategies could influence the situation. This part makes sure that insights generated by AI constitute more than simply numbers. They are also useful tools for getting better results. It makes operational planning more effective, encourages patients get involved, while simultaneously making sure that everyone in the healthcare system makes better decisions.
7. *Visualization*: The visualization tools tend to be essential for making complicated predictions straightforward for people to comprehend and to utilize. They demonstrate the results of the model in simple manners, including charts, graphs, heatmaps, or dashboards. To ensure individuals are able to comprehend the data being displayed. These images have been created for different people, like medical professionals, insurance companies, hospital managers, or even the patients themselves. For instance, a healthcare professional might see a persons' medical anticipated expenses and health risks during the same time, whereas

an insurance executive might observe gathered forecasts for an entire population. Individuals can also filter data, contrast metrics, and maintain track of changes over time using these interfaces. The correct visuals can assist to find hidden patterns and make decisions faster and alongside additional details. The organization also makes things simpler to understand, thus making it simpler to articulate model choices and earn the confidence of consumers. With immediate visualizations, individuals who work in healthcare can take action on forecasting data right away, which makes medical and financial preparation more proactive and efficient.

8. *Feedback Loop*: The feedback loop has become an element of the system that helps this to learn and get more effective as time passes. As the model is implemented, it acquires new information such as real outcomes of treatment, patient responses, and revised financial records. It allows the models acquire knowledge again and get more proficient in the things they do. The actions of users and feedback, such as decision overrides and model errors, are captured as well to find ways that can enhance the system. The loop described above makes adaptive learning possible through permitting the framework evolve as healthcare trends, novel therapies, and policy changes emerge. The model additionally employs, the static historical data which renders this more relevant in the future. For instance, whenever a new treatment cuts down on hospitalizations for a condition by considerable amounts, the model can observe this trend and change its forecasts to match. In the rapidly changing fields of healthcare and finance, during which having the capability to change on an ongoing basis is important for success, this continual process of improvement in oneself has been very important.

5 Implementation Scenarios and Simulated Use Cases

5.1 Cost-Effectiveness Analysis for Different Demographics

Cost-effectiveness analysis (CEA) constitutes a very important tool for comparing healthcare interventions for different groups of people. It compares the expenses and outcomes of different treatments in order to find the best way for utilizing healthcare resources. CEA helps decision makers for taking decision for the best use of limited resources by looking at both the cost and health outcomes of different actions. This is especially helpful in groups of people that are complicated and different. As soon as doing a CEA with people from different groups. It is essential to take into account about the things that each group needs and the ways they are different from the other groups. Things such as age, gender, socioeconomic status, the prevalence of chronic diseases, and cultural differences all affect the ways individuals use healthcare and what ultimately happens to them as a consequence. For instance, adolescents can benefit from preventative measures like immunizations that could save money in the long run. On the other hand, older people might need more treatments and hospitalizations because these individuals are more likely to have chronic conditions like diabetes or high blood pressure. An intervention which can be cheap for one group of people might not work as well or be as cheap for another group. For example, a high-cost treatment could possibly be seen as cost-effective in a wealthy capital, but not in a rural or impoverished area were getting to a medical facility is challenging. CEA allows stakeholders to tailor interventions to meet the needs of specific groups of people, making sure that healthcare strategies are both effective and fair. This analysis is especially useful for customized a healthcare, where the treatments are tailored to each specific needs to get the best health results at the lowest cost. It ultimately helps the policymakers, healthcare providers, and insurers choose the interventions that will help each group the most while also making sure that the economy stays stable (Samala & Rawas, 2024).

5.2 Strategic Implications for Providers, Insurers, and Policymakers

The use of advanced predictive models and cost-effectiveness analysis in healthcare finance has big strategic effects on medical professionals (Sehrawat, 2023), insurance companies along with policymakers. It allows them make better decisions regarding the best way to distribute resources, plan care, and formulate policies. These models enable healthcare providers find people that are at high risk and estimate the treatment they could require in the near future, and these helps make overseeing care easier and more effective (Pandey et al., 2024). By knowing the quantity of money, they will make along with how risky their patients are for their health. The medical professionals can optimize the best use of their staff, treatment plans, and hospital resources that lowers costs and improves patient outcomes. Furthermore, customized treatment plans based on cost-effectiveness analysis allow providers to give care that can be more focused and financially sound. By employing these predictive models (Pandey & Pandey, 2025) helps insurers set more accurate premium prices and risk adjusted plans for insurance. Insurers can better manage their risk exposure by offering customized insurance packages that meet the needs of their policyholders determined by demographic data. This method not only helps businesses save money by making their plans more personalized, but it also makes customers more fulfilled. Insurers can focus on covering the most valuable interventions by using cost-effectiveness analysis. This will lower the number of claims and make the company more profitable. These tools give policymakers data driven insights that aid them make policies that make sure healthcare resources are distributed fairly and efficiently. Policymakers may develop programmes (David et al., 2023) that meet the specific needs of different groups of individuals if they have access to cost-effectiveness analyses and data on specific demographics. This means that public health programmes should focus on preventive care for people who additionally are at risk, promote treatments that are affordable, and make it easier for people with low incomes or who live in rural areas to get medical treatment. Predictive models additionally have the potential to assist policymakers plan for longevity by helping them predict exactly what will happen in the future with healthcare trends.

6 Conclusion

The healthcare finance has advanced, in part due to the better financial modelling, predictive algorithms, and customized healthcare data. This study developed an intelligent financial planning system that forecasts a healthcare cost and enhances the resource allocation by means of the predictive analytics. It was shown that machine learning models could improve financial forecasting, risk stratification, and cost-effectiveness analysis more accurate for various demographic categories. By combining the clinical, financial, and behavioural data. This framework helps healthcare providers, insurers, and the regulators to arrive at smart choices that help to improve health outcomes, while maintaining costs down. These new ideas will have significant consequences. Comprehensive financial planning based on predictive models could help make healthcare better by making it affordable and tailored to every person. Healthcare providers can cut costs in the long run and improve patient health by concentrating on preventing situations with elevated risks through accurate forecasting and risk categorization. Insurance companies can offer fairer prices and more complete coverage since they can make customized plans based on a patients expected medical path. These findings help policymakers make healthcare equitable and make the best use of available funds. AI in healthcare finance possesses a lot of potential as technology grows more advanced. AI could make healthcare financial planning more accurate and customized by making it easier to collect, process, and model data. Additional advanced technologies are going to demonstrate the manner in which to cut costs, improve patient outcomes, and make healthcare finance more sustainable.

References

Wachter, R. M., & Brynjolfsson, E. (2024). Will generative artificial intelligence deliver on its promise in health care? *JAMA, 331*, 65–69.

Zhang, P., & Boulos, M. N. K. (2023). Generative AI in medicine and healthcare: Promises, opportunities and challenges. *Future Internet, 15*, 286.

Zaballa, O., Pérez, A., Inhiesto, E. G., Ayesta, T. A., & Lozano, J. A. (2023). Learning the progression patterns of treatments using a probabilistic generative model. *Journal of Biomedical Informatics, 137*, Article 104271.

Tan, T. F., Thirunavukarasu, A. J., Campbell, J. P., Keane, P. A., Pasquale, L. R., Abramoff, M. D., Kalpathy-Cramer, J., Lum, F., Kim, J. E., Baxter, S. L., et al. (2023). Generative artificial intelligence through ChatGPT and other large language models in ophthalmology: Clinical applications and challenges. *Ophthalmology Science, 3*, Article 100394.

Ooi, K.-B., Tan, G. W. H., Al-Emran, M., Al-Sharafi, M. A., Capatina, A., Chakraborty, A., Dwivedi, Y. K., Huang, T. L., Kar, A. K., Lee, V. H., et al. (2023). The potential of generative artificial intelligence across disciplines: Perspectives and future directions. *Journal of Computer Information Systems,* 1–32.

Nova, K. (2023). Generative AI in healthcare: Advancements in electronic health records, facilitating medical languages, and personalized patient care. *Journal of Advanced Analytics in Healthcare Management, 7*, 115–131.

Miao, H., Li, C., & Wang, J. (2023). A future of smarter digital health empowered by generative pretrained transformer. *Journal of Medical Internet Research, 25*, Article e49963.

Ullah, E., Baig, M. M., GholamHosseini, H., & Lu, J. (2022). Failure mode and effect analysis (FMEA) to identify and mitigate failures in a hospital rapid response system (RRS). *Heliyon, 8*, Article e08944.

Malik, S., Tyagi, A. K., & Mahajan, S. (2022). Architecture, generative model, and deep reinforcement learning for IoT applications: Deep learning perspective. *Artificial Intelligence Based Internet of Things Systems,* 243–265.

Saravanakumar, R., TamilSelvi, T., Pandey, D., Pandey, B. K., Mahajan, D. A., & Lelisho, M. E. (2024). Big data processing using hybrid Gaussian mixture model with salp swarm algorithm. *Journal of Big Data, 11*(1), 167.

Bugaj, M., Kliestik, T., & Lăzăroiu, G. (2023). Generative artificial intelligence-based diagnostic algorithms in disease risk detection, in personalized and targeted healthcare procedures, and in patient care safety and quality. *Contemporary Readings in Law and Social Justice, 15*, 9–26.

Ghebrehiwet, I., Zaki, N., Damseh, R., & Mohamad, M. S. (2024). Revolutionizing personalized medicine with generative AI: A systematic review. *Artificial Intelligence Review, 57*, 1–41.

Preiksaitis, C., & Rose, C. (2023). Opportunities, challenges, and future directions of generative artificial intelligence in medical education: Scoping review. *JMIR Medical Education, 9*, Article e48785.

Samala, A. D., & Rawas, S. (2024). Generative AI as virtual healthcare assistant for enhancing patient care quality. *International Journal of Online and Biomedical Engineering, 20*, 174.

Sehrawat, S. K. (2023). Empowering the patient journey: The role of generative AI in healthcare. *International Journal of Sustainable Development Through AI, ML, and IoT, 2*, 1–18.

Pandey, B. K., Pandey, D., & Lelisho, M. E. (2024). Face mask identification with enhanced cuckoo optimization and deep learning-based faster regional neural network. *Scientific Reports, 14*(1), 29719.

Pandey, B. K., & Pandey, D. (2025). Securing healthcare medical image information using advance morphological component analysis, information hiding systems, and hybrid convolutional neural networks on IoMT. *Computers in Biology and Medicine, 185*, 109499.

David, S., Duraipandian, K., Chandrasekaran, D., Pandey, D., Sindhwani, N., & Pandey, B. K. (2023). Impact of blockchain in healthcare system. In *Unleashing the Potentials of blockchain technology for healthcare industries* (pp. 37–57). Academic Press.

AI-Driven Strategies for Enhancing Competitiveness in Healthcare Startups

Uvaldo Cuno-Chunga, Hernán Ramirez Asís, Jorge Manrique Cáceres, and Andree Jhaire Liñan Ramirez

Abstract The manner in which modern technology allows healthcare startups to be more competitive. An organization can improve patient care, speed up operations, and arrive at better strategic decisions by using predictive analytics, machine learning, and the natural language processing. Healthcare establishments can save cash while operating more efficiently by performing automated administrative tasks including billing and scheduling. Predictive techniques help find health risks ahead of time, enhance the accuracy of diagnoses, and encourage personalized treatment plans. The clinical decision support system helps healthcare providers by giving them actual time, data-driven information that helps them reach better decisions for their patients. The role of market intelligence, and these focusses the manner in which these technologies can keep up to date on trends in the industry, consumer behavior, and the competition. New businesses can use data to make smart decisions that help them remain ahead of changes in the market, keep up with novel offerings, and get an edge over their competitors. The need to use these technologies responsibly. To keep trust and responsibility while getting the most out of these new tools that will enhance patient care and operational efficiency. It is important to deal with ethical issues involving protecting data privacy, getting rid of biases, and obeying healthcare laws.

Keywords Healthcare startups · Machine learning · Predictive analytics · Clinical decision support · Digital transformation · AI

U. Cuno-Chunga
Universidad Cesar Vallejo, Lima, Perú
e-mail: ccunocu@ucvvirtual.edu.pe

H. Ramirez Asís (✉)
CENTRUM PUCP Business School, Surco - Lima, Perú
e-mail: hernan.ramireza@pucp.edu.pe

J. M. Cáceres
Universidad Nacional Santiago Antunez de Mayolo, Huaraz, Peru
e-mail: jmanriquec@unasam.edu.pe

A. J. L. Ramirez
Universidad Peruana de Ciencias Aplicadas, Lima, Perú
e-mail: u201914391@upc.edu.pe

D. Pandey et al. (eds.), *Smart Healthcare*,
https://doi.org/10.1007/978-981-95-8828-2_17

1 Introduction

The startup ecosystem in the current medical and health fields has changed a lot and grown a significant amount in the last ten years. An emerging company have arisen up, to provide immediate digital solutions owing to advances in technology. These businesses provide a wide range of services that include the virtual consultations, artificially intelligent diagnostics, wearable monitoring devices, and internet-enabled therapies. Perhaps the most important thing about this growing field is the fact that it covers a wide range of areas. A few concentrates on services that benefit patients, including remote care and assistance with mental disorders, whereas other people desire to streamline operations more efficient in areas like claims processing, appointment scheduling, and inventory management. A growing number of individuals are employing smartphone applications and smart wearables to help them live healthier lives and find potential health problems earlier. These are called preventive solutions. The fields of biotechnology and personalized medicine are opening up exciting new possibilities. Innovative companies are using big data, genetics, and machine learning to speed up drug discovery, develop treatments that are tailored to each patient, and cut down on the time and capital that are usually needed for clinical testing. Innovation is not limited to events in prominent technological regions. Countries in Asia, Europe, and Latin America are encouraging strong business activity in this field through implementing policies that are good for the economy, getting more investors interested, and making healthcare easier to obtain. Investing in health related businesses around the world has never been higher, particularly in areas like artificial intelligence, remote diagnostics, and mental health technologies. These groups have to deal with a lot of existing problems. Some of the most important challenges are getting around the complicated legal frameworks includes the keeping data safe, and building trust with patients and providers. It is especially important task to make sure that a new technology is safe and effective in a field, where the lives of an individuals are directly affected. There is a lot of competition between new startups and big companies, which makes it even more important to stand out and grow quickly. Emerging businesses have a competitive edge because their processes are quick, flexible, and focused on innovation. The COVID-19 pandemic has accelerated up the worldwide shift to virtual and technologically driven services. As digital tools become more common in everyday care, these programs will help make long-lasting improvements in quality and efficiency that will change the manner in which health systems work around the world.

1.1 Health Innovation Startup Ecosystem

In the last few years, healthcare and wellness innovation has become one of the most active areas for entrepreneurs. Innovative businesses have resolved problems with outdated technologies by improving them easier to comprehend, more customizable, as well as more efficient. The use of AI, mobile technology, and cloud computing facilitate the possible for small and flexible teams to build revolutionary solutions that is driving the current tide of novel concepts. There can be a lot of diversity in ecosystems. Artificial intelligence-enabled system checks, teleconsultations, and remote monitoring have all been transforming the manner in which patients receive medical attention. A number people are automating managerial duties to make billing, recordkeeping, and claims processing in the back end systems faster and better. These changes contribute to making the system adaptable and getting rid of bottlenecks. Precision and preventive medicine are both extremely interesting. Startups are companies that can use wearables, genetics, and data analytics to seek out health risks and tailor medications. This personalized approach leads to better results and lower ongoing treatment costs, which has become a big deal in both public and private care. This rush for innovation is not only taking place in Silicon Valley and other technological regions. There are many successful digital health entrepreneurs in Asia, Africa, Latin America, and Europe. This development is happening all over the world due to government programs, easier access to venture capital, and customers wanting better care. Investors have an appetite in machine learning platforms, mental health solutions, and telemedicine infrastructure with the potential to grow. But these businesses have a lot of problems to contend endure. They have to follow strict rules about data privacy and validation in clinical settings. As soon as adding new technology to care workflows, it is essential to trust both users and healthcare professionals. New companies and established businesses use digital tools, consequently it's imperative to be innovative and clear about the approach to stand out in a crowded market. The situation will get better in the future. The COVID-19 pandemic has accelerated up the digitization of health services and the widespread implementation of virtual care. The businesses that are driven by innovation are ready to change the way medical services are delivered, experienced, and improved as consumer habits change and technology advances (Alsheibani et al., 2018).

1.2 Artificial Intelligence (AI) in Healthcare Transformation

Artificial intelligence has transformed the manner in which modern medicine works by making healthcare smarter, faster, and more personalized. Figure 1 illustrates the way artificial intelligence (AI) is changing healthcare. AI is changing how doctors give treatment along with the way patients feel about it by making diagnoses more accurate and automating administrative tasks. AI will identify patterns, make predictions, and contribute to important decisions in both clinical and operational areas since the technology can look at large datasets in real time. AI is helping health systems become more efficient, accessible, and superior as the industry moves toward accountable and preventive care models. There are the main ways the fact that AI contributes to make this change take place.

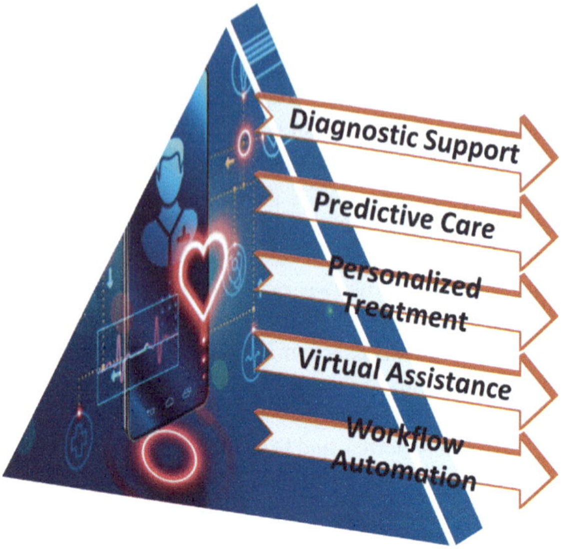

Fig. 1 AI's role in healthcare evolution

- *Diagnostic Support*: AI is changing the manner in which diagnoses are performed, particularly with regard to pathology and medical imaging. Algorithms developed using deep learning are capable of understanding X-rays, CT scans, and MRIs with a level of resolution that can be considered similar to or even better than the abilities of human experts. These tools aid in identifying diseases such as cancer, neurological disorders, and heart disease in their earliest stages. AI can find patterns in medical images that have dimensions that are too small for the human eye to recognize. This enables healthcare providers respond promptly, which leads to better medical results for the patients. AI systems may combine a patient's medical history, lab results, and even genetic data to help determine different diagnoses. The result not only decreases the number of mistakes in diagnosis, instead it also speeds up the process in places with a lot of patients, like emergency rooms. The radiologists are able to employ these tools as second readers as well or they can be utilized used on their own to help make decisions in places with limited resources. As AI becomes more common in diagnostic workflows, this is expected to facilitate work more straightforwardly, lower healthcare costs, and contribute to making sure that treatment can be provided with greater speed and precision (Arora et al., 2020).
- *Predictive Care*: AI enables healthcare providers to transition from reactive to proactive care through the use of predictive analytics. AI systems can forecast the chances of getting diseases like diabetes, heart attacks, or strokes by evaluating a lot of structured and unstructured information about patients, like Electronic Health Records (EHRs), wearable sensor outcomes, lifestyle factors, and even social components of health. These insights allow clinicians to formulate tailored

preventative measures and make data-driven clinical decisions prior to the manifestation of symptoms. Healthcare facilities additionally employ predictive tools to identify patients that are at high risk to be readmitted or having problems following surgical procedures. The reason for this additionally helps each person perform greater success, it additionally allows organizations use their resources more effectively and reduce down on unnecessary admissions. As people with chronic conditions, forecasting AI can help manage their medications better and keep an eye upon whether their disease continues to get worse from faraway locations. Being readily capable to predict medical needs additionally helps insurance companies and public health administrators plan substantial initiatives. So, artificial intelligence-driven predictive care has been a step toward an increased effective and sustainable methods to manage health (Bers et al., 2009).

- *Personalized Treatment*: The one of the most important things AI can do for healthcare is to customize treatment plans for each patient based on their profile. AI changes this by examining large datasets that include genomic information, patient history, lifestyle patterns, and clinical outcomes to develop treatment plans that are right for every individual. Traditional treatment plans frequently employ an approach that fits everybody. For instance, in cancer treatment, AI can help determine out which chemotherapy medications have been most probable to work for a certain mutation in the genome. The machine learning models examine into the way patients adapt to different therapies in mental health and modify suggestions for treatment based on that information. Personalized treatment rather than only improves efficacy instead also minimizes side effects and unnecessary interventions. AI additionally assists with deciding in real time by continually looking at data while tracking patients and offering changes to treatment plans to make them more successful. As AI becomes better at working with mobile devices and biosensors, this will make the situation possible for treatments to be truly dynamic and always changing. This progress could significantly enhance patient satisfaction, adherence, and subsequent health outcomes (Bessen et al., 2022).
- *Virtual Assistance*: Virtual assistants and chatbots generated through AI are changing the manner in which patients communicate with support services and get help from healthcare providers. These digital tools could assist resolve medical questions, schedule meetings, encourage to take your medicine, and give the health tips in real time. AI assistants are readily accessible 24/7, as opposed to regular customer service systems. This means that patients are constantly receiving the information and support they ought to require. Virtual agents are capable of keeping watch on symptoms, log data, and notify medical professionals know about any problems for people with chronic illnesses. AI chatbots in mental health use cognitive behavioral therapy (CBT) to help patients deal with anxiety, stress, or depression between therapy sessions. These tools additionally facilitate things easier for healthcare workers, who additionally can then focus on more important tasks. AI performs care of repetitive and administrative tasks, which frees up human resources for more important care tasks. Virtual assistants allow individuals get the help that they require quickly in areas with limited resources or

in rural areas. Virtual assistants are becoming smarter, more conversational, and more understanding as language models and speech recognition improve more accurate (Binowo & Hidayanto, 2023).

- *Workflow Automation*: Artificial intelligence helps make things simpler for hospitals and clinics by taking care of monotonous and mundane administrative duties. An artificial intelligence (AI) tools help with everything from the registering of patients and creating their medical records to billing and managing inventory. They also make mistakes less likely to occur. Natural Language Processing (NLP) has been used to turn conversations between healthcare professionals and patients into structured documentation, which saves time on paper work. The use of robotic process automation, or RPA, supports with tasks like handling insurance claims while maintaining health records up to relevant. This level of automation improves operations more accurate and faster, lowers costs, and lets clinical staff spend more time caring for patients. AI systems ensure that the right number of medications are continually on hand and that their expiration dates are documented correctly in pharmacy management. Artificially intelligent systems manage calendars smartly for scheduling appointments that cuts down on missing appointments and makes sure that providers are always readily accessible. As healthcare administration becomes more complicated, employing AI to automate workflows has grown more important for keeping operations functioning smoothly while additionally making sure that patients have a positive experience at every point of communication.

2 Competitiveness in Healthcare Startups

The healthcare startup ecosystem is a very rapidly evolving and the success of it depends on things like innovation, cost effectiveness and the ability to continue expanding. These companies always push boundaries with the new technologies, business models, and the compassionate solutions. In a competitive market, healthcare businesses need to be innovative to stand distinguish themselves. Innovative companies need to come up with new and high impact full ideas to address the problems with traditional healthcare systems. This could mean making an AI-driven diagnostic tools, telemedicine platforms, or personalized treatment plans. Furthermore, affordability is an important factor to think about it. The healthcare industry requires a lot of financing to run. So, that the new businesses have to find a way to provide good service and maintain the costs affordable. New businesses that offer affordable solutions without lowering the quality of care are more likely to succeed, especially in markets or groups that have yet to become very developed. At the same time, scalability is very important. A company may start by focusing on a niche solution or a regional market, but its long-term success depends on its ability to grow and serve larger, global markets. Startups need business models that can work in a lot of different markets, use technology to grow their operations, and work with established health systems to grow. The healthcare industry needs a lot of money for research, developing new technologies, following rules, and running the clinical trials. Getting money from venture capitalists, angel investors, or government grants is also consider as a very important, but it can be hard to do. Investors often hesitate due to the unpredictable nature of healthcare legislation, lengthy development timelines, and the high-risk environment. Regulation is a big problem that healthcare companies have to deal with (Blank & Dorf, 2020). The healthcare industry is one of the most regulated in the world. There are strict laws about the privacy of patient data, medical devices, and the clinical trials. Following rules like HIPAA in the USA or GDPR in the Europe can be hard and not following them can have a strong legal and the reputational consequences. The startups that want to use the disruptive technology may have to go through a long and the costly process to follow the rules. Getting into the market is a big challenge. Hospitals, insurance companies, and other established healthcare providers sometimes take over the market, making it hard for new businesses to gain trust and market share. Getting healthcare workers to accept new ideas, especially those that involve adding technology to old ways of doing things, can take a long time. The startup needs to show that its solutions are reliable, cost-effective, and better than current methods in measurable ways. Digital technologies like AI, machine learning, blockchain, and IoT devices offer new ways to improve processes, get better results for patients, and cut costs. The AI-powered solutions can use to automate an administrative task, which makes operations to run more smoothly. The wearable devices and IoT technology permit to keep an eye on the patients from a distance that makes the patients to more involve and lowers the number of times they have to go back to the hospital. These tools help healthcare professionals make decisions based on data by giving them real-time information so they can give more personalized care. Using blockchain technology to manage patient data could make it more open and secure, which is a very important issue in today's digital health world. Businesses can set themselves apart and come up with long-lasting, scalable solutions that solve the most pressing problems in healthcare by using these technologies. Technology helps healthcare startups get over a lot of problems while also letting them stay flexible, speed up innovation, and meet the growing need for care that is efficient, easy to get to, and focused on the patient (Chapman, 2006).

3 Artificial Intelligence in Healthcare

3.1 Key Technologies and Their Roles

Artificial intelligence (AI) encompasses a diverse range of technological advances, as depicted in Fig. 2, which emulate human cognitive processes. Machine learning (ML), natural language processing (NLP), as well as computer vision (CV) are changing the manner in which businesses work by making decisions easier, performing repetitive tasks, and making the user experience better. Machine learning algorithms enable systems learn from data by finding patterns that can be used for

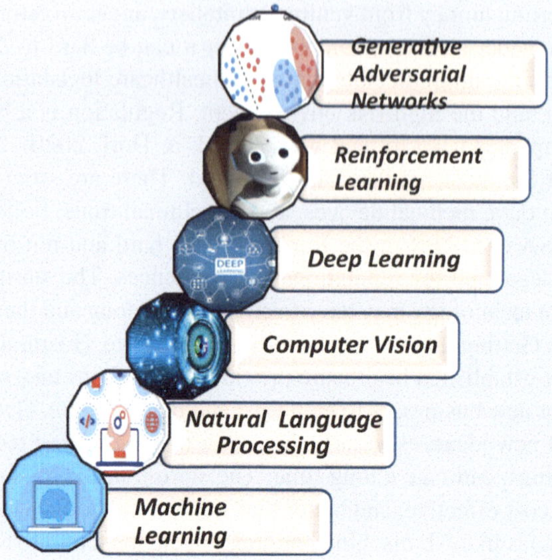

Fig. 2 Core AI technologies

creating estimations. Natural Language Processing (NLP) assists robots understand and speak human language. This allows things like chatbots and voice assistants attainable. Computer vision enables machines to comprehend and analyze visual input. This has contributed to progress in areas like medical imaging and autonomous automobiles. All of these technologies are driving innovation and making things work better in all areas. An artificial intelligence means that machines are made to think and act like people. AI includes many different technologies and methods that empower machines do things that usually require cognitive abilities including understanding, solving issues, reasoning, and perception. There are two main types of artificial intelligence—narrow artificial intelligence, which is made for specific tasks (like voice assistants), and general artificial intelligence that is meant to do any intellectual task that a person is capable of performing. AI is very important in fields like healthcare, finance, automotive, and customer service since it uses data analysis and automation to solve challenging issues (Chatterji et al., 2019).

1. *Machine Learning* (ML): Machine Learning (ML) is a subset of AI that enables computers to learn from data and improve their performance over time without being explicitly programmed. In ML, algorithms are trained using large datasets to recognize patterns and make predictions or decisions based on new, unseen data. There are three primary types of ML: Supervised Learning: The model is trained on labeled data (input–output pairs). Unsupervised Learning: The model works with unlabeled data to discover hidden patterns.
2. *Natural Language Processing* (NLP): Natural Language Processing (NLP) is a branch of AI focused on the interaction between computers and human languages. It enables machines to understand, interpret, and generate human language in

a way that is both meaningful and useful. NLP involves tasks like sentiment analysis, machine translation, speech recognition, and text summarization. It is essential in applications such as chatbots, virtual assistants, and voice-activated systems. NLP allows systems to process large volumes of textual data, making it possible to automate customer service, perform content analysis, and even translate languages in real-time (Chen, 2019).

3. *Computer Vision* (CV): Computer Vision (CV) enables machines to interpret and understand the visual world. By processing digital images or videos, CV systems can extract information, recognize objects, and make decisions based on visual inputs. This technology is used in facial recognition, autonomous vehicles, medical imaging analysis, and security surveillance. Machine learning, particularly deep learning, plays a significant role in advancing computer vision by improving object detection and image classification tasks. In healthcare, CV is applied to analyze medical images like X-rays or MRIs, assisting in the diagnosis of conditions such as cancer or neurological disorders.
4. *Deep Learning* (DL): Deep Learning (DL) is a specialized form of machine learning that uses neural networks with many layers (hence "deep") to analyze large volumes of data. This method is particularly effective in handling complex tasks like image and speech recognition, natural language understanding, and even autonomous driving. DL models require massive amounts of data and computational power but have proven to be highly accurate in areas such as speech recognition (e.g., virtual assistants), image processing (e.g., self-driving cars), and language translation (e.g., Google Translate). Deep learning models mimic the way the human brain works, enabling them to identify patterns in vast datasets.
5. *Reinforcement Learning* (RL): Reinforcement Learning (RL) is an area of machine learning where an agent learns to make decisions by performing actions in an environment and receiving feedback in the form of rewards or penalties. It is widely used in robotics, gaming, and autonomous vehicles. In RL, the system learns by trial and error to optimize its actions to achieve the best possible outcomes. For instance, in self-driving cars, RL helps the vehicle learn to navigate traffic, avoid obstacles, and make real-time decisions based on its environment. RL can also be applied in healthcare for optimizing treatment plans and personalized patient care.
6. *Generative Adversarial Networks* (GANs): Generative Adversarial Networks (GANs) are a class of AI algorithms that generate new data instances that resemble existing data. GANs consist of two neural networks: a generator, which creates fake data, and a discriminator, which evaluates the authenticity of the generated data. GANs are used for tasks such as generating realistic images, creating artwork, improving image resolution, and even generating synthetic medical images for training models in healthcare. The potential of GANs in generating realistic simulations has wide applications in training, research, and content creation (Chen & Zhu, 2008).

3.2 AI Tools and Platforms Relevant to Startups

AI tools and platforms help businesses establish themselves to operate more efficiently, and remain competitive at a low cost. As AI technology moves forward decisively. There are many platforms and tools that help startups produce and come up with new ideas whilst making it easier and cheaper to build artificial intelligence capabilities from the bottom. These tools enable new businesses add predictive analytics, automation, and personalized experiences without the user having to know anything about machine learning or data science. The search engine Google AI, Microsoft Azure AI, and Amazon Web Services (AWS) AI all have already developed models, infrastructures, and services for natural language processing (NLP), computer vision (CV), and machine learning (ML). These platforms have been flexible, scalable, and provide entrepreneurs the tools that are required to run AI models in the cloud rather than having to buy expensive hardware. These platforms also work well with additional technologies, which helps startups come up with and share ideas quickly. TensorFlow, Keras, and PyTorch have been widely used applications for machine learning and deep learning. By employing these free platforms, startups can build everything from simple predictive algorithms to complex neural networks. TensorFlow has become popular because it possesses a lot of community support, a substantial number of libraries, and it can run on mobile phones and embedded systems. OpenAI GPT-3 and Dialogflow (from Google Cloud) have been examples of NLP technologies that startups can use to add conversational AI. A person can get platforms that currently include chatbots, virtual assistants, and content generators built within them. OpenAI's GPT-3 can help the startups to develop an advanced language models that are capable of reading and writing like human beings for things like customer service, content creation, and the data analysis. The computer vision startups can employ the Clarifai and OpenCV to recognize images and videos. A person can use these tools to recognize the products, keep people safe, take medical images, and to drive the cars without having a driver. New entrepreneurs can make their own computer vision solutions with OpenCV's large library, and Clarifai's powerful API can analyze images and videos. DataRobot and H2O.ai have sophisticated automated machine learning tools that have made it possible for startups to use AI without needing to know how to perform data science. These tools make it easy for individuals that are not experts to rapidly develop AI-driven solutions by automating the creation and optimization of mathematical models. They are very helpful for businesses that cannot afford an excessive amount of money and need AI to help them predict sales, group customers, and find fraud. AI tools and platforms give entrepreneurs the freedom, scalability, and resources that they require to grow faster, save money, and stay competitive in a rapidly changing business world. These solutions (Child, 1972) enable startups focus on making new products and services while outsourcing the building of AI models, infrastructure, and scaling.

4 AI-Driven Strategies for Enhancing Competitiveness

4.1 Predictive Analytics for Patient Outcomes

The use of predictive analytical techniques for the treatment of patients are transforming healthcare. By giving more accurate methods to foresee the manner in which patients will respond. The techniques of predictive analytics employ advanced data analytics, machine learning to find patterns and trends in large amounts of healthcare information. These developments permit healthcare workers decide on smart choices to enhance care plans, and achieve better results for patients before problems yield progressively worse. Predictive models are capable of looking at patient data in order to figure out exactly how probable it is that they ought to will get sick via something like heart disease, diabetes, or a stroke. Healthcare professionals may intervene immediately by using preventive measures or personalized therapeutic strategies to reduce the severity of these illnesses when they can spot initial symptoms and risk factors. Machine learning algorithms are somewhat outstanding in analyzing complicated data and finding subtle connections which might not be apparent at initial glance. A significant application is predicting the chances of a patient coming back to the hospital. The use of predictive analytics can identify people that are significantly more likely to need to go returning to the hospital by investigating old health information that includes medical histories and treatment developments. This enables medical professionals to tailor following discharge plans and ensure subsequent treatment, thus decreasing readmission rates and improving patient satisfaction. Predictive analytics is necessary for improving the manner in which resources are being utilized (Cho & Lee, 1997). Hospitals may enhance efficiency while decreasing delays in care delivery by predicting patient volumes, emergency room visits, or surgical operations. This allows them to optimize staffing levels while additionally making sure that essential resources are always readily accessible. Models with predictive abilities can help individuals determine out the ways diseases spread as well as when outbreaks take place that can help lawmakers make decisions based on data to mitigate public health risks.

4.2 Disease Forecasting and Risk Assessment

The disease forecasting and the risk assessment constitute two important parts of predictive analytics in healthcare. It helps professionals find possible health risks and predict disease outbreaks via more accuracy. Predictive models are capable of looking at current and past data from a variety of sources, such as patient health records, environmental factors, and lifestyle information to figure out exactly how probable, it is that certain diseases are going to influence people or groups of people. Therefore, it makes simpler to intervene early, come up with more targeted prevention strategies and better manage healthcare assets. The models used in disease forecasting employ trends in data to predict the manner in which infectious diseases will propagate. Computers can use past data and environmental factors including temperature, humidity, and population movement to predict areas that will be in higher risk during flu season. This ability to predict allows healthcare professionals and public health officials take quick action, such as beginning vaccination campaigns or sending medical supplies to areas where cases are on increasing numbers. This could help reduce the spread of infectious diseases and mitigate their effects. On the contrary, the risk assessment emphasizes on finding people that have a more likely to get chronic diseases like diabetes, heart disease, or cancer. Predictive analytics could potentially be able to give each patient a unique risk score by looking at things like their genetic makeup, lifestyle, medical history, and socioeconomic factors that affect health. This makes it feasible to provide more personalized care as well as take preventative steps sooner, which can stop the disease from getting worse or lessen its detrimental effects. AI algorithms can predict the probability that a patient is to get diabetes by examining things like their BMI, family history, and activity levels. This can lead healthcare providers to suggest changes to the individuals' lifestyle or better monitoring of the patient. Anticipating diseases and assessing risks have been important steps in changing healthcare from a reactive to a proactive model. Healthcare professionals are able to make smart choices, ease the burden on healthcare systems, and enhance patient outcomes by preventing or minimizing the damage caused by illness at an early stage (Cho & Jung, 2004).

4.3 Automation of Administrative Processes

The automation of administrative duties is an important part of making healthcare settings more efficient and lowering the associated expenses. The administrative duties including billing, scheduling, processing claims, and keeping track of patient records frequently consume a lot of time and financial resources. The healthcare sector may make their business processes more efficient by performing these repetitive and tedious duties. This frees out staff to focus on tasks that are more significant, and ultimately contributes to better treatment for patients and service execution. For instance, AI and machine learning algorithms have been employed by artificially intelligent scheduling systems to find the best times for patients to make appointments based on their schedules, the healthcare professional availability, and the office hours. This reduces drastically the need for laborious tasks, lowers the number of scheduling errors, and makes patients more satisfied by making sure that appointments can be scheduled faster and more precisely. The tools for automation may take care of everyday data entry, check insurance information, as well as flag variations for review in payment and reimbursement processing. These systems improve coding and billing quicker and more precise that reduces down on mistakes made by individuals as well as makes the whole revenue cycle management more efficient. The automation of these tasks also speeds up the processing of payments, which helps medical professionals avoid delays that might adversely affect their financial situation. The automation also helps with the management of Electronic Health Records (EHRs).

Applications powered by AI are capable of updating and sort EHRs, ensuring sure that patient information is straightforward to locate, correct, and consistent across all systems. These tools are capable of a gathering and updating of the data from lab results, medications, or plans for treatment. This reduces considerably the time healthcare workers devote to entering data by themselves. They aid in making certain that compliance necessities have been fulfilled by processing and storing data in a manner that complies with rules like HIPAA. Chatbots and virtual assistants have been used to streamline conversations with patients, such as answering enquiries regarding appointments, prescriptions, and subsequent treatment. This can greatly reduce the load on staff, allowing them to focus on more complicated requirements for patients (Dowling & McGee, 1994).

4.4 Clinical Decision Support

The Clinical Decision Support (CDS) represents a group of a tools, systems, and the technologies that help a healthcare professional to arrive at smart, rational decisions that will help their patients get healthier. These systems employ AI, machine learning, and the data analytics to examine an enormous quantity of the patient data and give medical professionals immediate suggestions, alerts, and conclusions that assist them identify, treat, and manage a wide range of health problems. CDS systems seek to improve the quality of a medical services, cut down on errors, and make interventions as effective as possible. By combining patient history, clinical guidelines, and the most recent studies. One of the main benefits of CDS is the fact that, it makes diagnoses more reliable. AI algorithms are capable of looking at patient data such as symptoms, lab results, and medical images to help medical professionals figure out which conditions might be wrong. For instance, a system could end up with a list of possible diagnoses based on the symptoms of a person, medical history, and demographic information. This information can prove particularly beneficial in complicated cases or as doctors come across conditions they do not understand much about. It lowers the likelihood of providing a wrong diagnosis and helps patients get to feel better. CDS additionally becomes very important in developing plans for treatment that are right for every individual. These systems can offer the best treatment options by analyzing data from prior patients with similar profiles while additionally taking into consideration variables like age, other health problems, and medication history. This prevents healthcare providers from using an approach that is universal, which allows them give each patient more accurate care tailored to their requirements. CDS systems help keep drugs safe through the delivery of alerts in real time for potential interactions between drugs or dosage errors. For example, if a doctor suggests a drug that could interact with the patient's current medications, the CDS system may notify the medical professional understand this before the drug has been administered. This feature assists in lowering the number of adverse drug reactions that are a major cause of damage to patients in healthcare. An additional important part of CDS seems guidelines based on information. These systems make certain that healthcare providers possess access to the most current information through incorporating the most recent clinical research and standards of care in the process of making decisions. This makes sure that treatments are in line with exactly what medical researchers know right now, which improves the quality of care and contributes to better outcome for patients (Feroz et al., 2021).

4.5 Market Intelligence and Business Strategy

Market Intelligence and Business Strategy in healthcare includes employing data analytics, artificial intelligence (AI) (Kumarganesh et al., 2025), and machine learning. To gather, analyze, and use information about developments in the market, competition, customer behavior, and regulations. The healthcare sector is able to utilize this information in order to make smart choices, predict the manner in which the market is going to develop, establish rules to foster growth and sustained profitability. Market information gives businesses the power to quickly adapt to changing economic circumstances, enhance their products and services, as well as render their businesses more efficient in order to stay ahead of the competition. By looking at developments among consumer and patient populations is a vital component of market intelligence. AI tools (Pandey et al., 2024) are capable of looking at enormous quantities of data from patient encounters, surveys, and public health information to identify trends in the way individuals act. This helps healthcare professionals comprehend which services are in demand, the things patients are seeking, and the best way to tailor their offerings in order to meet those requirements. Predictive analytics (Pandey et al., 2021) might demonstrate that additional individuals need telemedicine that might motivate medical organizations to invest in virtual care services to satisfy their requirements. Healthcare organizations can differentiate each other apart from the competition and provide more customized, flexible services by keeping an eye on consumer behavior. The market intelligence systems can keep updated concerning what competitors are doing by looking at data from a variety of sources, including industry reports, social media, and customer reviews. This gives us information about the manner in which other healthcare providers are positioned in the market. The techniques they use and how prospective customers see their businesses. By keeping a watch on their competitors, healthcare businesses can determine what is effective and what does not in their strategies, modify their services, and discover new ways to expand their business. The modifications in regulations and policies possess a big effect on the way healthcare companies plan their business. Market intelligence systems may maintain an eye on and predict changes to healthcare laws, policies, and payment methods. Changes in healthcare regulations, such as new insurance policies or rules about telemedicine, might have a big impact concerning the way healthcare providers do their occupations. Businesses can change their business models in advance of time to comply with new rules and take advantage of fresh possibilities by making sure they stay aware of changes in legislation. Technologies based on AI (Saravanakumar et al., 2024) could assist with making informed choices by finding fresh market possibilities and predicting potential dangers. Healthcare businesses can use massive databases and immediate market information to make smart choices about investments, partnerships, and growth. Healthcare organizations may employ market intelligence to help them make better decisions about their approaches and lower their risks when they decide to move into novel markets, start new service lines, or buy novel technologies (Sreedhar et al., 2025).

5 Conclusion

Artificial intelligence has transformed the level of competition of a healthcare startup. The AI-powered predictive analytics, disease forecasting, and clinical decision support systems might assist startups arrive at choices based on data that improve diagnosis, patient outcomes, and business processes. Automating scheduling and billing helps things run more efficiently and reduces costs, so business owners are able to concentrate on growth. Market intelligence tools assist new businesses find trends, examine their rivals, and make their business strategies more successful. The healthcare startups, which employ AI need to carry it out in phases. Before picking AI tools, new companies ought to figure out their business goals. Making investments in scalable AI platforms like machine learning and natural language processing can help startups improve their healthcare, operational efficiency, and business strategy. Healthcare professionals and data scientists require to work together to implement AI technologies in medical settings. Emerging businesses should put data protection and HIPAA compliance before anything else if they want to earn the trust of healthcare consumers and other interested parties. As healthcare uses AI tools more frequently, startups must to use them in a fair, ethical, and transparent manner. Data privacy, biases in AI models, and complying with the rules constitute each part of this process. Using AI in a responsible way builds confidence within patients and improves treatment instead of putting safety or fairness at potential hazards. Startups should work with politicians and legitimate organizations to create AI healthcare frameworks, which benefit everyone and make our communities healthier.

References

Alsheibani, S., Cheung, Y., & Messom, C. (2018). Artificial intelligence adoption: AI-readiness at firm-level. *PACIS, 4*, 231–245.

Arora, S., Li, Y., Youtie, J., & Shapira, P. (2020). Measuring dynamic capabilities in new ventures: Exploring strategic change in US green goods manufacturing using website data. *The Journal of Technology Transfer, 45*, 1451–1480.

Bers, J., Dismukes, J., Miller, L., & Dubrovensky, A. (2009). Accelerated radical innovation: Theory and application. *Technological Forecasting and Social Change, 76*, 165–177.

Bessen, J., Impink, S. M., & Seamans, R. (2022). The cost of ethical AI development for AI startups. Paper presented at 2022 AAAI/ACM Conference on AI, Ethics, and Society, Oxford, UK, May 19–21; pp. 92–106.

Binowo, K., & Hidayanto, A. N. (2023). Discovering success factors in the pioneering stage of a digital startup. *Organizacija, 56*, 3–17.

Blank, S., & Dorf, B. (2020). *The startup owner's manual: The step-by-step guide for building a great company*. John Wiley & Sons and Springer Science & Business Media.

Chapman, M. (2006). Building an innovative organization: Consistent business and technology integration. *Strategy & Leadership, 34*, 32–38.

Chatterji, A., Delecourt, S., Hasan, S., & Koning, R. (2019). When does advice impact startup performance? *Strategic Management Journal, 40*, 331–356.

Chen, H. (2019). *Success factors impacting artificial intelligence adoption: Perspective from the telecom industry in China*. Old Dominion University.

Chen, J., & Zhu, X. (2008). A research on the relationship between academic entrepreneurs and enterprise performance: A three-dimension model. *Frontiers of Business Research in China, 2*, 155–169.

Child, J. (1972). Organizational structure, environment and performance: The role of strategic choice. *Sociology, 6*, 1–22.

Cho, D., & Lee, D. (1997). A new paradigm in strategy theory: Ser-M. *Monash MT Eliza Business Review, 1*, 82–98.

Cho, D., & Jung, J. (2004). The existence and usefulness of mechanism on international growth. In *Korean Strategy Management Academic Conference Presentation Proceedings* (pp. 329–402). Seoul: Korean Strategic Management Society Conference Paper Collection.

Dowling, M., & McGee, J. (1994). Business and technology strategies and new venture performance: A study of the telecommunications equipment industry. *Management Science, 40*, 1663–1677.

Feroz, A. K., Zo, H., & Chiravuri, A. (2021). Digital transformation and environmental sustainability: A review and research agenda. *Sustainability, 13*, 1530.

Kumarganesh, S., Murugesan, M., Ganesh, C., Santhiyakumari, N., Thangavel, M., Jayaram, K., Sagayam, K. M., Pandey, B. K., & Pandey, D. (2025). Hybrid plasmonic biosensors with deep learning for colorectal cancer detection. *Plasmonics, 20*(7), 4895–4909.

Pandey, B. K., Pandey, D., & Lelisho, M. E. (2024). Face mask identification with enhanced cuckoo optimization and deep learning-based faster regional neural network. *Scientific Reports, 14*(1), 29719.

Pandey, B. K., Pandey, D., Wariya, S., & Agarwal, G. (2021). A deep neural network-based approach for extracting textual images from deteriorate images. *EAI Endorsed Transactions on Industrial Networks and Intelligent Systems, 8*(28), e3.

Saravanakumar, R., TamilSelvi, T., Pandey, D., Pandey, B. K., Mahajan, D. A., & Lelisho, M. E. (2024). Big data processing using hybrid Gaussian mixture model with salp swarm algorithm. *Journal of Big Data, 11*(1), 167.

Sreedhar, C., Suresh Kallam, G. S., Pradeep Ghantasala, S., Anthoniraj, S., Kumarganesh, K., Sagayam, M., Pandey, B. K., & Pandey, D. (2025). Enhancing healthcare data security using RFE and CRHSM for big data. *Computers in Biology and Medicine, 190*, 110063.

Human Resource Management in AI-Driven Hospitals: Challenges and Solutions

Norma Ramírez-Asís, Edwin Hernan Ramirez, Carmen Cardenas Lara, Jorge Manrique Cáceres, and Martha Esther Guerra-Muñoz

Abstract The latest innovations for managing the workforce are changing the way healthcare works. The changing roles, problems and solutions of smart systems and digital tools in managing people in hospitals and clinics. As the health tech industry uses technology to improve operations, it needs digital integration specialists and leaders. These jobs help make sure that new technologies are in line with the goals of the company, make changes easier and boost performance. A lack of trained multitasking staff, a resistance to change and a fragmented organizational culture are all major barriers to this change. To deal with problems, hospitals need to keep their staff up to date on their skills, encourage them to adapt and make multidisciplinary teams with both healthcare and technical skills. If not used in a fair and open a way digital technologies could unintentionally keep biases and unfairness going. Specifically designed strategic solutions that give workers the tools they need to work with technology instead of being replaced by it. A strategy for changing the workforce that is fair and sustainable focuses on future training, diversity and investments in inclusiveness. This method gets the workforce ready for the future by helping them adapt to changes and making patients better and operations run more smoothly.

N. Ramírez-Asís
Seguro Social de Salud del Perú, EsSalud, Lima, Perú

E. H. Ramirez (✉)
Universidad Autonoma del Peru, Lima, Peru
e-mail: eramireza18@autonoma.edu.pe; elva.ramirez@essalud.gob.pe

C. C. Lara
Universidad Católica de Trujillo Benedicto XVI, La Libertad, Peru
e-mail: c.cardenas@uct.edu.pe

J. M. Cáceres
Universidad Nacional Santiago Antunez de Mayolo, Huaraz, Peru
e-mail: jmanriquec@unasam.edu.pe

M. E. Guerra-Muñoz
Universidad Popular del Cesar, Valledupar, Colombia
e-mail: marthaguerra@unicesar.edu.co

D. Pandey et al. (eds.), *Smart Healthcare*,
https://doi.org/10.1007/978-981-95-8828-2_18

Keywords Digital transformation · Workforce management · Technology integration · Healthcare innovation · AI · HRM

1 Introduction

The incorporation of advanced digital intelligence into healthcare systems is revolutionizing the delivery, management and optimization of medical services. This change is more than just using new tools. It means a big change in how healthcare professionals use gadgets how they understand data and how they get good results for patients. Intelligent systems are making processes easier, more accurate, and more personalized from diagnosis to administration. These technologies are becoming more and more useful for diagnostic purposes in clinical settings. Such as image recognition algorithms can read X-rays, MRIs and CT scans with amazing accuracy and they can often find patterns better than human specialists. Automatic speech and text recognition tools are also helping to make sense of huge amounts of unstructured data from medical records, clinician notes and lab reports. These apps help with early diagnosis, cut down on mistakes made by people and help people make better decisions. The advantages also apply to patient care and management. Predictive tools look at past health data to find problems that might happen, like readmissions or bad reactions, so that preventive steps can be taken. Digital assistants are being used to talk to patients about making appointments, reminding them to take their medications, and following up with them. This makes it easier for patients to get in touch with their doctors and stay involved in their care. These kinds of tools make it easier for clinical staff and make the whole care experience better. There are also big changes happening in the way that administrative and operational tasks are done. Effective automation is making things like processing insurance claims, scheduling staff and keeping track of inventory more efficient. This not only cuts down on the administrative expenses but it also lets hospitals use their resources better and lower their operating costs. The growth of digital intelligence in healthcare also means that we need to rethink the roles of workers. The skilled are increasingly required to work alongside automated systems, necessitating new skills and collaborative approaches. In this these technologies to work well together and there needs to be a balanced ecosystem in which machines do tasks that are heavy on data or repetitive and human workers focus on the more ethical and caring aspects of their jobs.

1.1 Human Resource Management in AI-Driven Settings

The human element is still very important to the success of hospitals that use advanced technologies. In addition, advanced tools automate clinical diagnostics, administrative tasks, patient interactions and managing staff in this new setting becomes both a challenge and a necessity. The role of human resource leadership has changed from traditional duties to include helping with digital transformation, developing the workforce and making sure that the company is run ethically. The labor market is changing quickly. As routine jobs become automated and roles shift toward decision support, data analysis and collaboration between humans and AI. The employees need to learn new skills. This means that we need a progressive plan for hiring, training and helping people move up in their careers. It is very important to improve digital literacy, flexibility as well as the ability to work with people from different fields. Especially for healthcare workers who use automated systems in real time, it is very important to make it easier for staff to get help during this transition. The use of smart technologies may cause uncertainty, fears about losing jobs and resistance. The right change management makes it easy for transitions to happen without any problems. This means clear communication, thorough planning and constant involvement with staff. An organization can build a sense of ownership and trust by getting employees involved early in the process of adopting new technologies and stressing how these technologies improve their jobs rather than replacing them. A vital duty entails preserving the human dimension of care. The algorithms can make things work better. They cannot show compassion, empath or moral judgment. The workers should be encouraged and helped to keep these important qualities. The assessment of performance must include both technical skills and interpersonal skills as well as behavior that puts the patient first. In situations where data is important, openness and ethics must be upheld. The right platforms often use employee data to keep an eye on productivity, predict trends or set up shifts. To protect patient data, information must be kept private and its misuse avoided. It is essential that everyone understands how to use it and that fair policies are implemented, which generates a culture of trust and responsibility. In modern hospitals, human resource specialists are more than just managers. They help new ideas come to life. They play a strategic role in making sure that the workforce stays skilled, flexible and motivated by matching human potential with new technology. They make sure that the digital advancement of healthcare stays focused on people by promoting a culture of learning, protecting well-being and pushing for ethical integration (Çalışkan, 2010; Yamin et al., 2024).

2 Reimagining Human Capital in AI-Driven Hospitals

2.1 Traditional to Digital Workforce Competencies

The shift from traditional healthcare models to artificially intelligent systems has caused a big change in the skills and abilities that healthcare professionals need to have. Today workers need to be able to work in a digital environment where automation, machine learning and data analysis in real-time affect everyday tasks. A technical understanding is no longer limited to medical procedures and patient care. In traditional medical facilities skills were mostly about being able to do things manually, making good clinical decisions, talking to patients and following standard procedures. These skills are still essential but in an artificially intelligent world. They need to be combined with new digital skills. Clinicians are now expected to use predictive analytics to read generated by algorithms diagnostic suggestions, work with robotic surgical tools or use digital dashboards that keep track of patients vital signs. The nurses may use smart monitoring systems and cloud-based platforms to coordinate care. Whereas administrative staff are using virtual assistants and automated scheduling systems more and more. The digital transformation also requires people to be able to read data and use systems. The medical community need to know how smart tools get their results Especially when it comes to important things like diagnosis or treatment planning. This awareness makes sure that people make responsible choices and helps keep people accountable even when they share tasks with autonomous systems. The soft abilities are also being redefined. The conventional ways of communicating and leading are changing to include things like remote collaboration, managing virtual consultations and digital etiquette. Empathy has always been an important part of healthcare, but now it needs to be shown through digital channels. This means that emotional intelligence and adaptability are more important than ever. In conjunction together across fields has become the norm. These professionals work closely with data scientists, AI developers, cybersecurity experts and health informatics experts. This requires not only being open to different points of view and also having a common vocabulary and understanding of how digital processes work. Receiving competent to work with non-medical professionals to come up with solutions is becoming an important skill. Upskilling and ongoing learning are no longer things we do when we need to. They are things we must do. Healthcare organizations must cultivate an environment in which learning is integrated into daily operations and employees are encouraged to obtain certifications in digital health, AI ethics, or data security (Ehnert et al., 2016; Esan et al., 2024).

2.2 Identifying and Nurturing AI-Compatible Roles

When hospitals start using smart technologies, they need to rethink how they do their jobs and how they are set up. To make the switch to artificially intelligent healthcare go smoothly, it's important to find roles that naturally lend themselves to automation and data-driven tools and then build on those roles. Employment opportunities that work with AI are jobs that change as technology does. The radiologists used to look at pictures by hand but now they use diagnostic algorithms. They use artificially generated insights to validate put things in context and make tough choices instead of being replaced. The field of clinical information specialists are needed to check electronic health record data, make sure the data is correct and connect medical staff and technology teams. The individuals who work in healthcare, are good with data, and know how to use digital systems are in high demand outside of clinical roles. Digital health coordinators, AI workflow analysts, and virtual care facilitators need to know what patients want and what the system can do. The integration specialists make sure that everything runs smoothly and that communication between people and machines is as good as possible across departments. In order to encourage these kinds of jobs, hospitals need a strong talent strategy. Initially mapping out roles is important. This means looking at how smart systems change jobs that already exist and figuring out which tasks are most likely to be done by machines. With automating boring administrative tasks like entering data or making appointments, staff can move up to supervisory or analytical positions. The nurses can now run platforms for AI-assisted triage or monitoring patients from afar. Second, companies should pay for training that is specific to each role and that involves people from different departments. Each function needs its own programming instead of general digital upskilling. The doctors may need to learn how to read algorithmic output and understand the limits of artificial intelligence. While administrators may need to learn how to manage automated systems and follow the rules, they should also think about your career options again. Make it clear how new skills can lead to more opportunities for advancement to encourage workers to change. Mentorship, internal mobility, and links to academics can all help this ecosystem. The future of healthcare depends on using advanced tools and changing the way people work to use them. When carefully creating artificial intelligence compatible employment opportunities hospitals can build a healthy and strong workforce for the future (Manzoor et al., 2019).

2.3 A New Paradigm in Care Delivery

The use of smart systems in hospitals is creating a new way of caring for patients where technology and human knowledge work together instead of separately. The goal of this collaborative approach has not to replace healthcare workers however to help them provide more accurate, timely and personalized care. The redefinition of roles is what this change is all about. The physicians are no longer the only ones who make decisions. Instead, they work with digital tools that help with diagnosis, treatment planning and monitoring. Some image analysis software can show radiologists where to look on scans so they can focus on more complicated cases that need more careful interpretation. In emergencies, predictive tools can look at current information to find patients who are likely to get worse. This gives medical teams an early warning system and more time to act. This partnership works especially well for tasks that are repetitive or need a lot of data. The software can quickly process thousands of data points such as lab results, vital signs or medication history. Fortunately, only people can provide the empathy and moral judgment that machines cannot. This synergy makes care faster and better. This is especially important in high-pressure situations where quick decisions are necessary. Artificial intelligence assistants can keep track of vital signs or make appointments for nurses and patients, giving nurses more time to focus on caring for patients with compassion and direct care. This balance makes sure that the healing process stays focused on the human connection even as operational efficiency gets better. In order collaboration to work, everyone needs to know their limits and be on the same page, healthcare workers need to know what the systems they use can and cannot do. This way, they can make smart decisions about automated suggestions instead of just following them. The developers and engineers also need to talk to doctors all the time to make sure that tools are made with everyday needs in mind. To successfully execute this cooperative model work, hospitals need to spend money on training people from different fields and encourage a culture of respect between people and digital tools. The professionals should be able to question and challenge what the system says and they should also be able to use their full potential. All individuals need to trust both the technology and the people who use it. This new way of thinking is not about picking between people and machines. It is about making care systems that work together so that the results are safer, faster and more humane. The future of medicine gets closer to its true mission of healing using intelligence and heart as human compassion meets computational power (Ehnert et al., 2014; Wikhamn, 2019).

3 Strategic Transformation of HR Functions

The tools for automation can make tasks like payroll, recruiting, and managing employee data easier, which frees up HR teams to focus on more important things. Artificial intelligence can also improve the hiring process by scanning resumes and matching candidates with the best roles. This makes the process more efficient and fairer. As shown in Fig. 1, the adding technology to HR tasks is necessary to modernize processes. Technology lets HR teams get precise information about how well the workforce is doing and how engaged they are, which they can use to make smart choices. The move toward technology not only makes operations run more smoothly but additionally also brings HR in line with the companies bigger goals and making it a bigger part of reaching overall success.

- **Digital Talent Acquisition**: As the need for digital skills expands the way people find and hire new employees has changed a lot. The Human Resources department is now looking for people who not only have technical skills but also know how to work together in digitally enhanced workplaces. Because of this change, it is now more important to hire people who have worked with data analysis, system integration, and digital health before. These are all important skills in a tech-driven healthcare setting. Supplementary hiring strategies now use digital tools like social media, online job boards and automated recruitment platforms to find a wider range of candidates. These platforms can even use analytical data to guess how well a candidate will perform over time, which helps HR teams make better hiring decisions. The changes in hiring make sure that healthcare organizations have a staff that can help them move their operations online (Hong & Liu, 2007).

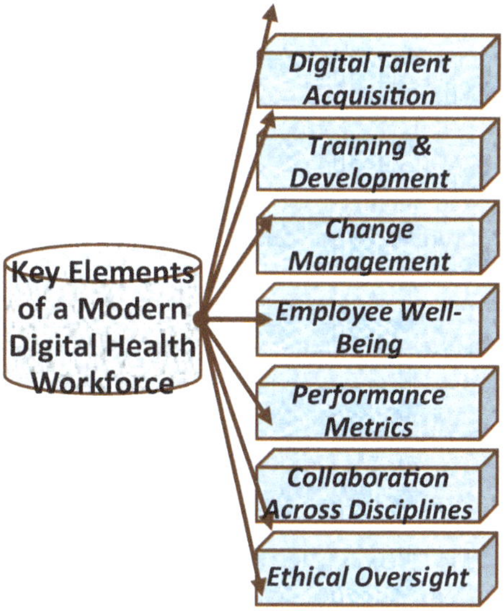

Fig. 1 Key elements of a modern digital health workforce

- **Training and Development**: The healthcare sector are putting a lot of effort into training and development as they learn how to use new technologies. The staff needs to keep learning all the time so they can keep up with tools and systems that change quickly. The Human Resources department is very important in creating training programs that teach more than just basic technical skills. These programs should also teach how to work with data, use digital tools and work with people from different fields. The personalized development tracks are becoming more important because they let employees focus on areas like telemedicine, artificial intelligence diagnostics or health informatics. The Human Resources department helps employees stay relevant and competitive in a changing job market by making personalized learning paths. This ongoing development makes sure that healthcare workers are not only able to keep up with fresh technologies and also know how to use them to improve patient care and make operations run more smoothly (Kam et al., 2010).
- **Change Management**: The public are often afraid of losing their jobs or don't know how to use new technologies, which makes it hard to put them into use. To get past these problems, you need to use good strategies for managing change. The human resources department is in charge of making this change happen by clearly explaining the benefits of digital tools and addressing employee worries through training, workshops and open forums. It is important to create a culture of innovation where people see technology as a tool to help them instead of a threat. The Human Resources department can build trust and make people more open to change by getting employees involved in the process and letting them give feedback. The Human Resources department needs to focus on encouraging the workforce to be flexible and adaptable. They need to help them understand that

using technology is necessary to stay competitive and keep providing excellent care to patients.

- **The health of employees**: The fast pace at which technology is being used in healthcare settings can make employees more stressed as they learn how to use new tools and systems. The Human Resources department needs to put the health and happiness of employees first to make sure that the workforce stays engaged, productive and mentally healthy during this change. The staff can better deal with the difficulties of adjusting to a digital environment if they have access to mental health resources, counseling services and work-life balance programs. The Human Resources department should also be proactive in finding out what causes burnout and fixing it by offering flexible work hours, job rotation or cutting down on repetitive tasks. Making sure that employees feel supported during this change will not only help keep good employees but it will also make everyone happier at work, which will lead to better results for both staff and patients (Song & Wang, 2009).
- **Performance Metrics:** The standard performance metrics which look at productivity and clinical outcomes. This needs to change to show how people and technology work together. In a world where technology is everywhere. It is just as important to judge an employee's ability to learn new technologies as it is to judge their old skills. The Human Resources department should come up with performance indicators that show how well employees use digital systems. Perhaps these could include how well they use systems powered by AI or how well they can manage and understand data outputs. These assessments should include soft skills like adaptability, creativity and emotional intelligence because they are important for working in a hybrid environment. A full performance review system that includes these metrics will make sure that workers are not only technically skilled but also emotionally ready to do well in a workplace that has changed to digital.
- **Working together across fields**: As hospitals use more advanced technologies. It is important for people from different fields to work together. The Human Resources department is a key part of building a culture of collaboration by making it easier for healthcare workers, IT professionals, data scientists, and engineers to talk to and work with each other. To encourage people from different fields to work together makes sure that digital tools are used to their full potential in clinical settings. The Human Resources department can help with this by setting up events to strengthen teams, making multidisciplinary working groups and encouraging sessions where people can share what they know. These efforts not only improve the technical implementation of new systems but they also make sure that employees learn how to work well with others in a diverse and digitally integrated setting. Encouragement for healthcare providers and tech experts to work together makes the organization better able to come up with new ideas and meet the changing needs of the healthcare industry.
- **Ethical Oversight**: As businesses rely more and more on data and digital tools. The HR must make sure that ethical standards are always followed. This means keeping patient and employee data safe, making sure privacy is respected and making clear rules about how to use sensitive information. The Human Resources

department should work closely with the legal and compliance teams to make sure that all of the company's technology meets regulatory standards and that employees know how to handle data in an ethical way. When working with healthcare data, which is often sensitive and heavily regulated. This duty is even more important. The Human Resources department should encourage an ethical mindset in the company by encouraging talks about the ethics of artificial intelligence, bias in algorithms and how to use technology responsibly. Utilizing the clear rules and making sure everyone knows what is going on helps build trust between employees and patients. It makes sure that everyone follows the rules.

4 Human Capital Hurdles in Tech-Driven Hospitals

4.1 Shortage of Cross-Functional Talent

As the healthcare industry relies more on advanced technologies. The need for the people with skills in more than one area has grown. Since they need a unique mix of technical skills and knowledge of their field. These professionals are hard to find and very valuable. Such as healthcare providers now need professionals who can connect clinical care with technology. These professionals should know both the details of medical procedures and how digital systems work. It is very hard to find enough of these people. In the past, healthcare roles were mostly about taking care of patients and doing administrative work. But as the field becomes more digital. There is a greater need for professionals from different fields who can manage and integrate complex systems. To make sure that healthcare organizations can smoothly switch to new technologies, they need employees who know how to use data analysis, artificial intelligence, healthcare informatics, and clinical practice.

The rapid changes in healthcare make it even harder to find people with these skills. Many professionals already working may have one set of skills but not know much about new fields like machine learning or data science. On the other a situation people with a technical background may not fully understand how healthcare is delivered, which makes it hard for them to work well with medical teams. Training alone is not enough to close this gap. The problem gets worse because there are so many people looking for jobs. There are not enough qualified candidates for organizations to hire, which is driving up the cost of hiring. To fix this, healthcare organizations need to take a strategic approach. This includes training current employees, working with schools and colleges and coming up with ways to keep employees so that they can thrive in a digital world (Challoumis, 2024).

4.2 Technological Anxiety and Resistance to Change

The healthcare sector is using more advanced technologies in their work, which often makes staff afraid and resistant to change. This is especially true for professionals who are used to traditional methods and may be scared by how quickly digital transformation is happening. The fear of becoming obsolete because of automation or the uncertainty of using new technologies could create big psychological barriers that hurt both personal performance and business success. There are many reasons for this resistance. A common worry is the lack of clarity about job security. The employees may be worried that automation or artificial intelligence could take over their jobs, which would mean layoffs or less responsibility. The employees may feel inadequate or incompetent if they do not know how to use new systems. Especially if they don't have the right technical skills. This sense of helplessness can lead to anxiety, which makes people resistant to change. Some workers might look closely at how well new technologies work or what their ethical effects are. The worries about the reliability of digital tools, data privacy and the chance of biased algorithms make people distrustful and hesitant. This lack of trust can make it hard for healthcare professionals and IT teams to work together, which can slow down the adoption of useful new ideas. Leaders need to have a plan for dealing with technology anxiety. It is essential to articulate the role of technology in enhancing rather than replacing the human contributions. The training and support can help the transition go more smoothly by making employees surer that they can use the new systems well. The promotion of a culture of continuous learning where individuals are encouraged to adapt and evolve with the evolving surroundings and can reduce resistance and increase confidence in the technology (Chinda & Omorogieva, 2024).

4.3 Fragmentation of Work Culture and Team Cohesion

As healthcare organizations use digital tools and automated systems. The traditional way of working often breaks down. As employees rely more on technology for things like keeping an eye on patients, processing data and making diagnoses, the amount of physical and interpersonal communication within teams may go down. This change might cause people to become disconnected from each other, which would hurt the sense of unity that usually comes from working together in person. In a technologically advanced setting, healthcare professionals might spend more time using technology than talking to their coworkers. Healthcare professionals, nurses and office workers who used to work together in hospital wards or offices may now be alone. Each relying on their own digital devices and systems to do their jobs. This separation enhancing operational efficiency, may foster feelings of alienation and reduce collaboration as individuals focus more on personal responsibilities rather than collective goals. Adding cross functional teams made up of healthcare professionals and IT experts could make team dynamics worse. These groups may have trouble communicating well because they speak different languages, have different priorities and have different levels of expertise. The medical community may encounter challenges due to technical jargon or face difficulties in engaging with IT specialists who lack clinical knowledge. When people in different departments do not understand each other, it can make it harder for them to work together to create it harder to solve problems and create silos in the business. To fix this problem, healthcare organizations need to intentionally create a culture of teamwork and open communication. To encourage regular direct conversations, team building exercises and training across disciplines can help employees get to know each other better and break down barriers. Making sure that everyone understands what each department does and how it helps the organization as a whole makes sure that everyone is working toward the same goals (Tsai, 2001).

5 Innovative HR Solutions and Approaches

New approaches in workforce management focus on using technology to speed up processes, make better decisions and get employees more involved. Figure 2 shows some of these tactics such as using advanced data analytics to make better decisions, creating personalized learning platforms to help students learn and using digital tools to hire students and keep track of their progress. This technology is also being used more and more to cut down on administrative work, which lets human resources teams focus on strategic goals like developing talent and keeping employees happy. Adding wellness programs, flexible work schedules, and diversity programs are other things that help new ideas come about. In addition, do these solutions make operations run more smoothly, but they also make the workplace more welcoming, flexible and interesting for employees.

1. **The Digital HR Ecosystem**: A Digital HR Ecosystem shows how different technologies and strategies work together to make HR processes better. Artificially intelligent recruitment tools, employee engagement platforms, data analytics for decision-making, and wellness programs are just a few of the important parts of this ecosystem that work together. Artificial intelligence can make the hiring process easier by looking at resumes, figuring out if a candidate is a good fit and even doing the first interviews. The staff engagement tools keep track of morale and give HR real-time feedback that helps them find ways to make things better. This approach uses big data analytics to figure out things like turnover rates, improve performance management and make personalized plans for employee development. The programs for wellness can also work with digital health tools to give employees tools to help them take care of their mental and physical health. These technologies are often connected. So data can move easily between them. This lets human resources departments be more strategic and give each employee a unique experience.

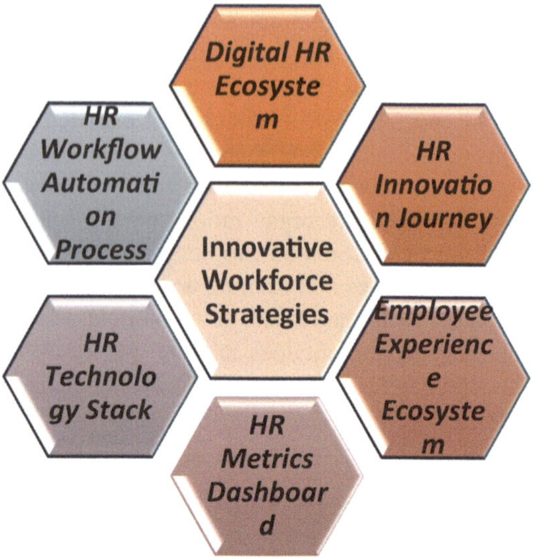

Fig. 2 Innovative workforce strategies

2. **The HR Innovation Journey**: The Human Resources Innovation Journey shows how HR practices have changed from manual, paper-based processes to a modern, digitally driven HR environment. At first the HR tasks like hiring, managing employees and evaluating their performance were done by your hands often using paper records. As technology became more common, companies started using basic HR software to help them with administrative tasks. This made it easier to keep records. The HR departments started using AI and automation to hire new employees, analyses data, and manage performance as digital tools got better. This made things much more efficient and accurate. Now that the journey has reached the stage of personalized experiences, employees get customized learning paths, flexible work schedules and wellness programs that are specific to their needs. In the future, HR will use fully integrated systems that use predictive analytics and artificial intelligence to not only make operations more efficient but also create more engaged and empowered employees. This ongoing change in human resource procedures shows how technology is becoming more important in improving the experience of both employees and employers.
3. **Employee Experience Ecosystem**: The Employee Experience Ecosystem shows the different stages of an employees' time with a company and how human resources can help improve satisfaction and productivity at each stage. The journey starts with hiring in which AI powered tools help human resource departments find the right people by looking at resumes and doing first interviews. The next comes initial introduction which includes personalized digital training programs that teach new employees about the companies' policies and culture. When the continuous development phase, employees can use personalized learning platforms to learn new skills that will help them reach their career goals. The pulse surveys and real-time sentiment analysis are two ways that

companies can keep track of how engaged their employees are. Finally, the retention efforts focus on wellness programs like access to virtual therapy or fitness apps and systems that reward people for their achievements. The Human Resources department can make sure that employees are happy and motivated to stay and grow with the company by making the whole process from hiring to keeping employees as smooth and personalized as possible.

4. **Dashboard for HR Metrics**: A Human Resources Metrics Dashboard shows key performance indicators (KPIs) in a way that helps HR departments make decisions based on data. These dashboards pull together information from different parts of HR to show how well recruitment is working, how engaged employees are, how effective training is and how many employees are staying with the company. For instance, the metrics like turnaround time and expense per hire can be used to measure how well hiring methods are working. The Human Resources department can keep an eye on morale and find areas that need improvement by using pulse surveys and feedback scores to measure employee engagement. The effectiveness of training can be measured by how many people finish it, how well they remember what they learnt and how well they use what they learnt at work. Final retention metrics like turnover rates and employee satisfaction can help HR teams' spot problems early and come up with ways to keep employees from leaving. This data-driven, real-time approach helps HR make sure that its work is in line with the companies' goals, which help the company as a whole succeed.
5. **HR Technology Stack**: The HR Technology Stack is the set of digital tools and platforms that HR departments use to effectively manage their employees. This stack usually has a few levels each of which handles a different HR task. The HR Information System (HRIS) is at the heart of it all. It keeps track of employee information and handles administrative tasks like payroll and benefits. There are also specialized tools around this core that include talent acquisition platforms that use AI to speed up the hiring process and learning management systems (LMS) that give employees personalized training and development opportunities and performance management tools that keep track of employees' progress and give them feedback. Employee wellness apps and engagement platforms also help HR departments support mental health, encourage engagement and promote happiness. The last three analytics tools bring all of these parts together by giving decision-makers and planners statistical information that help them make decisions and plan their strategies. By putting these tools together, you can make an HR system that works well and helps both employees and the company.
6. **The HR Workflow Automation**: The technique uses digital tools to make repetitive and tedious assignments easier, so, HR professionals can focus on more important projects, such as artificially intelligent applications that scan resumes, rank candidates and even do initial assessments are used in candidate screening. This cuts down on the time and effort needed for manual reviews by a lot. The automation is also helpful for onboarding as new employees get automated welcome emails, digital forms, and training modules that help them through the process. The automated tools that let managers and employees set and track

goals in real time make it possible for continuous feedback loops in performance management. Automated surveys and sentiment analysis tools that give HR immediate feedback on how employees feel can also help keep them engaged. This lets HR deal with problems right away. HR departments can make things run smoothly as well as make fewer mistakes and make sure that all employees have the same experience by automating these tasks.

6 HRM in AI-Driven Healthcare

6.1 Integration Specialists and Digital Health Leaders

In order to develop hospitals learning organizations, they need to create a culture where learning, sharing information and adapting are all part of everyday life (Fong et al., 2011). A learning hospital creates an environment where everyone, from doctors to nurses to administrative staff is always working to improve patient care, operational efficiency and the overall performance of the organization (Haq et al., 2023). To create this kind of environment, hospitals need to set up ways for their staff to keep learning throughout their careers, such as professional development programs (Saravanakumar et al., 2024), continuing education classes, and opportunities for staff to work together across disciplines. The systems for knowledge management that let people share best practices, research results and current clinical insights are the most important part of a learning hospital. These systems give medical staff access to recent information and evidence-based protocols, which help them make better decisions. The hospitals can encourage teamwork by holding regular workshops, seminars and case discussions where healthcare workers can share their knowledge and experiences. The hospitals can fill in knowledge gaps, improve decision-making and improve patient outcomes by encouraging a culture of learning together. For expansion, it is important to create a culture that values feedback. The healthcare sector should encourage a way for staff, patients and leaders to give each other feedback and make sure that suggestions are put into action to make things better. Frequent performance reviews, patient feedback surveys, and team debriefings can help with this. The educational hospitals help people at all levels develop their leadership skills, which allows them to take charge of their own professional growth. The development of leadership teaches people at all levels how to handle change and lead teams toward common goals. The best hospitals are all about combining technology and new ideas. Hospitals can improve patient care, streamline processes and reduce mistakes by using digital tools like electronic health records (EHRs), telemedicine and data analytics. A hospital can use technology to give their staff the tools they need to stay up to date on medical and industrial advances, which improve the delivery of healthcare.

6.2 *Building Hospitals as Learning Organizations*

As healthcare organizations start using more advanced digital tools and structures new jobs are opening up at the intersection of technology, human resources and digital health management. The artificial intelligence and human Resource Integration Specialists and Digital Health Leaders are very important for making sure that new technologies are used in healthcare settings. These experts are in charge of making sure that technical skills match healthcare goals in order to make operations more efficient and improve patient outcomes. The artificial Intelligence (Sahani et al., 2024) and Human Resource Integration Specialists work to connect old fashioned human resource practices with new technologies. Part of their job is to find ways that digital tools can make the hiring, training and performance management processes better. These experts use technology to make things like automated hiring, employee sentiment analysis and predictive workforce management easier. This frees up HR teams to focus on more strategic tasks like developing talent and getting people involved in the organization. They also work to make sure that technology is used in an ethical way by dealing with problems like data privacy and bias in algorithms. The digital health field (Muralidhar et al., 2024) on the other a situation is in charge of the strategic integration and optimization of digital health technologies like telemedicine, electronic health records (EHRs) and data analytics platforms. These leaders make sure that digital tools make clinical workflows stronger help doctors take better care of patients, and help people make decisions that are based on facts. They also help train hospital staff on how to use new technologies effectively and make sure that their work is in line with the hospital's larger goals. Such as improving patient outcomes and lowering costs. They need to work closely with IT teams, doctors and administrators to make sure that their work fits into healthcare delivery systems without getting in the way of how things are already done. The two careers are important for the future of healthcare because they will help digital technologies (Sreedhar et al., 2025) become more common in managing the workforce and caring for patients.

6.3 *Ethical and Inclusive AI-HRM Ecosystems*

To create, use and keep fair, open and responsible solutions in workforce management, systems that are ethical and open to everyone are necessary. The internet is being used more and more in hiring, performance reviews, and employee engagement. So, it is important that these tools are not making biases or inequalities in the workplace worse. The ethical systems make sure that decisions about managing employees are fair, diverse and open to everyone. One of the biggest problems with creating an ethical workforce management ecosystem is dealing with bias in digital models. There is a chance that these systems will show past biases in hiring or promo tions because they are trained on historical data. These systems can make existing biases worse and lead to unfair results if they are lacking in the right protections. One example is that a hiring system might unintentionally favor candidates from certain genders, ethnic groups or schools. To stop this from happening, it is important to regularly check the algorithms for bias and fix any problems and to train systems on a variety of datasets that show a wider range of experiences and backgrounds. Regularly open and honest is also important for making an ethical ecosystem. Employees will trust digital tools more if they can see how decisions are made clearly and simply. It is important for employees to be able to understand and question decisions about promotions or performance reviews if they think they were treated unfairly. This openness promotes responsibility and makes sure that digital systems are used properly. An inclusive environment means that everyone who works there, no matter how good they are with technology, should be able to use these systems. There are many tools for managing a workforce must be easy to use and have interfaces that everyone can utilized. The regular training sessions are important for helping employees feel more confident and work well with new technologies (Kumarganesh et al., 2025). The organization can make a fair, open and diverse system that encourages positive engagement and builds trust among employees by putting ethics and inclusion first.

7 Conclusion

The healthcare sector human resource management is hard because there are not enough people with multiple skills, people are reluctant to evolve and the work culture might spread out. An employee to use new systems and processes is one of the hardest things to do. This is usually because they are afraid of becoming obsolete or not being able to use technology. An additional issue is that there are not enough skilled workers who can connect technology with managing people. Effective solutions to these problems include ongoing training, a culture of adaptation and clear lines of communication that make it easy for people to work together and share information. As technology becomes more common in managing people, a more humane approach is needed. Instead of getting rid of their human parts, healthcare companies should make them better. By putting people first, hospitals and healthcare systems can use technology to help healthcare workers get better at their jobs. For employees to be able to use new technology without feeling like they are being left out, there needs to be a balance between automation and personal connection. To help the healthcare workforce adjust to a new digital world. It needs a plan that is both fair and lasting. This necessitates the amalgamation of technological advancements and human transformation strategies. This process includes offering training programs that are easy for everyone to access and that give workers the skills they need to succeed in a changing digital world, encouraging diversity and inclusion during workforce transformation and customizing technology solutions to meet the needs of employees. Future strategies for changing the workforce must include ongoing learning, new ideas and developing leaders.

References

Çalışkan, E. N. (2010). The impact of strategic human resource management on organizational performance. *Journal of Naval Sciences and Engineering, 6*, 100–116.

Yamin, M. A., Almuteri, S. D., Bogari, K. J., & Ashi, A. K. (2024). The influence of strategic human resource management and artificial intelligence in determining supply chain agility and supply chain resilience. *Sustainability, 16*, 2688.

Esan, O., Ajayi, F. A., & Olawale, O. (2024). Managing global supply chain teams: Human resource strategies for effective collaboration and performance. *GSC Advanced Research and Reviews, 19*, 013–031.

Ehnert, I., Parsa, S., Roper, I., Wagner, M., & Muller-Camen, M. (2016). Reporting on sustainability and HRM: A comparative study of sustainability reporting practices by the world's largest companies. *International Journal of Human Resource Management, 27*, 88–108.

Manzoor, F., Wei, L., Bányai, T., Nurunnabi, M., & Subhan, Q. A. (2019). An examination of sustainable HRM practices on job performance: An application of training as a moderator. *Sustainability, 11*, 2263.

Ehnert, I., Harry, W., & Zink, K. J. (2014). *Sustainability and human resource management: Developing sustainable business organizations*. Springer.

Wikhamn, W. (2019). Innovation, sustainable HRM and customer satisfaction. *International Journal of Hospitality Management, 76*, 102–110.

Hong, J., & Liu, B. (2007). Logistics development in China: A provider perspective. *Transportation Journal, 46*, 55–65.

Kam, B. H., Tsahuridu, E. E., & Ding, M. J. (2010). Does human resource management contribute to the development of logistics and supply chain capabilities? An empirical study of logistics service providers in China. *Research and Practice in Human Resource Management, 18*, 15.

Song, H., & Wang, L. (2009). The status and development of logistics cost management: Evidence from Mainland China. *Benchmarking: An International Journal, 16*, 657–670.

Challoumis, C. (2024). Building a sustainable economy-how AI can optimize resource allocation. In *Proceedings of the XVI International Scientific Conference*. Copenhagen, Denmark, 17–20 December 2024.

Chinda, C. N., & Omorogieva, A. A. (2024). Reward system and employee commitment. *American Journal of Multidisciplinary Bulletin, 1*, 13–23.

Tsai, W. (2001). Knowledge transfer in intraorganizational networks: Effects of network position and absorptive capacity on business unit innovation and performance. *Academy of Management Journal, 44*, 996–1004.

Fong, C. Y., Ooi, K. B., Tan, B. I., Lee, V. H., & Chong, A. Y. L. (2011). HRM practices and knowledge sharing: An empirical study. *International Journal of Manpower, 32*, 704–723.

Haq, M. Z. U., Asadullah, M. A., & Manzoor, F. (2023). The impact of human resource and information technology on supply chain learning and operational performance. *The Journal of Business and Industrial Marketing, 38*, 1927–1940.

Saravanakumar, R., TamilSelvi, T., Pandey, D., Pandey, B. K., Mahajan, D. A., & Lelisho, M. E. (2024). Big data processing using hybrid Gaussian mixture model with salp swarm algorithm. *Journal of Big Data, 11*(1), 167.

Sahani, S. K., Pandey, B. K., & Pandey, D. (2024). Single-valued signals, multi-valued signals, and fixed point of contractive signals. *Mathematics Open, 3*, 2450002.

Muralidhar, L. B., Lakshmi, K. V. N., Swapna, H. R., Rupani, J., Nethravathi, K., Pandey, B. K., & Pandey, D. (2024). Impact of organizational culture on the level of corporate social responsibility investments: an exploratory study. *Circular Economy and Sustainability, 4*(3), 2267–2285.

Sreedhar, C., Suresh Kallam, G. S., Pradeep Ghantasala, S., Anthoniraj, S., Kumarganesh, K., Sagayam, M., Pandey, B. K., & Pandey, D. (2025). Enhancing healthcare data security using RFE and CRHSM for big data. *Computers in Biology and Medicine, 190*, 110063.

Kumarganesh, S., Murugesan, M., Ganesh, C., Santhiyakumari, N., Thangavel, M., Jayaram, K., Sagayam, M., Pandey, B. K., & Pandey, D. (2025). Hybrid plasmonic biosensors with deep learning for colorectal cancer detection. *Plasmonics, 20*(7), 4895–4909.

Ensuring Data Privacy and Security in Smart Healthcare: A Fuzzy Logic Approach

Sony Kulshrestha and Ruchi Kulshrestha

Abstract The use of adaptable logic-based frameworks has greatly improved data privacy and security in healthcare places, especially as more and more people depend on IoT and networked technologies. This framework can handle the complexities of cyber security in healthcare by giving people the ability to make decisions that are flexible and smart. The traditional binary logic systems work well in simple situations but they do not work well with healthcare data because it is often unclear and uncertain. The latest logical systems offer a solution by transforming definitive inputs into varying degrees of fact thereby enabling more precise security measures that can adjust to evolving threats. The basic ideas behind fuzzification, rule-based inference and defuzzification help explain how these processes make continual and flexible security solutions possible. In the future, medical information technology and the Internet of Things will need to generate and transmit a lot of private data. These versatile frameworks make it easier to find vulnerabilities and determine vulnerabilities more quickly. Using this approach strengthens security policies and makes them better able to deal with a variety of safety issues such as data breaches and unauthorized access. It is very important for keeping patients trust and privacy. The safety measures make healthcare safer by making it easier to make smart security choices and stay up to date on emerging cyber risks. The significance of integrating intelligent security measures with ethical data governance to safeguard sensitive medical information while ensuring system design remains responsible and ethical.

Keywords Fuzzy logic · Healthcare security · Data privacy · IoT systems · Cybersecurity · Risk assessment · IoT

S. Kulshrestha (✉)
Department of Law, Manipal University Jaipur, Jaipur, India
e-mail: sonykulshrestha@gmail.com

R. Kulshrestha
Department of English, Radhe Hari Govt. PG College, Kashipur, India

D. Pandey et al. (eds.), *Smart Healthcare*,
https://doi.org/10.1007/978-981-95-8828-2_19

1 Introduction

The use of digital technologies had made a big difference in the healthcare industry in the past few years. The healthcare industry is quickly moving away from hospitalized care and towards a more distributed, smart and focused on the patient approach. This includes things like remote diagnostics, wearable devices and real-time patient monitoring systems. The smart technology like the Internet of Things (IoT), artificial intelligence (AI), machine learning (ML), big data analytics and cloud computing make this change possible. These technologies work together to make what we now call smart healthcare. This is a connected system where medical devices, health information systems, and healthcare professionals all work together to give patients timely, accurate and personalized care. The biggest and the most revolutionary things about this change is that wearable sensors and mobile health (mHealth) apps can keep an eye on patients all the time. They are not in a hospital. These technologies gather a lot of physiological and behavioural information such as heart rate, glucose levels, activity patterns and how well people follow their medication plans. Subsequently this information is sent to healthcare providers in real time or saved on cloud servers for later analysis. These kinds of ongoing data-driven insights not only help with early diagnosis and preventive healthcare but they also help doctors make better decisions and improve health outcomes. At the same time, smart hospitals have started to use automation, robotics and intelligent systems for things like surgery, diagnosis, inventory management and helping patients find their way around. Tools based on AI are being used to look at complicated datasets like genomic and medical imaging data. These tools help doctors find patterns that the human eye might not be able to see right away. The integrated health information platforms make it easy for departments, hospitals and even national health systems to talk to each other and share information. This makes it easier to take a more holistic approach to patient care, but as these new technologies change how healthcare is delivered. They also make things more complicated especially when it comes to data governance. As the amount and types of personal health data being created and shared grow at an alarming rate, worries about data privacy, security and ethical use are more important than ever. Unauthorized access, data breaches and identity theft are big threats to both patient safety and the trustworthiness of smart healthcare systems. As a result, making sure that digital health information is handled safely and ethically is now a basic requirement for the design and implementation of any smart healthcare project. This section goes into more detail about these problems and suggests using fuzzy logic to deal with privacy and security issues in smart healthcare systems.

1.1 Data Privacy and Security

In the current digital healthcare world in which electronic health records (EHRs), wearable technologies and remote patient monitoring have all important parts of patient care, data privacy and security are more important than ever. The medical record is one of the most private types of personal information. This often includes a full picture of their medical history, genetic makeup, mental health and even their lifestyle. Medical data if not handled correctly and they can not only hurt finances of individuals or image but it can also directly affect their physical and mental health. This means that on smart healthcare applications it is a basic moral and legal duty to keep this information private, safe and accessible. Thus, smart healthcare systems grow and connect more devices and platforms in general the need for strong privacy and security measures becomes even more important. Every point where data is collected or sent, whether it is through wearable sensors, mobile apps, or cloud-based databases, could be a weak point (Shafique et al., 2020). If someone gets unauthorized access to this data. It could lead to bad things like insurance fraud, medical identity theft or even tampering with medical devices. Also, if patients feel that their data is not being handled safely or openly. They may lose faith in healthcare systems and not want to use helpful technologies or share important health information. The regulatory bodies have set up a number of laws and frameworks to protect patient data. This includes the Health Insurance Portability and Accountability Act (HIPAA) in the USA and the General Data Protection Regulation (GDPR) in Europe and national policies in many other countries. These rules require healthcare providers and technology vendors to follow strict rules about the informed consent, data minimization, data encryption, access control and breach notification. However conventional security models frequently find it difficult to keep up with the ever-changing and diverse nature of smart healthcare systems where data is always moving, devices are always being informed and threats are always changing. Therefore, there is a growing need for security solutions that are smart, flexible and aware of their surroundings and can make subtle decisions in complicated situations. The use of fuzzy logic and other methods that are good at handling uncertainty and variations in input data are especially good for this problem. They allow many factors in real time like device trust levels, access frequency and data sensitivity then give a responses that go beyond with simple security rules. This chapter will examine the utilization of intelligent systems to enhance data privacy and security within contemporary healthcare infrastructures (Serna, 2022).

1.2 Healthcare IoT Environments

The more healthcare IoT devices there have been the more vulnerable the ecosystem is to cyber threats, as shown in Fig. 1. The patient monitoring systems and wearable health trackers are examples of these devices that collect, send and store a lot of private information. The personal information of patients safe and build their trust. It is important to protect this data from unauthorized access, changes and loss. Since more devices have links the attack surface expands making it harder for healthcare companies to protect each endpoint. In order to safeguard healthcare systems efficiently we need more than just technological solutions like encryption and firewalls.

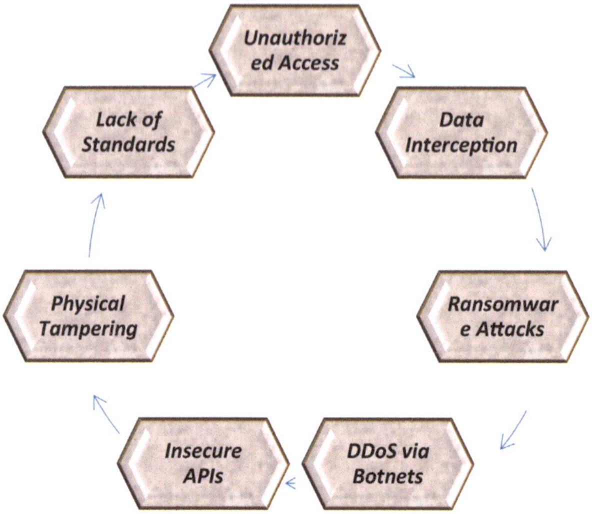

Fig. 1 Emerging threats in healthcare IoT environments

We also need a proactively designed complete strategy that includes regulation, user education and ongoing monitoring.

- **Unauthorized Access**: The majority of healthcare IoT devices had weak or old authentication protocols. The perpetrators can easily guess or crack default credentials to get in without multiple authentication methods or biometric validation. When the hackers get into the system as they can get to electronic health records (EHRs), change patient information or mess with how devices work, which puts patient safety at risk. For example, messing with an insulin pump or a heart monitor could put someone's life in danger. Because of either limited continuous surveillance or poor intrusion detection such breaches often go unnoticed. Thus, advanced healthcare facilities depend more on connected systems even one unauthorized access point can put the whole infrastructure at risk.
- **Data Interception**: Internet of Things equipment sends sensitive health data over networks that might not be fully encrypted all the time. The attackers often use tools to listen in on these conversations and get current medical information like blood pressure, heart rate and medication schedules. An individual can use this stolen information to blackmail, commit insurance fraud or sell it on the dark web. The danger is even worse in mobile or remote care settings where wireless transmission is more common. The intruders can more easily launch MITM (man-in-the-middle) breaches when there is no entire encryption or secure network protocols. This puts data integrity at risk and violates patient privacy without raising immediate suspicion (Buzdugan, 2020).
- **Ransomware Attacks**: Ransomware continues to remain one of the worst threats to the healthcare industry. It means locking up an organizations files or systems

and asking for money in exchange for the keys to unlock them. In smart healthcare settings attackers might also lock up IoT devices like imaging machines or patient monitors. As a result the hospitals have to stop working, procedures are cancelled and emergency responses are delayed. The majority of hospitals are seen as easy targets because their systems are old and they need to get care to people quickly, which makes it more likely that they will pay ransoms quickly. These incidents not only cost money but they also hurt public trust and make it harder to follow the rules.

- **Malicious Updates**: It is important to keep the firmware and software up to date to keep a system safe but when these updates are sent out without proper authentication or encryption. They can be used to attack. The hackers can use unsafe update channels to put bad code on medical devices. When a device has been breached it may send patient data to people who should not have it or do things that are not allowed. Such as a tampered infusion pump might give the wrong amount of medicine. It is hard to tell when these attacks happen because the devices usually keep working normally from the users' point of view. The risk is higher because there is no audit trails or validation checks during updates. This shows how important it is to have secure update protocols (Scott, 2022).
- **DDoS via Botnets**: The intruders can take control of healthcare IoT devices with weak security and use them to make botnets that consist of big networks of infected devices that attackers can control from afar. These botnets can launch Distributed Denial of Service (DDoS) attacks that flood hospital networks with too much traffic and making them unavailable to real users. During these kinds of attacks the important services like cloud-based health records, diagnostic platforms and telehealth systems might stop working. In addition, being able to get to patient data or use clinical tools can have a direct impact on patient care. The medical IT teams are very worried about botnet attacks because the number of connected devices is increasing which means that the attack surface is also growing.
- **APIs that are not secure**: Application programming interfaces are important for letting different systems and devices in smart healthcare settings share data. But if APIs are not well designed or protected then they can let attackers get to sensitive data and features. The hackers can use these weaknesses to get around access controls, steal private patient information or even add harmful commands to backend systems. Application programming interfaces that do not have rate limiting, input validation or the right ways to authenticate users are especially easy to hack. Many healthcare apps and IoT platforms rely heavily on APIs. So, these flaws can lead to widespread breaches, data corruption and operational failures, especially when they are used with third-party services or mobile apps (Richardson et al., 2021).
- **Physical Tampering**: IoT devices used in homes or outpatient settings are often left alone which makes them easy to tamper with. The attackers can take apart, clone or switch out these devices to get to the data they hold or change how they work. Such as someone could steal a heart monitor that can wear and use it to get authentication tokens or install malware. Utilizing a short amount of time with these kinds of devices can let attackers get unencrypted data or install harmful

firmware. Physical breaches are harder to find than network attacks especially outside of hospitals. This is a big problem for healthcare IoT security strategies (Minnaar & Herbig, 2021).

- **No Standards**: The healthcare IoT landscape has devices from a variety of businesses as well as each one uses a different way to communicate, protect data and update itself. Since there are no standards, protection is not the same on all devices. Some devices may use new encryption and authentication techniques. While others may still use old software and default passwords. As a result of that the security posture is broken up into pieces that are hard to keep an eye on, manage or patch in the same way. Healthcare providers have to make up their own rules for interoperability, compliance and security because there are not any clear ones. These rules may not work. This difference creates many weak spots in the chain that attackers can use to their advantage.

2 Conceptual Foundations of Privacy and Security in Healthcare

2.1 *Ethical Principles in Handling Health Information*

This is very important for healthcare providers to handle health information ethically because it is private and sensitive. The rules of ethics create a set of rules for how to handle patient data in a way that protects their privacy, integrity and trust. The basic ethical ideas of autonomy, beneficence, non-maleficence and justice are important for handling health information in a careful and responsible way. Independent living stresses the right of people to control their own health information. The general public must be fully informed about how their data will be used who will have access to it and the risks that come with sharing it. A clear understanding of consent is a crucial component of this principle, ensuring that patients understand and voluntarily agree to the collection and use of their health information. Both beneficence and non-maleficence are two of the most important rules of healthcare ethics. The field of healthcare ought to be employed to improve patient welfare, inform medical decisions, maximize treatment outcomes and encourage research for enhanced healthcare solutions. At the same time the main steps must be taken to keep people from getting hurt. This includes keeping people who should not have access to personal health information from getting it. In order to ensuring that the data is correct and protecting against mistakes that could lead to wrong diagnoses or bad treatment. It is accurate and equal access to healthcare resources and health information is necessary for justice. It makes sure that no one is unfairly hurt or discriminated against because of their private health information. This method is very important for stopping the misuse of private health information to shame or push certain groups to the edge, which helps create an environment of equality and inclusion. It is important to uphold these moral principles in order to protect peoples' rights and keep peoples trust in healthcare systems. Clear rules, protecting privacy and making sure that health information is used in a way that is open and honest are all important steps towards improving ethical data management practices (Alam & Benaida, 2022; Ma & McKinnon, 2022).

2.2 CIA Triad in Medical Data

The CIA Triad Confidentiality, Integrity and Availability are three important parts of keeping medical data safe. These rules tell healthcare organizations how to keep private patient information safe from theft, corruption and loss. In the modern healthcare industry where, more and more data is stored and sent digitally. Conforming to the CIA Triad is very important for keeping trust, making sure patients are safe and following rules like HIPAA. Confidentiality means keeping private patient information safe from people who should not be able to see it or share it. This means making sure that only certain people like medical professionals or researchers with clear permission can see personal health information. The most typical methods to keep information private were encryption, role-based access control and data masking. A breach of confidentiality can have serious repercussions such as stealing someone is identity, violating their privacy and losing their trust. The concept of integrity is all about making sure that health data stays accurate and reliable throughout its entire life cycle. A medical record must not be changed or damaged while they are being stored, sent or processed. Any unauthorized changes or damage to patient records whether done on purpose or by accident can lead to wrong diagnoses, wrong treatments or delayed care. In order to make sure that health records are accurate and trustworthy techniques like hashing, digital signatures and audit trails are used to check data integrity. The availability makes sure that authorized people can get to medical data when they need it especially in emergencies. The medical profession needs quick access to patient information to make smart choices. A system failure, cyberattacks or natural disasters can cause downtime or data loss which can delay treatment and hurt patients. For continuous access to data available they need backup systems, disaster recovery plans and redundancy measures. The presence of the CIA Triad to the management of healthcare data not only protects private information but also makes the healthcare environment safer, more efficient and more trustworthy (Mukati et al., 2021).

2.3 Trust Models and Stakeholder Roles

The trust models are crucial in managing healthcare data and ensuring the secure, ethical exchange of information between stakeholders in a healthcare system. The trust is a foundational element for cooperation in healthcare, particularly as medical data becomes increasingly shared across different platforms and organizations. These models help define how trust is established, maintained and verified within the healthcare ecosystem, ensuring that all parties involved patients, healthcare providers, insurers and third party service providers act in accordance with established standards of privacy, security and integrity. The Public Key Infrastructure (PKI) is a common way for people to trust each other in healthcare. This uses digital certificates and encryption keys to verify users and devices. A private key infrastructure makes sure that data sent between parties is safe and that identities are checked which lowers the risk of fraud or data breaches. The Blockchain approach is another trust model that is becoming more popular because it is decentralized. It also makes sure that all transactions involving medical data are recorded in a ledger that cannot be changed that stops tampering and makes audit trails clear. Patients, healthcare providers, insurers and regulatory bodies are all important players in keeping trust in healthcare. The patients need to know that their private health information has safe and used in a fair way. Effective consent procedures, openness about how data is used and strong data privacy policies help build this trust. The medical profession is responsible for keeping patient information safe making sure that only authorized people can access it and using it in a way that follows ethical guidelines. The insurance companies are also responsible for managing and protecting data but they must make sure that patient information is only shared when it is needed for claims and reimbursement in accordance with strict rules. The Health and Human Services (HHS) in the USA and the General Data Protection Regulation (GDPR) in Europe tend to be two examples of regulatory bodies that set up legal frameworks and standards to protect medical data and make sure that everyone follows them. As someone adds these roles to good trust models can be sure that healthcare systems work safely, morally and efficiently (Zhang & Lu, 2021).

3 Smart Healthcare Systems

3.1 Sensors, Devices, Networks, and Cloud Infrastructure

A smart healthcare system is built on a complex network of sensors, devices, networks and cloud-based platforms. The device patches, implantable chips and environmental monitors are all types of sensors that constantly measure things like heart rate, blood pressure, glucose levels and oxygen saturation. These small, low power modules often have accelerometers, temperature sensors and biochemical receptors that change analogue signals into digital data streams. Applying them on or in the patient makes it possible to track vital signs in real time which allows for early interventions and personalized treatment plans. Supplementary sensors are smart medical devices like intelligent infusion pumps, robotic surgical arms, portable ultrasound scanners and diagnostic apps for smartphones. In addition to providing therapy or doing assessments. These types of devices also have local processing capabilities that let them find problems, notify carers and change operation parameters on their own.

The gateways and edge-computing units often collect data from sensors, filter it and encrypt it before sending it on to the next step. The channels of communication are what hold this ecosystem together. The Bluetooth Low Energy (BLE), Zigbee and Near-Field Communication (NFC) are short-range protocols that connect sensors to edge gateways. Wi-Fi, LTE and new 5G networks provide the bandwidth and low latency needed for high-definition imaging, remote surgery, and continuous monitoring. A network reliability, quality of service (QoS) and integrated security features like VPN tunnelling and SDN (software defined network) make sure that data packets get to their destination on time and without being damaged even in crowded or noisy areas. The cloud platform supports data storage, advanced analytics and the ability for different institutions to work together. The electronic health records or EHRs, are stored on scalable cloud platforms, which also use machine learning models to sort patients by risk and make telehealth consultations easier through secure portals. They are flexible enough to handle spikes in data volume like during mass screenings and they work with frameworks that follow the rules to keep audit logs, enforce access controls and handle encryption keys. The edge cloud hybrids make performance even better by keeping time sensitive calculations close to home and moving heavy analytics and long term storage to centralized data centers. These core components work together to create a strong, flexible base that drives the ongoing development of personalized, predictive healthcare (Greco et al., 2020).

3.2 Data Flow and Storage in Healthcare IoT Systems

The transfer of information and storage are very important parts of healthcare IoT systems that make sure medical monitoring, diagnostics and treatment systems work efficiently. These systems gather a lot of information from many different types of devices, such as wearables, implantable sensors and remote monitoring gear. The sensors start the data flow by collecting information about the patient like their heart rate, blood pressure, glucose levels and movement patterns. Afterward these data points are sent to a central processing unit or edge device for initial analysis and storage through communication networks like Bluetooth or Wi-Fi. The local device or gateway that sits between the sensor and the cloud generally serves as the first place where the data is processed. This step makes sure that only useful data is sent that cuts down on the amount of data sent to the cloud and makes the best use of bandwidth. In this juncture data may also be encrypted or anonymized to protect privacy before being sent for more analysis. Such as a wearable device could look at a patients' heart rate data in real time and only send an alert to the doctor if the rate goes below a safe level. The data is stored in the cloud system after it goes through the edge devices. The use of cloud storage is a great way to handle big datasets in healthcare because it is scalable, flexible and can be accessed from anywhere. The authorized healthcare providers can access data stored in the cloud. This allows their homes watch in patients from faraway places and give them personalized assistance. There are regulations that cloud storage services must adhere to like HIPAA or GDPR. This maintains patient information safe and private. The healthcare based on internet of things may additionally utilized hybrid storage methods which mix local and cloud storage. This enhances performance and makes sure that important information is always there. This technique finds a middle ground between the need for processing data at the same time and storing it for a long time. That makes healthcare operations more efficient and improves patient care (Puri et al., 2021).

4 Principles and Its Role in Cybersecurity

4.1 Fuzzy vs. Traditional Binary Logic

The conventional method binary logic and fuzzy logic differ significantly in how they handle information and uncertainty. The concept of precise sets is what binary logic is based on. In this system the opinions are either true or false that are represented by 1 and 0, respectively. This method works well when the information is clear and exact. In the case of Boolean algebra, for example, "the light is on" is either true (1) or false (0). The operations with these kinds of statements follow rigid guidelines, which always lead to clear true/false answers. The fuzzy systems as a whole on the other hand, let truth values range from 0 to 1, which makes them more flexible and less certain. In lieu of a strict true/false structure, the level of truth can change that makes it easier to make decisions. A temperature reading, for instance, might not just be "high" or "not high," but instead be 0.7 on a scale from 0 to 1 that would mean that it is only partially true. The primary difference is in how each system deals with uncertainty. A binary logic requires a strict separation that makes it good for tasks that need exact results. The fuzzy systems on the other hand show how complicated everyday circumstances can be. A membership system can help them measure and show how true something is. This is especially helpful when the data is missing or not very clear. The binary code logic works best for problems that are clearly defined. On the other hand, the fuzzy systems are better for systems that have to deal with uncertainty like a cybersecurity. Due to threats and risks are not always easy to put into groups. These environments often need to be flexible. The fuzzy system can better handle changing and unpredictable situations than traditional binary methods because they allow for intermediate states (Othman et al., 2022).

4.2 Security Decision Uncertainty and Imprecision

As a result, security environments are always changing and are very complicated. It is hard to deal with uncertainty and imprecision in cybersecurity. The standard security frameworks often rely on clear binary procedures for making choices that may not work well when threats are unclear or changeable. In order to handle this type risk more flexible strategies are needed to deal with the uncertainty that comes with real-life situations. The incremental risk assessments are a good way to deal with imprecision. In these assessments, threats are not just labelled as "secure" or "insecure," but are instead given a range of possible risk levels. In lieu of quickly labelling a network as compromised because of one strange event. The system may look at a number of threats based on how serious, frequent and reliable different signs are. This makes it easier to make better decisions when the threat level is unclear. Implementing automated reasoning systems is a big part of this approach. These systems make decisions by looking at a series of criteria that are not just binary. Instead of defining an attack by a single criterion (like a specific signature). A system can look at a number of things such as user behaviour patterns, unusual network traffic and system weaknesses. These criteria although not providing definitive answers and are combined to create a comprehensive risk assessment that helps make security decisions that are more informed. The adaptable systems are important for cybersecurity because they can change in response to changes in the environment in real time. Threats can change quickly and an adaptive security model can change its defences when it gets new information. Instead of using fixed thresholds there is systems that can change their assessments all the time. This keeps decisions up to date as things change. These strategies help to make better and more complicated decisions about cybersecurity. This is especially true when it is hard to measure risks, like in big internet of things or complex cyberattacks that happen on multiple levels. The security industry can better protect against threats that do not fit neatly into categories by accepting uncertainty and viewing risks along a path (Rawat et al., 2022).

4.3 Fuzzy Logic in Healthcare Environments

The uncertainty and imprecision must be handled when making medical decisions. The information that is incomplete, unclear or changes often does not work with binary systems. The medical field can process data on a spectrum thanks to advanced techniques makes analysis more flexible and accurate. The use of fuzzy reasoning in healthcare is shown in Fig. 2. While making a medical diagnosis the doctors may have to look at symptoms and test results that do not fit into neat categories. This method helps find diseases that have similar signs. Specific treatment looks at even unclear data such as genetics, lifestyle and environment. The adaptive systems handle incomplete or noisy data in medical imaging and risk assessment. With constantly checking on health conditions. These systems make diagnosis, treatment and outcomes better. This method makes healthcare better when quick and accurate decisions are needed.

- **Diagnosis Support**: The use of fuzzy reasoning is very important for diagnosing medical conditions, especially when symptoms and test results are not completely clear. It helps doctors make smart choices by looking at data that is not clear or complete. This is because it can help doctors figure out if someone has cancer, diabetes or heart disease by looking at symptoms that are unclear or similar to

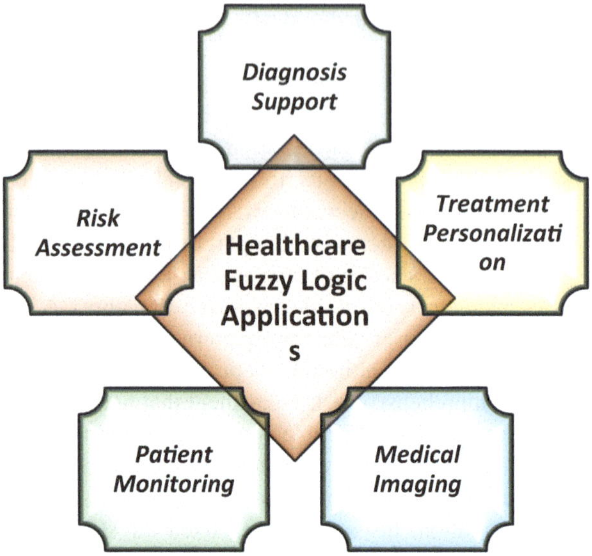

Fig. 2 Healthcare fuzzy logic applications

those of other illnesses. The fuzzy system is more flexible when figuring out how sick someone and offer more accurate results when the data is not clear.

- **Personalization of Treatment**: The use of fuzzy logic can be used to make treatment plans more personal because it takes into account a number of specific to the patient factors that may not be easy to measure. The use of fuzzy logic can suggest treatment plans that are better suited to each persons' needs by looking at their medical history, current health conditions and lifestyle factors. Such fuzzy systems might look at the size of the tumour, the patients age and any other health problems they have to suggest the best treatment for cancer. This leads to better treatments that have fewer side effects because fuzzy systems can work with incomplete or imprecise data to make better decisions.
- **Medical Imaging**: The use of fuzzy logic is widely used in medical imaging to make sense of unclear or noisy images like CT scans, MRIs, and X-rays. The medical profession can use fuzzy algorithms to improve the quality of images, find problems and better separate images. The use of fuzzy logic can help find areas of interest when looking for tumours even when the picture is not clear or there are small signs of disease. This ability makes diagnoses more accurate. Especially when the images are low resolution or the patient is moving that makes it easier to understand the results.
- **Patient Monitoring**: The fuzzy logic interprets vital signs like heart rate, blood pressure and oxygen levels in real time for giving results that are more flexible and accurate. Due to the fact that patient data can be noisy or change over time and fuzzy systems help find problems by looking at the data in a way that is always changing. For instance, the fuzzy logic can determine how abnormal a heart rate

is instead of just labelling it as "normal" or "abnormal." This lets healthcare providers respond appropriately and making sure that intervention happens when it needs to or even if the data is not completely clear.

- **Risk Assessment**: The clinical decision support system uses fuzzy logic to figure out how risky a patient is. A fuzzy system looks at a lot of different things when figuring out how likely it is that someone will get diabetes or heart disease. These things include their family history, their lifestyle and their current health. These variables might not always be clear or exact but fuzzy logic lets us make risk models that take into account uncertainties and make better predictions. The fuzzy systems help healthcare professionals understand potential health risks better by putting them on a timeline. This helps them stop or lessen diseases before they fully develop.

4.4 Fuzzy Logic for Adaptive Security Mechanisms

The adaptable security measures use the ability to deal with uncertainty and imprecision in situations that change. The traditional security systems often rely on clear binary opinions. However, in everyday situations the risks to security are rarely so straightforward. These systems can evaluate risk and security status on a continuum by allowing more flexible evaluations instead of just labelling events as threats or safe. Such as contrary to labelling network traffic as "malicious" or "safe," adaptive systems can look at a number of factors to figure out how likely a threat is, which gives a more accurate picture of security. Absolutely one of the best things about these systems is how flexible they are. The risks associated with cyberspace are always changing and security models that do not change may not be able to deal with new types of attacks. The adaptable security systems can respond to changes in real time by constantly changing their defences based on new information. This is especially useful in situations like IoT or cloud networks, where weaknesses can appear out of nowhere. As a result of these systems can provide faster and more relevant security responses. The adaptable systems make it easier to make decisions that are more complex. These systems do not just follow a set of rules. Instead of this they look at a number of things such as how users behave, how active the network is and how serious any problems that are found are. This multifaceted strategy makes sure that the response is tailored to the specific situation of the attack, which leads to more effective and accurate security measures. These types of structures are harder to hack because they are more flexible and can make better decisions. This capacity to change security procedures as conditions change means that even in unstable or very complicated situations overall protection is better. This technique makes security strategies work better overall by making sure that the right level of response is used to deal with the risks (Sarosh et al., 2022).

5 Fuzzy Logic Framework for Data Privacy and Security

5.1 *Fuzzification and Rule-Based Inference Engine*

The fuzzy nature is the process of turning clear, exact data into fuzzy values so that a system can work with data that is not always clear or certain. This process turns traditional binary or discrete values like "secure" or "insecure," into degrees of membership in the context of data privacy and security (Sreedhar et al., 2025). Fuzzy authentication, for example, allows the system give each data access request a level of certainty like 70% authorized or 30% unauthorized, instead of just saying it is "authorized" or "unauthorized." This makes it easier to make decisions that are more nuanced, which makes the system better at handling complicated, everyday circumstances where certainty is often not possible. The supervised inference engine gets the fuzzified data and processes it to make security decisions. This engine runs on a set of rules that were made by experts in data security. These rules are meant to look at different inputs and situations that could affect the privacy and security of data (Pandey & Pandey, 2025). Such rules could say things like: "If the user's location is suspicious and the access request comes from an unknown device then give it a high risk level." The inference engine uses these rules to make decisions based on fuzzified inputs that help with security actions. The machine learning engine uses fuzzy inference mechanisms to combine different fuzzy inputs and use logical operators (like AND and OR) to figure out the most likely outcomes. As results are defuzzied which means they are turned back into a clear value so that decisions can be made, such as whether to give or deny access, warn the user of suspicious activity or add more security measures. This method makes sure that the system can adapt and work with situations where the data is incomplete or uncertain. The security systems can look at possible risks in a more detailed and flexible way by using fuzzification and rule-based inference. This makes them better at protecting against data breaches and unauthorized access.

5.2 *Defuzzification and Action Trigger Mechanism*

This technique turns fuzzy values into clear and useful results. The rule-based inference engine has to turn the results of processing fuzzy inputs into exact actions. This change is necessary to make security decisions in real systems. Since giving access, turning down a request or sending out alarms all need clear instructions. Defuzzification is makes decisions about data privacy and security into things that can do. If the user is trustworthy and fuzzy logic might give an 80% chance of allowing their access request. This process changes this number into an action like letting someone in or marking the request for review. The centroid approach, which finds the fuzzy sets centre of gravity to get a clear value and the mean of maxima, which finds the average of the fuzzy set's maximum values, are the two most common ways to defuzzified. The action trigger mechanism turns on after defuzzification. In this system defuzzied results set off security actions. If the system thinks that the request made by a user for access is likely illegal then the action trigger may block access or require more than one form of authentication (Vijayalakshmi et al., 2025). The system might mark the request for review or send it up to a security administrator. The action trigger mechanism helps the security system deal with risk and uncertainty. It gives precise control over security measures, which lets the system quickly respond to new threats and change its rules. This flexibility makes data privacy and security better by stopping illegal access and breaches.

5.3 Integration with Healthcare IT and IoT Systems

The fuzzy logic-based security measures make it easier to protect real time data and manage risks in healthcare IT and IoT systems. Healthcare facilities produce a lot of data from patient records, medical devices and IoT sensors. These devices are often connected by complicated networks. The data is always changing and comes from a lot of different sources that could make it hard for traditional security measures to work. Intelligent fuzzy-based frameworks can help healthcare IT and IoT systems better identify and respond to security risks, which improves data privacy and system reliability. The use of fuzzy logic makes healthcare IT systems like EHRs and hospital management systems safer by looking at user access requests, keeping an eye on system logs and finding unusual behaviour. A healthcare worker who wants to get to patient data from an unknown device or location can be checked for risk and given access based on rules that have already been set. The fuzzy system may change how it evaluates risk based on the time of day, the users role and how they have accessed the system in the past. This stops breaches by only letting authorized users see sensitive data. The method of fuzzy logic can be used with IoT devices like smart wearables, patient monitoring systems, and connected medical equipment to keep an eye on threats all the time. IoT devices are used by a lot of people, but they usually don't have any security (Singh et al., 2025), so they are easy to attack. The system can dynamically encrypt communications or cut off hacked devices from the network by using fuzzy logic to guess when IoT devices will be hacked. The use of fuzzy logic also helps the system deal with new threats. The healthcare industry is susceptible to emerging attack vectors, necessitating real time learning and adaptation of security protocols. The adaptive security methods in healthcare IT and IoT systems protect against new cyber threats and make sure that different healthcare technologies work together smoothly.

6 Conclusion

The use of fuzzy logic makes healthcare data more secure by helping to solve tough problems in situations that are uncertain and changing. Fuzzification, rule-based inference and adaptive mechanisms help healthcare systems figure out how risky something is, make tough security choices and deal with new threats as they come up. This method makes healthcare IT and IoT security better by dealing with data that is missing or unclear. The security measures that are specific to healthcare data offer better protection, more options and a quicker response to cyber threats. The use of fuzzy reasoning helps keep healthcare data safe by dealing with how unpredictable the current healthcare system is. Transformation of exact data into flexible and useful insights helps people make better choices. The fuzzing and rule-based systems can take into account how users act, requests for access and device security, all of which have an impact on data privacy. This flexibility helps healthcare companies keep sensitive patient information safe as cyber threats increase. It also encourages granular security that help to makes systems more resilient and lowers the risk of data breaches and unauthorized access. As healthcare systems use advanced security measures. It is very important to have ethical data governance. It is hard to find a balance between using new technologies to improve results and keeping patient data safe. To make sure that security systems are open, accountable and fair. They must be designed and built with ethics in mind. The use of fuzzy logic improves security without breaking the rules of ethics. It makes solutions that protect privacy and the integrity and trust of healthcare. For data governance to be sustainable, smart systems and strong ethical standards will need to work together.

References

Alam, T., & Benaida, M. (2022). Internet of things and blockchain-based framework for Coronavirus (COVID-19) disease. *International Journal of Online and Biomedical Engineering, 18*, 82–94.

Buzdugan, A. (2020). Integration of cyber security in healthcare equipment. In *Proceedings of the 4th International Conference on Nanotechnologies and Biomedical Engineering: Proceedings of ICNBME-2019* (pp. 681–684). Chisinau, Moldova, 18–21 September 2019; Springer International Publishing.

Greco, L., Percannella, G., Ritrovato, P., Tortorella, F., & Vento, M. (2020). Trends in IoT based solutions for health care: Moving AI to the edge. *Pattern Recognition Letters, 135*, 346–353.

Ma, K. W. F., & McKinnon, T. (2022). COVID-19 and cyber fraud: Emerging threats during the pandemic. *Journal of Financial Crime, 29*, 433–446.

Minnaar, A., & Herbig, F. J. (2021). Cyberattacks and the cybercrime threat of ransomware to hospitals and healthcare services during the COVID-19 pandemic. *Acta Criminologica: African Journal of Criminology & Victimology, 34*, 155–185.

Mukati, N., Namdev, N., Dilip, R., Hemalatha, N., Dhiman, V., & Sahu, B. (2021). Healthcare assistance to COVID-19 patient using internet of things (IoT) enabled technologies. *Materials Today: Proceedings*, in press.

Othman, S. B., Almalki, F. A., Chakraborty, C., & Sakli, H. (2022). Privacy-preserving aware data aggregation for IoT-based healthcare with green computing technologies. *Computers & Electrical Engineering, 101*, Article 108025.

Pandey, B. K., & Pandey, D. (2025). Securing healthcare medical image information using advance morphological component analysis, information hiding systems, and hybrid convolutional neural networks on IoMT. *Computers in Biology and Medicine, 185*, 109499.

Puri, V., Kataria, A., & Sharma, V. (2021). Artificial intelligence-powered decentralized framework for Internet of Things in Healthcare 4.0. *Transactions on Emerging Telecommunications Technologies*, e4245.

Rawat, R., Mahor, V., Garg, B., Chouhan, M., Pachlasiya, K., & Telang, S. (2022). Modeling of cyber threat analysis and vulnerability in IoT-based healthcare systems during COVID. In *Lessons from COVID-19* (pp. 405–425). Academic Press.

Richardson, R., North, M. M., & Garofalo, D. (2021). Ransomware: The landscape is shifting-a concise report. *International Management Review, 17*, 5–86.

Sarosh, P., Parah, S. A., & Bhat, G. M. (2022). An efficient image encryption scheme for healthcare applications. *Multimedia Tools and Applications, 81*, 7253–7270.

Scott, C. R. (2022). *Comparing cybercrime in banking and healthcare sectors*. Ph.D. Thesis, Utica University, Utica, NY, USA.

Serna, S. (2022). *The increase of Ransomware attacks within the healthcare and education sector*. Ph.D. Thesis, Utica University, Utica, NY, USA.

Shafique, K., Khawaja, B. A., Sabir, F., Qazi, S., & Mustaqim, M. (2020). Internet of things (IoT) for next-generation smart systems: A review of current challenges, future trends and prospects for emerging 5G-IoT scenarios. *IEEE Access, 8*, 23022–23040.

Singh, S., Madaan, G., Swapna, H. R., Singh, A., Pandey, B. K., George, A. S., & Pandey, D. (2025). Unleashing the power of AI and data analysis: Transforming insights into action. In *Interdisciplinary approaches to AI, internet of everything, and machine learning* (pp. 1–24). IGI Global Scientific Publishing.

Sreedhar, C., Kallam, S., Ghantasala, G. P., Anthoniraj, S., Kumarganesh, S., Sagayam, K. M., Pandey, B. K., & Pandey, D. (2025).Enhancing healthcare data security using RFE and CRHSM for big data. *Computers in Biology and Medicine, 190*, 110063.

Vijayalakshmi, S., Pandey, B. K., Pandey, D., & Lelisho, M. E. (2025). Innovative deep learning classifiers for breast cancer detection through hybrid feature extraction techniques. *Scientific Reports, 15*(1), 22212.

Zhang, C., & Lu, Y. (2021). Study on artificial intelligence: The state of the art and future prospects. *Journal of Industrial Information Integration, 23*, Article 100224.

Ethical Implications of AI in Mental Health Diagnosis

Sony Kulshrestha and Ruchi Kulshrestha

Abstract The incorporation of artificial intelligence (AI) in mental health care presents considerable promise to improve patient outcomes. Due to earlier diagnosis, tailored treatments and more efficient care delivery. However, its widespread adoption in this area raises a lot of important ethical questions that need to be answered in order to make sure it is used correctly. Security and privacy are very important because these systems often deal with sensitive information mental health. Therefore, the patient information needs to be kept safe with strict security methods. Algorithmic biases are a big problem since they might hurt some demographic groups more than others just because of the biased datasets or wrong models. The patients must completely know how these systems work and what they could mean for their care in order to supply informed permission. This poses significant challenges. These concerns need to be alleviated. It is important to have people watch over things. So that technology helps rather than replaces human judgment. These systems also need to be open and have strong data protection rules in place. The human-in-the-loop methods keep doctors involved in the decision-making process. This approach ensures that system recommendations are put into context and to be analyzed. Finally, it is important to create proactive ethical frameworks to make sure that these tools meet high standards of ethics, accountability and patient safety. These technologies can improve the mental health care. While still following ethical guidelines and protecting patient rights if they attain a balance between innovation and accountability.

Keywords AI in mental health · Ethical concerns · Privacy · Algorithmic bias · Informed consent · Accountability · Data protection · Human oversight

S. Kulshrestha (✉)
Department of Law, Manipal University Jaipur, Jaipur, India
e-mail: sonykulshrestha@gmail.com

R. Kulshrestha
Department of English, Radhe Hari Govt. PG College, Kashipur, India

D. Pandey et al. (eds.), *Smart Healthcare*,
https://doi.org/10.1007/978-981-95-8828-2_20

1 Introduction

The use of artificial intelligence in mental health is the use of computer systems that can learn, reason and make decisions to help people understand, diagnose and treat mental health illnesses. These technologies analyses a vast amount of biological, behavioral and psychological data to identify patterns associated with disorders such as schizophrenia, anxiety and depression. A smart systems help doctors by mimicking cognitive processes like pattern recognition and predictive reasoning. This makes it possible to make diagnoses faster and more accurately. Instead of just using traditional diagnostic interviews or questionnaires modern systems use information from several places such as speech patterns, wearable sensors, social media activity and electronic health data. This data integration allows them to find the tiny changes that could mean the start or progression of the mental health problems. Often before they are obvious to the human eye. This field's tools operate continuously providing real-time monitoring and insights that traditional methods struggle to provide. One of the best things about these systems is that they can handle vast and complex datasets well. By finding connections between the different elements. They make it feasible to build highly personalized diagnostic profiles and treatment plans. The virtual therapists and conversational agents that use machine learning make it easier for people to receive basic mental health treatment by removing barriers like expense, stigma or geographic remoteness. Remember the purpose of smart diagnostic technologies is to assist mental health professionals not to supplant their expertise. Their role is to reduce errors, expedite procedures and ensure data-driven care delivery. There are also many problems with using this technology in mental health therapy although. For instance, in order to maintain the human connection necessary for psychological recovery, protecting privacy and upholding justice can be challenging. A thorough and critical understanding of the concept and intended purpose of these technologies is essential to ensure ethical and effective implementation in the mental health sector.

1.1 Growing Relevance and Trends

The importance of artificial intelligence in mental health has been growing a lot in the last few years. There is a global rise in mental health problems. There is an urgent need for solutions that can be used on a larger scale and more effectively. The COVID-19 pandemic and increasing social pressure are two of these factors. In the past few years. This is artificial intelligence has become a lot more important in mental health. This is because mental health issues are getting worse all over the world. We need more effective treatments that can be used on a larger scale. The COVID-19 epidemic, rising social pressures and more people being aware of their mental health have all made it more important to have mental health facilities that are easy to get to. The traditional healthcare systems have had a hard time keeping up since they are often overwhelmed by the number and complexity of cases. This gap has sped up the use of smart technologies that can help with early detection, personalized treatment and ongoing patient monitoring. One of the most intriguing trends is the rise of digital mental health platforms that use machine learning models to provide risk assessments, mood tracking and therapeutic interactions. The uses mobile applications, wearable devices and online therapy platforms are increasingly integrating intelligent features to provide real-time feedback and tailored support. These tools not only make it easier for people to get care especially in distant or underserved places but they also let people stay anonymous. Which might encourage those who might not otherwise seek help because of stigma? The advanced improvements in natural language processing (NLP) have further sped up this change by letting systems use text and speech analysis to understand complicated human emotions. Emotional AI is getting better at picking up on little changes in tone, language patterns and facial expressions. This opens up new ways to monitor mental health without being intrusive. At the same time the predictive analytics is used to identify people who might be at risk of serious mental health issues before obvious signs appear and allowing for early intervention. Another trend that is growing is the partnership of digital businesses, healthcare providers and schools to make solutions that are led by ethics and have been tested in real-world situations. The clear and understandable processes are becoming increasingly important, prioritizing patient safety and trust. Regulatory bodies and professional organizations are also starting to set rules to make sure that new ideas in this domain are still fair, ethical and useful (Alhuwaydi, 2024).Ensure and increased awareness around psychological well-being have led to greater demand for accessible mental health services. The traditional type of healthcare systems are often overwhelmed by the volume and complexity of cases have struggled to keep pace. This type of gap has accelerated the adoption of intelligent technologies that can support early detection, personalized intervention and continuous patient monitoring. One of the most notable trends is the development of the digital mental health platforms that incorporate enhanced machine learning models to offer risk assessments and mood tracking as well as therapeutic conversations. The available mobile applications, wearable devices and online therapy platforms are increasingly integrating intelligent features to provide real-time feedback and the tailored support. These tools not only enhanced access in case of remote or underserved areas. But such kind system also offers anonymity. Encouraging individuals who might otherwise avoid seeking help due to stigma. The advancements in natural language processing (NLP) have further fueled this evolution by enabling systems to interpret complex human emotions through text and speech analysis. The enhanced emotional AI is capable of recognizing subtle shifts in tone, language patterns and facial expressions is becoming more sophisticated and opening new possibilities for non-invasive mental health monitoring. In parallel the predictive analytics is being used to identify individuals at risk of severe mental health episodes before symptoms become critical and allowing for preventive interventions. Another emerging trend is the collaboration between technology companies, healthcare providers and academic institutions to create ethically guided and clinically validated solutions. There is a growing emphasis on building transparent and explainable systems that prioritize patient safety and trust. The regulatory bodies and professional organizations are also beginning to establish guidelines to ensure that innovation in this area remains ethical, equitable and effective (Alhuwaydi, 2024).

2 AI in Mental Health Diagnosis

2.1 Early Detection of Mental Health Conditions

An early detection and treatment of mental health problems can improve outcomes and reduce long-term impacts. The intelligent technologies are increasingly used to detect subtle signs of mental health problems. Especially when traditional procedures are ineffective. By looking at behavior patterns, speech characteristics, social media activity, physiological signals and clinical records. These systems can detect early signs that regular clinical exams miss. One of the big advantages of these systems is that they can watch and make sense of enormous amounts of data in real time. Unlike going to the doctor, digital monitoring lets check someone mood, behavior and cognitive performance every day. The main changes in sleep patterns reduced social interaction and the way someone talks or chooses words can all be signs of depression, anxiety or bipolar disorder. The smart algorithms can quickly spot these kinds of differences. Which leads to evaluations and actions? It is critical that risk estimates may be tailored to each person. The advanced machine learning algorithms can predict mental health issues by looking at a person's history, environment and biology instead of using universal diagnostic criteria. This personalized approach enhances early detection and preventive measures as well as raising service quality. This technology can also help reduce the stigma around mental health support by finding problems early. Most people who do not want to consult a mental health professional may be able to obtain care before their symptoms get worse with discreet and non-invasive monitoring. To promote mental health, schools, companies and hospitals are incorporating these tools into wellness programs. Early detection has great potential but these systems must be applied ethically to protect privacy and avoid false positives that could cause worry. Responsible use of cognitive diagnostic tools can convert mental health care from reactive to preventive, enhancing individual and public health (Alowais et al., 2023).

2.2 Improved Accessibility to Mental Health Services

Factors such as location, cost, stigma and a shortage of qualified professionals have always limited access to mental healthcare. Smart technology is starting to solve many of these problems by coming up with new ways to make mental health care more accessible, inexpensive and easy for a wide range of people. Many people can obtain support using digital platforms that use machine learning and other similar technologies. This approach makes it easier for people to get treatment outside of traditional healthcare settings. These platforms offer chat-based counseling, mood tracking and cognitive behavioral therapy (CBT) activities around the clock. They are generally much cheaper than treatment in person. This kind of program is especially helpful for people who live in rural or underserved areas. These programs are particularly beneficial for individuals residing in rural or underserved areas, where access to mental health experts is limited. Additionally, providing support through smartphones and computers is beneficial. They cut down on the need to travel and wait. This greatly simplifies the process of obtaining mental health care. Another main part of making things more accessible is the chance to reach out to marginalized and disadvantaged populations, who might not want to use traditional services because of stigma, cultural obstacles, or fear of prejudice. Digital interventions can supply people with a stronger sense of privacy and anonymity. This can encourage more individuals to seek assistance when they encounter difficulties. Some systems also support multiple languages and offer culturally specific content. This main feature makes these systems even more useful for a wider range of people. More and more schools, businesses and community groups use AI-powered mental health tools to help their members before they need them. These programs help make mental health care a part of everyday life; make it easier to talk about mental health; and lower the barriers to getting treatment. The smart systems may also prioritize cases according to how urgent they are. This is a crucial step. This ensures that those in greater danger receive help promptly. It is still essential to ensure that accessibility doesn't mean giving up more quality. To ensure that digital mental health treatments are safe, effective, fair and ethical, it is necessary to implement designs, conduct clinical validation and perform ongoing monitoring. These elements must be carefully applied to the system. These technologies have the potential to transform mental health care delivery and enhance accessibility to the support system (Balcombe, 2023).

2.3 Consistency and Reduction of Human Error

A significant advantage of employing intelligent technology in mental health diagnosis is their capacity to deliver consistent assessments and mitigate human error. The conventional diagnostic methods however successful and frequently affected by subjective elements including clinician experience, emotional state, cultural background and implicit biases. These human factors may result in evaluation inconsistencies and at times, misdiagnosis or delayed intervention. In contrast the computational systems employ uniform standards and analytical precision across all instances. This is providing a consistency that is challenging to attain manually. The automated tools can systematically examine huge volumes of patient data, accounting for numerous variables concurrently and devoid of weariness or emotional bias. The advanced machine learning models trained on numerous clinical cases can identify nuanced trends that may be missed in a conventional clinical interview. They can identify early warning signals, monitor symptom progression and discriminate between diseases with overlapping characteristics. Such as separating bipolar disorder from major depressive disorder a task that even experienced physicians may find difficult. These solutions mitigate the danger of supervision resulting from task pressures. In bustling healthcare settings where the practitioners oversee multiple patients concurrently. The likelihood of overlooking essential details may rise the development of new system. An intelligent system assists clinicians by identifying potential issues, proposing differential diagnosis and encouraging additional inquiry when necessary. This decision support system not only improves diagnostic precision but also enables mental health professionals to concentrate more on therapeutic interaction with their patients. It is crucial to acknowledge that although these systems help reduce specific types of errors. They are not flawless. Their precision is significantly influenced by the quality of the training data and the strength of their design. The biases included in the training data may be inadvertently sustained. Resulting in novel diagnostic mistakes if not meticulously addressed. Consequently, the human supervision is crucial for validating results, interpreting intricate circumstances and making ethical decisions according to particular requirements. When utilized judiciously sophisticated diagnostic tools can markedly enhance the dependability of mental health evaluations, diminish inconsistencies in patient treatment and facilitate prompt and more efficacious interventions (Balcombe & Leo, 2021; Baskin et al., 2021).

2.4 Data-Driven Insights and Predictive Capabilities

The use of modern technologies in mental health care has made it possible to obtain data-driven insights and make predictions about the future of mental health outcomes. In the past type diagnosis and treatment planning relied heavily on patient self-reported types and physician observations. While these methods are helpful. They are sometimes limited by subjective interpretations and inconsistent data collection. Many intelligent systems are a big change because they constantly collect and analyze large amounts of different data to detect patterns that would otherwise remain hidden. These systems can look at information from electronic health records, wearable sensors, social media activities and even biological signs to create thorough profiles of a person's mental health over time. The advanced algorithms can detect subtle alterations in behavior or physiology that may indicate the onset or exacerbation of mental health issues. These changes might include changes in how to sleep, how to talk or how the individual heart rate varies. These insights provide clinicians with a more thorough and impartial basis for diagnosis and intervention. Long before clinical indicators are fully obvious, predictive analytics can reveal people who are at high risk of developing disorders like depression, anxiety or suicidal thoughts. It is better to do this than to wait until symptoms are severe enough to make a diagnosis. This early warning system lets people make efforts to avoid getting sick. This can significantly impact the progression of the illness and enhance its long-term consequences. The aggregated data can also highlight trends across groups of people. Which can help with planning for public health and deciding how to use resources?

For example, analyzing mental health data during global crises like the COVID-19 pandemic has taught us about new stressors and groups of people who are more likely to be affected. This has led to tailored support programmers. Most people worry about privacy, informed consent and the chance of being taken advantage of since predictive skills are so powerful. It is crucial to uphold people's trust while maximizing the potential of new technologies. It is crucial to ensure that data collection and analysis are open, safe and respectful of peoples' rights. When applied correctly, data-driven insights and predictive modeling could alter how mental health is treated by making interventions. The process should be earlier, more tailored to each individual and more successful (Carr, 2020).

3 Ethical Considerations and Dilemmas

3.1 Privacy and Confidentiality

The integration of the many intelligent technologies into mental health care brings significant concerns regarding privacy and confidentiality. These technologies often rely on large amounts of sensitive personal data and raising significant concerns about privacy and confidentiality. Safeguarding this confidential information is critically important. A dataset of mental health, including diagnoses, treatment histories and behavioral patterns, is among the most sensitive categories of information. Misuse or unauthorized access could have severe consequences for individuals. It is not merely a legal responsibility to ensure that strong privacy measures are in place. But it is important for keeping patients trust and getting them to adopt this advanced technology. To make sure that sensitive data is handled safely and responsibly. Most mental health professionals and technology developers need to work together to set clear rules and guidelines. The widespread use of artificial intelligence systems is gaining momentum. The need for uniform and transparent standards around data privacy becomes increasingly important to avoid breaches and protect vulnerable individuals. Unauthorized access leads to hacking and data breaches are the biggest threat to the security of sensitive mental health data. Most cybercriminals have a strong desire to steal health data from digital platforms. If they succeed, they could gain access to confidential patient data. This theft could lead to identity theft, discrimination, or even financial harm. It is crucial for mobile health apps and telehealth platforms to ensure the safety of health data. They need to use the best encryption technologies and security protections that are available. Cloud computing is not centralized, which poses security risks. When data is stored in different places, it can be more likely to be attacked by hackers. Sharing data with third parties is another concern. A lot of mental health apps and systems use data from outside sources, such as wearable or social media sites. If not adequately regulated, this can lead to data-sharing agreements that violate patient privacy. This is especially true when the third parties engaged do not have to follow the same strict privacy rules. To lessen these dangers, it is important to make sure that data is anonymized and transported securely. It is challenging to keep mental health technology systems anonymous because the data is very personal. Anonymization methods like data masking can lower the chance of personal identification. Although they are not perfect. Some advanced analytics methods like machine learning, can still find people even when direct identifiers are taken away. This risk is heightened when data is integrated with other type of existing datasets. This possibility of reidentification is especially high worrisome. In terms of the mental wellness. If people find out about their illnesses by accident. They may encounter stigma, discrimination, or emotional pain. Staying anonymous can be hard. When services need to talk to different healthcare systems. Personal information may be necessary for thorough treatment planning. In such situations, it becomes difficult to find a balance between the need for thorough data access and privacy protection. Another important part is making sure that people provide their informed consent. People need to know exactly how their data is used, stored and shared. To lessen these problems, there have to be clear and open policies, and users should be able to control their data (Chalyi, 2024; Chen & Esmaeilzadeh, 2024).

3.2 Bias and Discrimination

To ensure that intelligent technology is used fairly and openly as well as responsibly in mental health treatment and diagnosis. Clear ethical rules and guidelines are currently needed. These technologies promise to make mental healthcare more effective, but they also raise ethical questions about fairness, equity and algorithmic bias. As AI solutions become more common in hospitals, it's important to use them in a way that is safe and builds trust. The ethical frameworks must address risks such as reinforcing cultural biases or inadvertently perpetuating disparities in care. These rules should also make it clear that AI systems should be accountable that patients should give their consent and that algorithmic decision-making should be open. Clear rules can help people use mental health technology responsibly as well as cut down on ethical issues. The use of artificial intelligence may yield unjust or discriminatory outcomes due to inadequate training data as well as biased algorithms or flawed design decisions. This is especially worrying when it comes to mental health. Where systems that are biased may give wrong diagnoses or wrong treatments based on race, gender or social class. A lot of AI systems learn from old data, which can show how healthcare is biased. An AI model based on data from a dominant racial or socioeconomic group might not be able to correctly diagnose or treat people from minority groups. Such bias can lead to wrong diagnoses of mental health issues and delays in treatment. Care that is not culturally competent. Patients are often unfairly grouped or excluded from helpful therapies. An algorithmic bias could make health care differences worse. The advanced AI systems that misdiagnose or overlook the issues faced by specific groups may exacerbate their marginalization in the healthcare system. To make sure that AI systems are fair and treat all patients equally, we need strict audits, various data sets and open development processes. If not properly controlled, AI in mental health care could have a bigger effect on groups that are already at a disadvantage, such as racial and ethnic minorities, disabled people and those with low incomes. Smart technology could make mental health care unfair for some groups, worse or better, depending on how the systems are built and used. Artificial intelligence (AI) technologies that were built and tested on data from wealthy and mostly white groups may not work well for other groups of people. These limitations could make diagnoses and some treatments less efficient and care for marginalized patients worse. Artificial intelligence programs may hurt or alienate vulnerable people who need more customized, human-centered care if they do not take cultural contexts and life experiences into account. However, if we design and implement these systems with fairness and inclusivity in mind. AI has the potential to simplify access to care. An intelligent technology can help people with mental health issues who do not have a lot of money or competent staff by giving them flexible and affordable solutions. We must include marginalized groups in the development method and design the procedures to meet their needs in order to fairly share these benefits (Chintala, 2022).

3.3 Informed Consent

The consent form is a basic moral rule in healthcare. It makes sure that people understand exactly what their treatment means and are making choices based on all the information available to them about the process and its risks. When it comes to artificial intelligence in mental health care. The premise of informed consent gets more complicated. The patient needs to know not only what their condition is and what treatments will be offered but also how intelligent technologies are being used in order to gather, analyze and act on their personal data. Easy to understand, readily available and simple to understand acceptance practices are very important for protecting those receiving treatment privacy and freedom while still giving them control over their mental health care choices. AI systems in mental health frequently utilize advanced data collection methods, machine learning algorithms and automated methods for making decisions, all of which are intricate to elucidate and comprehend. In connection with that healthcare providers and technology developers have to make sure that patients really understand what they are agreeing to. Some of the biggest problems with getting informed consent for artificially intelligent mental health treatments is that the technology is very complicated. AI systems work through complex algorithms and data processing methods that many patients may not be able to understand. This is distinct from traditional forms of nursing that can be easily explained using medical terms and direct interactions. This is why explaining how machine learning models are used to evaluate mental health, forecast risk or suggest interventions necessitates a degree of technical proficiency that many individuals may lack. This complexity can make it hard for patients to make truly informed decisions because they might feel overwhelmed or confused by technical explanations. A patient may not fully understand what it means to be involved with systems driven by AI if the process of giving consent is not made easier or put into context. This could mean that their consent is not really informed (Cohen, 2019). Some patients may depend on clinicians to explain these processes in a clear and meaningful manner but clinicians may not always be able to explain the subtleties of AI technology in a way that is easy to understand. To keep ethical standards and confidence it is crucial to make sure that patients get information that is clear and useful. AI system developers need to work closely with healthcare providers to make sure that people of all levels of technological literacy can understand how their technologies work. A patient should always be able to give informed consent, which means they should be able to make their own decisions without being forced or pressured. In the context of artificially intelligent mental health care. However, patients may feel lightly pressured to consent due to the perceived benefits of AI tools. Such as the convenience of virtual therapy or the promise of more quickly and more accurate diagnoses. Patients may feel like they have to take part in artificial intelligence interventions just because they are the standard or because they are afraid of not being able to get care if they refuse to participate. To make sure that consent is truly voluntary and important patients need to feel safe asking questions, voicing worries and understanding the full scope of their involvement. This means giving patients that they have choice to say no or take back their own consent at any time without affecting their care in any way. To make sure that permission is free and also need to be honest about any risks. Such as the possibility of data breaches, mistakes or the limits of AI systems. The patients ought to be afforded the opportunity to comprehend the utilization of their data and the precise function of AI in their mental health care. The consent forms must be fully complete and without ambiguity covering not only the process and technology but also the rights of patients to privacy and data protection. It is important to stress the importance of ongoing consent. Where patients can choose whether or not to use certain features or systems as they learn more about them. This is an important part of keeping an ethical approach to AI-based system in the mental health care. We uphold the principles of the autonomy and dignity by making sure that the consent is both voluntary and meaningful in term and condition. This gives patients the power to make informed choices about the role of AI in their mental health journey (Bruijn et al., 2022).

3.4 Accountability and Responsibility

As technologies powered by AI become more common in the field of mental health, it is very important to think about who is responsible for mistakes and what role different people should play in making sure these systems are used responsibly. The smart system can help with medical care and results for patients but they also make people worry about who is to blame when something goes wrong. An inaccurate diagnosis or unsuitable treatment recommendation in the realm of mental health can yield severe, occasionally transformative, repercussions. This means that it is very important to make sure that there are clear lines of responsibility so that the benefits of

AI can be realized without putting patient safety or ethical standards at risk. To make and use AI tools in mental health care, developers, physicians and institutions need to work together. Each group is responsible for making sure that these systems are produced, erected and used in an ethical manner with the right checks and balances in place. When an AI makes a mistake in mental health treatment one of the hardest things to figure out is who is responsible. To protect patients and make sure that developers and clinicians are treated equitably the rules about who is responsible for AI mistakes in mental health care need to be clear. This is up to developers to make sure that the algorithms that run these systems are correct, well tested and free of bias. But developers are frequently unable to observe every possible outcome or change in practical patient data, which makes the issue of liability complicated. Physicians yet they have an ethical obligation to utilized these tools as an adjunct to rather than a substitute for, their professional judgment. If doctors fail to carefully check AI suggestions before following them. They could be partly to blame for mistakes. From an institutional point of point of view organizations that use AI systems need to make sure that these technologies are properly integrated into clinical workflows with the right oversight and protections. Institutions need to set up rules for checking the results of AI and making sure the system keeps working, such as regular audits and ways for patients to give feedback. In the end these stakeholders must share duties with clearly defined roles and responsibilities to make sure that patients are safe and that AI is used in a safe and ethical way. Developers, professionals and institutions are all important to making sure that AI is used safely in mental health care. The people who make AI systems are in charge of making them, testing them and making them better all the time. They need to make sure that their algorithms are based on data that is accurate, diverse and free of bias. They also need to test the systems regularly to make sure they work in everyday scenarios. The developers also need to write clear instructions on how the system works and make sure that clinicians who will use it get enough training. To be sure that the artificial intelligence method for making decisions is clear helps doctors understand why it made certain recommendations and gives them the information they need to make good choices. Clinicians must use AI suggestions in the treatment and diagnosis they receive. But they should always use their own judgment. They need to look at AI suggestions in light of the medical history of the individual, tastes and other personal factors. Clinicians should not depend exclusively on AI outcomes. Since they should utilize these tools to augment their clinical decisions. This partnership makes sure that AI is a helpful tool and not a replacement for the human knowledge. The institutions are in charge of making sure that AI systems are used properly in their clinical settings. Institutions must ensure the ethical use of these tools and provide clinicians with the necessary training and support. They should also take the initiative to establish policies governing AI application including data privacy protocols, accountability guidelines and patient consent procedures. To find errors of judgment, biases or unintended effects and make sure that AI systems stay useful and safe over time. They need to be checked and evaluated regularly (Ellahham et al., 2020).

4 Legal and Regulatory Considerations

The legal and the regulatory framework governing the application of AI in mental health treatment is complex and varied. As AI systems become more important for diagnosing and treating mental health problems. It is important to deal with big issues like data protection, accountability, intellectual property and regulatory problems that cross borders. The legal frameworks must protect confidentiality between patients. It is clear who is responsible for errors and set clear standards for approving AI tools. Figure 1 shows the legal and regulatory issues. Legal scrutiny is needed all the time because of worries about things like algorithmic bias, openness and how AI should be used with human making decisions. As technology improves, rules need to change to keep patients safe and encourage new ideas in mental health care.

- Data Protection: AI technologies used in mental health care work with private patient information. The reason why this is so important to keep that data safe. Laws like GDPR and HIPAA set rules for how data should be collected, maintained and shared to protect the privacy of patients. These rules say that patients must give clear permission for their data to be used, archived and shared with other people. Encryption, safe storage methods and regular audits are all necessary to keep data safe from breaches and unauthorized access. Following these rules not only keeps on the right side of the law. But it also builds trust with patients, which makes it easier to use AI for treatment and diagnosis.
- Responsibility and Accountability: This is hard to know who is to blame when something goes wrong with AI in mental health. If a mistake takes place like a wrong diagnosis or treatment suggestion, developers, medical personnel and institutions all need to know exactly what their jobs are. The law needs to make it

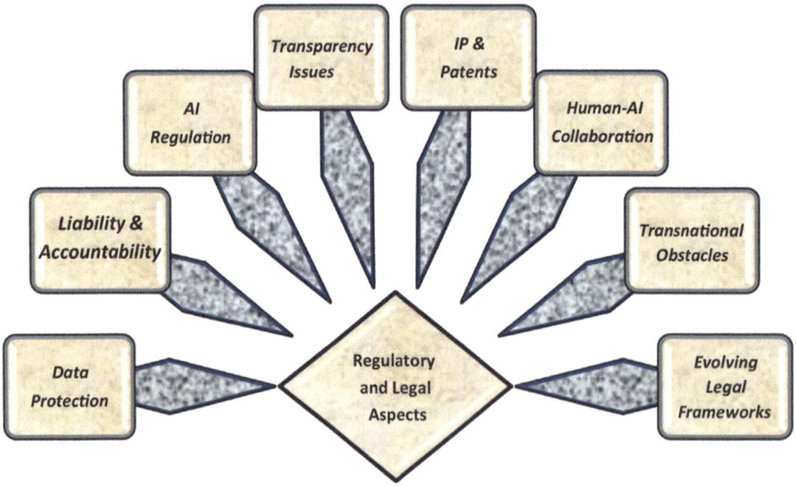

Fig. 1 Regulatory and legal aspects

clear who is responsible for the scheme: the clinicians who use it or the institutions that put it in place? When AI systems are used to help make decisions instead of replacing judgment from a physician. This is especially hard. Clinicians also need to be careful not to let AI suggestions take the place of their professional responsibilities. Especially when it comes to patient safety and standards of care.

- AI Regulation: The FDA in the USA while the EMA in Europe are two significant organizations that keep an eye on artificial intelligence (AI) used in mental health care. All of these organizations say that artificial intelligence cannot be used until it has passed strict tests for safety and effectiveness. This implies that there is proof that the technology works well in many different situations and is not placing patients in too much danger. Everyone still needs to keep an eye on AI tools to see how well they work when people use them. This is also important to change the rules from time to time to keep up with how AI is getting better. The reason for this keeps them up to date and ready to deal with new problems that come up as technology changes.
- Issues with openness: Patients and healthcare professionals must be aware of the way to make suggestions. It should be clear and open how AI makes decisions. A law might say that AI systems used in healthcare have to explain their decisions in a way that is easy to understand. This transparency makes individuals more likely to trust systems operated by AI as both doctors and patients can better judge how accurate and reliable artificially intelligent suggestions are. Patients and doctors may not trust AI systems if they do not understand how they work. Algorithmic transparency makes it easier to hold people accountable if something goes wrong because it lets people trace the decision-making process back to its source.
- IP and Patents: Using AI to make tools for mental health raises questions about intellectual property (IP) rights, especially when AI systems come up with new ideas or inventions. The conventional patent laws which were made with human inventors in mind, do not do a good job of addressing the role of AI in the process of coming up with new ideas. There are legal issues about who owns the rights to patents that were made by AI. The company that owns the AI, or the AI system itself? As AI becomes more common in diagnosis and treatment, these uncertainties could make it harder to sell AI technologies in healthcare. The laws about intellectual property need to change to reflect AI's role in new ideas while still making sure that ownership is fair (Koutsouleris et al., 2022).
- Human-AI Collaboration: In mental health care, an AI should always be thought of as a tool that helps people make decisions, not as a replacement for them. Lot of legal frameworks must clearly define the roles and responsibilities of clinicians working with AI. This means making sure that AI is used properly in clinical workflows and that doctors still have the last say over how to care for patients.AI systems should help with diagnosis, treatment ideas and data analysis. Yet doctors should always make the final decisions so that patients get the care that is best for them. Legal rules should also say what kind of training and skills clinicians need to use AI tools correctly. So, they can understand AI results and make smart choices.

- Transnational Obstacles: AI systems for mental health care are often made in one country but used in many others, which can cause legal problems. Different places may have different rules about privacy, data protection and healthcare, which could make it harder to use and set up AI tools. International cooperation is needed to make sure that AI-powered mental health tools follow the rules in each country. Data sovereignty issues arise as data transfers between nations become increasingly prevalent. This means that the laws of the country where the data is collected must be followed. Even if the data is stored or processed in a different country. The world needs to come together to make rules that protect patients while also letting AI in healthcare grow and change.
- Changing the Law: As AI gets better and better. The laws and rules that are already in place need to change to deal with new problems. We need new laws to keep up with AI technologies that are faster than the ones we have now. Regulatory bodies need to keep up with changes in AI technology and change their rules when they need to. This could mean that AI systems need to be more open, easy to understand and always watched over. Future rules should find a balance between encouraging new ideas and making sure that AI technologies stay ethical, responsible and in line with human concerns about health care and safety. Regular changes to the law will help mental health care professionals stay on top of the problems that AI brings up.

5 Ethical Training for AI Developers

5.1 Bias Auditing and Correction

Artificial intelligence (AI) programs that are biased can make existing inequalities worse and lead to wrong or harmful outcomes especially in sensitive areas like mental health. These systems depend so much on information any biases in the training data can cause the results to be wrong. The bias auditing is an important step in finding and fixing these differences. It means looking through the datasets and algorithms used to train AI systems in a systematic way to find any bias that could lead to unfair or discriminatory results. Auditing usually looks at a few distinct variables like gender, race, a particular socioeconomic and other demographic factors. AI model that is trained mostly on data from one demographic group may not work well for people from other groups. This could lead to wrong diagnoses or treatments that do not work. The identification of these biases through careful testing and analysis helps make sure that the system works fairly for people of all backgrounds. After biases have been found the model and data must be changed to fix them. The easiest way to fix this is to train the algorithm again using datasets that are more diverse and representative of the people it serves. Another way is to change how the model makes decisions so that it takes into account any biases that have been found that will lead to fairer results. The programmers can also add fairness constraints to algorithm to make predictions less affected by biased data. The purpose of the bias auditing and correction is to make AI systems that are more equitable and open to everyone. This process is ongoing because biases may not always be obvious immediately. The effectiveness of the system can change when new data is added. By including bias auditing in the development process. The developers can make AI systems that are stronger and more reliable, which can help with mental health diagnosis and treatment without making harmful biases worse (Lee, 2018).

5.2 Promoting Transparent Algorithms

As a mental health care apps to be trustworthy, accountable and fair. It is important to promote transparency in algorithmic systems (Leimanis & Palkova, 2021). The open systems let both doctors and patients know how decisions are made. Ensuring that suggestions do not come across as black-box solutions. This includes making it possible to understand and access how these systems operate as well as giving clear explanations of how data inputs are processed to produce results. Such transparency builds trust by letting people look closely at and confirm the process of making decisions (Singh et al., 2025). In mental health diagnostics, where choices have had a big impact on the health of patients. It is very important for doctors to know why they make certain suggestions. The openness enables professionals to interpret recommendations and incorporate them into their clinical judgment, facilitating the identification of errors or limitations (Chinnasamy et al., 2025). So, when a system suggests a treatment. Doctors should be able to follow the logic and data points that led to that suggestion. This will help them make better decisions. Providing clear documentation about how these systems work can help make them more open to the public. This could include information about the data sources and how accurate they are, and any problems they might have. Making technology less mysterious helps people feel more comfortable using it in mental health care, which is good for both patients and clinicians. Before being implemented the regulatory bodies may also require developers to meet standards for transparency. As these technologies get stronger it will be very important to keep things open and honest to make sure that ethical standards are followed and that there is no bias or misuse in clinical settings (Duraisamy et al., 2025). By putting transparency first innovators can make tools that are more reliable and useful. This will help people make superior choices and keep patients safe and confident.

5.3 Human Oversight in Decision-Making

Human oversight is crucial in AI-driven decision-making processes, especially in mental health care, where judgments significantly affect patients, as illustrated in Fig. 2.

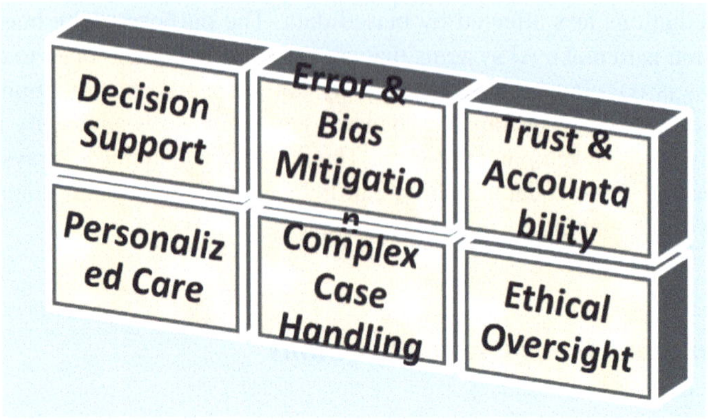

Fig. 2 Integrating human-in-the-loop approaches

Artificially intelligent technology offers considerable knowledge but it cannot replace the complexity and sensitivity that human professionals offer. Clinicians have to be present for interpreting suggestions, tailoring treatment and ensuring decisions are ethical. The contribution of human judgment to the process reduces the risks of mistakes, prejudices and misinterpretations that can happen when computers do the work. This partnership between artificial intelligence and human expertise makes sure that patients get care that is truthful, unbiased and that is tailored to their needs.

- **Decision Support:** It is important for humans to keep an eye on things so that clinicians can still make important decisions and use their professional knowledge to understand and change artificially intelligent insights. An algorithm can point out patterns and make suggestions. But doctors and nurses know more about the patients overall situation like their emotional state, family dynamics or lifestyle, which an automated system might miss (Chandraman et al., 2025). This human touch is necessary to provide care that takes into account all aspects of the health of a client and makes sure that decisions are based on facts and are unique to each person.
- **Error and Bias Mitigation**: The human being in the loop protects against mistakes or biases that could be in algorithmic systems. Clinicians are better able to spot inconsistencies, errors or biases in the data and results. Artificial intelligence might unintentionally favor some demographic groups or ignore minority populations because the data sets they use do not appear representative. Through peering over these outputs. The qualified doctors can find mistakes or harmful patterns and take steps to fix them, which will make treatment fairer and more accurate for all patients.
- **Trust and Responsibility**: A lack of a clinician helps make decisions builds trust and openness. Patients are more likely to trust suggestions when they know that a qualified professional has looked them over and approved them. This trust also

applies to clinicians. Who benefit from being able to evaluate, verify and comprehend the algorithms reasoning prior to making decisions. Including people makes sure that people are responsible for the results. If a decision has an unsatisfactory then the clinicians are still responsible. This creates a feedback loop that makes the system better while keeping patient safety at the top of the list.

- **Personalized Care:** The artificial intelligence can suggest treatment plans based on statistical trends but human oversight makes sure that each plan has tailored to the needs of each patient. A doctor change or ignore artificial intelligence suggestions based on what they know about each patients' history, habits and situation. This makes it possible to provide care in a more flexible and caring manner taking into account things like mental health history, cultural background and personal goals. By combining artificial intelligence speed with human insight as well as care becomes more complete and personalized.
- **Handling Complex Cases:** While a patient had a lot of different mental health issues or conditions that are happening simultaneously in order human oversight is even more important. Artificial intelligence systems are great at looking at big sets of data. But they might have trouble with cases that do not fit into typical patterns or that need a deeper understanding of things like trauma or culture. When these problems come up then clinicians can step in and change the artificial intelligences outputs to better meet the needs of each patient. This makes sure that the care given is relevant, timely and has the right amount of detail for more difficult cases.
- **Ethical Oversight:** When using advanced artificial intelligence in mental health, moral and ethical issues are very important. The general public make sure that algorithms follow basic ethical principles like respecting patients' rights to privacy, freedom and informed consent. Clinicians must ascertain whether the algorithms recommendations align with the patients' values, preferences and well-being. While also considering the broader ethical implications of technology utilization in healthcare. They can also talk about their fears that an algorithm might unintentionally cause bias or harm making sure that care stays morally sound and follows both medical standards and patient rights.

5.4 Strengthening Data Protection and Security

The information privacy and confidentiality are very important when using artificial intelligence in mental health care. These kinds of networks are especially at risk of data breaches because they store private information like diagnoses, treatment plans and mental health histories. In this information to be useful it must be private, freely accessible and accurate. This is important for keeping patients' trust and following the law and morals. To improve data protection, it is crucial to put in place strong security measures to keep data safe from breaches, illegal access as well as other threats. Using encryption is an important part of making things safer. Even if someone who should not have access to it gets their hands on it in order encrypting patient data while it is in transit and at rest makes sure that they cannot use it. This method is very important for protecting a sensitive data when it is sent over networks or stored in cloud-based systems. Using multi-factor authentication (MFA) to get into artificial intelligence systems adds another layer of security. This makes sure that only authorized users can talk to the system. A further significant step is to do regular security audits and vulnerability assessments. The medical profession should stay one step ahead of possible attacks by regularly checking their security measures and fixing any problems they find. These audits also make sure that the company is following all relevant data protection laws like the Health Insurance Portability and Accountability Act (HIPAA) in the US and the General Data Protection Regulation (GDPR) in Europe. These laws set strict rules for how to protect health information. Artificial intelligence (Hasan et al., 2025) professionals and healthcare workers must learn the best ways to keep data safe. This is important for developers and clinicians to know how to handle data safely and how important it is to keep patients privacy safe. The healthcare industry can reduce the risk of human error which is still one of the main causes of data violates by fostering a culture of security awareness.

6 Conclusion

There are a lot of ethical questions that come up when using artificial intelligence in mental health treatment that need to be answered in order to use it safely and effectively. Security and privacy algorithmic biases that could harm vulnerable groups and informed consent are significant challenges. This is very important to be able to hold artificial intelligence accountable for mistakes and make decisions without human input. We also need to think about data security, fairness of algorithms and openness. By fixing these types of issues, we can ethically use artificial intelligence in mental health care. The artificial intelligence could change the way mental health is treated. Although responsibilities need to be balanced. It is important to keep ethical standards in line with how quickly technology is changing. Innovation should not put patients' safety or rights at risk. To keep the equilibrium technology developers, healthcare workers, regulators and patients all need to work together. This plan makes AI technologies useful, creative and ethical by putting the health of patients first. If used correctly AI can make mental health treatments better without breaking any rules. To navigate the challenging ethical landscape with artificial intelligence in mental health treatment, proactive ethical frameworks are essential. People who work in technology, healthcare, ethics and the law should all work together to create these frameworks. Frameworks must deal with moral issues, set standards for openness, make sure people are responsible and keep peoples' privacy safe. These types of frameworks should have audits, ethical training for developers and healthcare providers and policy-making to keep up with technology. These frameworks will make sure that artificial intelligence keeps making mental health care better by following ethical guidelines and putting the needs of patients first.

References

Alhuwaydi, A. M. (2024). Exploring the role of artificial intelligence in mental healthcare: Current trends and future directions—A narrative review for a comprehensive insight. *Risk Management and Healthcare Policy, 17*, 1339–1348.

Alowais, S. A., Alghamdi, S. S., Alsuhebany, N., Alqahtani, T., Alshaya, A. I., Almohareb, S. N., Aldairem, A., Alrashed, M., Saleh, K. B., Badreldin, H. A., et al. (2023). Revolutionizing healthcare: The role of artificial intelligence in clinical practice. *BMC Medical Education, 23*, 689.

Balcombe, L. (2023). AI Chatbots in digital mental health. *Informatics, 10*, 82.

Balcombe, L., & De Leo, D. (2021). Digital mental health challenges and the horizon ahead for solutions. *JMIR Mental Health, 8*, Article e26811.

Baskin, A. S., Wang, T., Miller, J., Jagsi, R., Kerr, E. A., & Dossett, L. A. (2021). A health systems ethical framework for de-implementation in health care. *Journal of Surgical Research, 267*, 151–158.

Carr, S. (2020). 'AI gone mental': Engagement and ethics in data-driven technology for mental health. *Journal of Mental Health, 29*, 125–130.

Chalyi, O. (2024). An evaluation of general-purpose AI Chatbots: A comprehensive comparative analysis. *InfoScience Trends, 1*, 52–66.

Chandraman, M., Santhiyakumari, N., Shree, K. V. M., Murugesan, M., Kumarganesh, S., Rishabavarthani, P., Thiyaneswaran, B., Martin Sagayam, K., Pandey, D., Pandey, B. K., & Sahani, S. K. (2025). Enhancing Cardiovascular disease analysis in healthcare systems with hybrid random forest and neural network algorithm. *Engineering Reports, 7*(9), e70373.

Chen, Y., & Esmaeilzadeh, P. (2024). Generative AI in medical practice: In-depth exploration of privacy and security challenges. *Journal of Medical Internet Research, 26*, Article e53008.

Chinnasamy, P., Subashini, B., Ayyasamy, R. K., Kiran, A., Pandey, B. K., Pandey, D., & Lelisho, M. E. (2025). Blockchain based electronic educational document management with role-based access control using machine learning model. *Scientific Reports, 15*(1), 18828.

Chintala, S. K. (2022). Data privacy and security challenges in AI-driven healthcare systems in India. *Journal of Data Acquisition and Processing, 37*, 2769–2778.

Cohen, I. G. (2019). Informed consent and medical artificial intelligence: What to tell the patient? *The Georgetown Law Journal, 108*, 1425.

de Bruijn, H., Warnier, M., & Janssen, M. (2022). The perils and pitfalls of explainable AI: Strategies for explaining algorithmic decision-making. *Government Information Quarterly, 39*, Article 101666.

Duraisamy, M., Thangavel, M., Lalitha, S., Jayaram, K., Kumarganesh, S., Martin Sagayam, K., Pandey, B. K., Pandey, D., & Sahani, S. K. (2025). Development of an Ion-sensitive field-effect transistor device for high-performance diagnostic and clinical biomedical applications. *Engineering Reports, 7*(4), e70126.

Ellahham, S., Ellahham, N., & Simsekler, M. C. E. (2020). Application of artificial intelligence in the health care safety context: Opportunities and challenges. *American Journal of Medical Quality, 35*, 341–348.

Hasan, A., Nassa, V. K., Pandey, D., Pandey, B. K., George, A. H., & Shahul, A. (2025). The EEG is an introduction to attention perception. *Concepts and Applications of Brain-Computer Interfaces*, 93–122.

Koutsouleris, N., Hauser, T. U., Skvortsova, V., & De Choudhury, M. (2022). From promise to practice: Towards the realisation of AI-informed mental health care. *The Lancet Digital Health, 4*, e829–e840.

Lee, M. K. (2018). Understanding perception of algorithmic decisions: Fairness, trust, and emotion in response to algorithmic management. *Big Data & Society, 5*, 2053951718756684.

Leimanis, A., & Palkova, K. (2021). Ethical guidelines for artificial intelligence in healthcare from the sustainable development perspective. *European Journal of Sustainable Development, 10*, 90.

Singh, S., Madaan, G., Swapna, H. R., Singh, A., Pandey, B. K., George, A. S., & Pandey, D. (2025). Unleashing the power of AI and data analysis: Transforming insights into action. In *Interdisciplinary approaches to AI, internet of everything, and machine learning* (pp. 1–24). IGI Global Scientific Publishing.

The manufacturer's authorised representative in the EU is Springer
Nature Customer Service Centre GmbH, Europaplatz 3, 69115 Heidelberg,
Germany. If you have any concerns regarding our products, please
contact ProductSafety@springernature.com

Printed and bound by CPI Group (UK) Ltd, Croydon, CR0 4YY
20/10/2026
02236471-0011